DEADLY HARVEST

The Intimate Relationship
Between Our Health & Our Food

GEOFF BOND

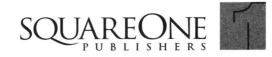
SQUAREONE
PUBLISHERS

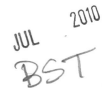

The information and advice contained in this book are based upon the research and the personal and professional experiences of the author. They are not intended as a substitute for consulting with a health care professional. The publisher and author are not responsible for any adverse effects or consequences resulting from the use of any of the suggestions, preparations, or procedures discussed in this book. All matters pertaining to your physical health should be supervised by a health care professional. It is a sign of wisdom, not cowardice, to seek a second or third opinion.

COVER DESIGNER: Jeannie Tudor
EDITOR: John Anderson
TYPESETTER: Gary A. Rosenberg and Theresa Wiscovitch

Square One Publishers
115 Herricks Road
Garden City Park, NY 11040
(516) 535-2010 • (877) 900-BOOK
www.squareonepublishers.com

Library of Congress Cataloging-in-Publication Data
Bond, Geoff.
  Deadly harvest : the intimate relationship between our health & our food /
Geoff Bond.
    p. cm.
  Includes bibliographical references and index.
  ISBN-13: 978-0-7570-0142-0 (pbk.)
  ISBN-10: 0-7570-0142-4 (pbk.)
  1. Nutritionally induced diseases--Prevention. 2. Diet. 3. Nutrition. 4.
Reducing diets. 5. Health. 6. Medical policy. I. Title.

RA784.B6643 2007
613.2--dc22

                              2006037460

Printed in the United States of America

10   9   8   7   6   5   4   3   2   1

Contents

To my children—
who carry the torch down the generations
"I see you stand like greyhounds in the slips,
Straining upon the start. The game's afoot:
Follow your spirit . . .!"

Acknowledgments

This book is the culmination of a long journey. Many people have helped me along the way and it is my pleasure here to single out some of them for special mention.

An early, and essential, influence was that of my quietly determined, selfless grandmother, Anna. At her knee, we learned to respect our bodies and to keep close to nature. She taught us to think critically about what we put in our mouths and to get plenty of fresh air, exercise, and sunshine. She pluckily challenged the dietary doctrines of her day. She was decades ahead of her time and, as pioneers do, had to suffer much uncomprehending banter. Thanks to her influence in my childhood over half a century ago, I have lived a life brimming with good health. If I have seen further than most, then it is only because, as a small boy, I used to sit on Anna's shoulders. She would be immensely proud.

My insights would not have been possible without the peculiarities of upbringing that created in me an untamed questioning, a delight in discovery, and a distaste for humbug. Thank you, then, to my undoctrinaire parents who taught me to be honest to the evidence and to hold fast in the teeth of dogma-driven opposition.

I am indebted to my wife Nicole. This book had a long and difficult gestation and she was always there with her encouragement and support. Like the faery's child, she found me the manna dew, which sustained and nourished my firmness of purpose. Nicole vetted the early proofs: thanks to her I made major improvements to comprehensibility and readability. With the enthusiasm of the convert, she works tirelessly to publicize the life-saving knowledge contained in these pages. With her French background, Nicole is an enthusiastic cook. She has delighted in developing ways of preparing delicious food in conformity with the Savanna Model. The reader will find a sample of these recipes in Chapter 7.

This book would not have been possible without the confidence of my publisher, Rudy Shur, of Square One Publishers. In his words, "You have a great rough diamond, we have to release the brilliant stone inside." Thanks to his patient guidance, we transformed the ugly duckling into a swan. Thanks also to my editor, John Anderson, who shaped the final drafts and refrained from excising too many of my flights of fancy.

I am indebted to the many expert reviewers whose opinions, encouragement, and advice have improved the relevance, usefulness, and scientific accuracy of the text: Rita Stec, MD, president of the Walter T. Stec Memorial Foundation of Indian Wells, California; Elber S. Camacho, MD, medical director of the Comprehensive Cancer Center, in Palm Springs; Dr. Günter Nöll, of Vienna, Austria, biochemist and authority on edible wild plants; and Caroline Mansfield, ND, director of The Naturopathic Clinic, in London. If, in spite of their efforts, there remain any deficiencies or differences of opinion, then these are mine alone.

Many visionaries helped me on my way in the early days: Christopher Brown MD who wrote the excellent foreword to my first book, Joe Schuchert of Kelso Corporation who, with Emmanuel Kampouris as chairman of American Standard, brought my ideas to their workforce, and Steven Gundry, MD, Medical Director of The International Heart Institute of Palm Springs. Many readers and followers have encouraged me with their enthusiasm over the years. It is invidious to single out any one of them. However, I must mention Dr. James Melton, visionary and speaker, for his sage guidance—and Frédéric and Jeanne Bouvet who, persuaded from the very earliest days, produced the first Bond Effect child, Alexandre, using my precepts all the way from inception, through pregnancy to upbringing.

If you are one of the many meritorious contributors whom it has not been possible to cite, just know that you are, like Henry V's unsung heroes, "freshly remember'd" and that your influence lives on in this work. To all of you, and to all of those as yet unsung, my heartfelt thanks.

Introduction

A zookeeper puts signs in front of the cages saying, "Please do not feed the animals." Have you ever thought about that? If you feed lions on popcorn or gorillas on pizza, they get sick and die. The zookeeper knows that there is a particular feeding pattern that is right for each of these creatures. We now realize that there is a particular feeding pattern appropriate for human creatures as well.

A new science has come into being to explore this fascinating subject: nutritional anthropology. It is the spellbinding story about what it means to be human—in nutritional terms. It provides an extraordinarily powerful understanding of how, by eating in harmony with the way our bodies are designed, we can rejoice in the best possible health and relish the prospect of a long life.

We accept that lions and gorillas have bodies, digestive systems, and feeding patterns that are adapted to the environment in which they live. Lions, who live by catching and eating fleet-footed antelope, have razor-sharp claws, needle teeth, and powerful stomach acids. Gorillas, who live by chomping through vast quantities of vegetation, have massive molars and long colons. Lions' bodies are designed to work on the food that lions eat and gorillas' bodies are designed to work on the food that gorillas eat. Yet we imagine, incorrectly, that humans are made to eat anything.

What feeding environment are human bodies designed for? Nutritional anthropology shows that there is a very precise specification for the human diet, developed by our human ancestors over millennia, and our bodies are designed to work according to those instructions and no others. It is an adventure story, stretching across the globe and into the distant past, to discover what humans were designed to eat. The past is the future: modern-day humans have changed very little, genetically speaking, and we are still living in bodies that nature designed to thrive in that far off time. Examining our ancestors' way of life provides powerful clues to how we should be living today. These remarkable insights show how, in many surprising and unsuspected ways, we can make critical, life-transforming adjustments. The way humans have been eating and living for many thousands of years has not been ideal. In this book, you will learn how we discovered this and come to understand what we can do to improve and enrich our own lives right now.

Our first goal is to open your mind to a whole new way of thinking about the fuel that your body needs. Once this reality is accepted, we can move forward to learning how to practice this way of feeding in today's world. The news is good—we live in a society where there is a huge variety and abundance of food available from all corners of the globe at any time of the year. We just have to learn how to choose wisely.

One of the most troubling aspects of our busy lives is the constant bombardment of conflicting messages directed at us by the health and food industries. In this book, we show you the way to peace of mind. The insights of nutritional anthropology empower you to judge for yourself. They bring clarity to the confusion and allow you to select with confidence which claims to accept and which to reject. After all, our ancestors knew they were living in a dangerous, treacherous, and unpredictable jungle. They had the skills to survive: they knew which mushrooms were poisonous and which berries were safe. This book can help teach you the skills to survive in today's supermarket jungle.

The insights of nutritional anthropology get at the root causes of the "diseases of civilization": cancer, heart disease, stroke, diabetes, obesity, arthritis, osteoporosis, Alzheimer's disease, and many more. These diseases are not inevitable, they are optional. These are lifestyle diseases, which can be avoided and put into remission. By understanding the principles of nutritional anthropology and eating in accordance with our naturally adapted lifestyle, you will be able to choose the right foods to eat and know why. You can improve your health to be better able to combat any disease and live longer. Your body will find its natural ideal weight, either losing or gaining according to its needs. You will be able to take control of your eating habits and thus your life.

These are powerful claims, but as a scientist I am not given to flights of fancy or guesswork. All the information in this book is based on evidence-driven science. These insights are new, because the various pieces of the puzzle have only recently been put together. For example, peering deep into our DNA is one of the exciting new tools for unlocking the secrets of our genetic heritage. And there are many other fields that are yielding fascinating new insights about how human beings are "designed" to live. This book gathers this scattered, cutting-edge information and synthesizes it into a coherent whole.

But this is not just theory—the ideas work. Over the past decade, thousands of individuals have been empowered by this information. I have personally worked with many of them to understand the nature of disease, to take control of their eating habits, and to help them live a healthier lifestyle. Many people's lives have been transformed by the insights of nutritional anthropology.

The Journey Ahead

The first part of the book explains nutritional anthropology—how we know what it means to be a human being, particularly in nutritional terms. We highlight the consequences of our divergence from the ideal eating pattern. The middle part of the book deals with how, as humans, we moved away from our naturally adapted environment, feeding patterns, and lifestyle, and looks at the science supporting our claims. Then, based on these insights, we develop an "Owner's Manual" for how we should be feeding ourselves and show you how to put it into action today. Finally, we present an overview of specific diseases and how these relate to the ways we eat and live.

• Chapter 1 describes the remarkable discoveries of nutritional anthropology: about where we came from and how our ancestors made their living there.

• Chapter 2 describes how, over many millennia, more and more foods have become part of our diets (not always for the best) and describes how governments, somewhat arbitrarily, provide dietary guidelines.

• Chapter 3 reviews how we eat today and hints at the surprising health consequences.

• Chapters 4 and 5 go backstage to look at the science behind these assertions, bringing in evidence from other areas of scientific enquiry that satisfyingly complete the picture.

• In Chapter 6, we pull all the pieces of evidence together to define the "Owners Manual," the naturally adapted eating pattern for the human species.

• Chapter 7 sets out the route map for feeding ourselves in today's world. It gives practical advice, strategies for different situations, and a step-by-step approach for easily putting the principles into practice.

• Chapter 8 shows how we can make adjustments in our lives—to bring them in line with our naturally adapted lifestyle—that can help our well-being. Stress, exercise, spirituality, kinships, family relationships, differences between the sexes, parenting, and other topics are explored.

• Chapter 9 looks at the connection between what we eat, lifestyle factors, and the "diseases of civilization." Returning to our naturally adapted feeding patterns can greatly improve our health and well-being.

This book's fusion of healthy eating with healthy thinking could not be more important, dealing as it does with the absolute fundamentals of human nature. It feels good to know at last that you have a coherent and focused road map for humbug-free bodily nutrition. It is a relief to be clear about where you have to go, and you'll feel better about yourself for taking control of your destiny.

You will find the secret to what it means to be a human being living in close connection with our natural lifestyle. Everyone can use these ideas to enhance their image, inside and out. It contains the easy-to-learn skills of how to harmonize your eating with human genetic programming. We *can* make adjustments to our ways of eating, our ways of thinking, and our lifestyle so that they coincide as closely as possible with our inherited natural traits: they are the key to a healthy and harmonious life. In this book, we dub this process—of aligning our lives with the way nature intended—the "Bond Effect."

1. What is Nutritional Anthropology?

Much of what we think we know about food has filtered into our minds through our upbringing, our cultural conditioning, and commercial advertising. We absorb still other ideas from the not-so-subtle influences of the health industry, junk science, and the trendy wisdom of the day. Our individual theories are all different and no one could argue that any of them is the complete answer. The reason is simple—even the experts cannot agree. They are like the blindfolded men trying to guess that they are touching an elephant. One touches the trunk and thinks it is a snake, the next touches a leg and thinks it is a tree, and so on.

There is, however, a valid science that has emerged which lifts the blindfold and shows the whole picture. It sees across the barriers between many compartmentalized scientific disciplines and finds new, overarching knowledge in the patterns that are revealed. We sometimes forget that, just like all other creatures on this planet, we sleep, feed, excrete, beget offspring, and indeed bleed. If we are like animals in those respects, then we resemble them in the rest.

This new science studies how humans fit into this vast and complex mosaic of nature. We go back to our origins to understand our place in the scheme of things. We learn what it means to be human—as organic beings—interacting in a multitude of intricate ways with our native environment. Second, it uses a range of scientific disciplines to identify the kind of feeding pattern for which our bodies have evolved over millennia. We learn the kinds and proportions of plants and creatures we consumed, and we match this with what we know makes us ill or well today. Various peoples around the world practice a range of dietary patterns—these practices are not without consequences and we learn from those as well.

This science puts all of these clues together to identify the ideal feeding pattern for the human species. Why is this important? Very simply, we are making ourselves grievously sick and unnaturally shortening our lives by blindly ignoring our nutritional heritage. This new science lights our way to the remedy: it not only gives us the definitive specification for the human diet, it also teaches us how to put it into practice. It is comforting to know that this is not only possible but also easy, once we connect the dots.

What is this science? It links the study of human beings (anthropology) with the science of fueling the body (nutrition). That science is *nutritional anthropology*. It goes right to the heart of what it means to be a human being in nutritional terms.

THE "OWNER'S MANUAL" FOR THE HUMAN BODY

It is helpful to think of the human body as being an incredibly complex machine. This machine has a particular construction and functions in a particular way, yet, annoyingly, we do not have an Owner's Manual. We do not have the specification of the *fuel* that the machine was designed to run on. It is incredible to think that, up until now, so little thought has been given to the matter. We inhabit this wonderful community of minute cells that have come together for a common purpose—to create and sustain life in a human body—and each one of those cells requires to be fueled, but with what?

In this chapter, we start the hunt for the Owner's Manual by looking at four promising trails:

• We will go on a journey of discovery back to our ancestral human homeland and get to know the workshop where our bodies were forged.

• We will find tribes that, even in modern times, continue to live like our early ancestors.

• We will analyze fossilized bones to see what food nutrients contributed to their structure and we will examine fossilized teeth to see what kind of feeding pattern caused them to wear and scratch in a particular way.

• We will seek confirmation for what we discover by comparing our digestive system with other human-like creatures.

OUR ANCESTRAL HOMELAND

Where do we come from? The answer to this question is of capital importance because it tells us *where* we should look to find the Owner's Manual. There we will find the place where our bodies were fashioned. We need to understand this place's geography and natural history, so we can discover what *use* our ancestors made of it and how it shaped our ideal feeding pattern.

The great explorations of the 15th to 18th centuries found human beings living on every continent, with the exception of Antarctica. Human populations were living in a huge variety of climates, geographies, and cultures. In the 19th century, intrepid explorers discovered the chimpanzee and the gorilla in the jungles of tropical Africa. Their human-like form and eerily human behavior fascinated the people of the time. The great naturalist Charles Darwin (1809–1882) predicted, but could not prove, that humans (*Homo sapiens*) had their origins in tropical Africa too. No one had yet uncovered any ancient fossils in Africa to confirm this prediction.

Then, in relatively quick succession, anthropologists discovered ancient bones not in Africa, but in Germany in 1856 (Neanderthal), in Indonesia in 1891 (Java Man), and in China in the 1930s (Peking Man). They were all remains of humanlike species dating back 50,000 to one million years ago. These creatures had stone tools, made rudimentary ornaments, and daubed crude cave paintings. However, there was no center—these humanlike creatures seemed to be living all over Europe and Asia.

The picture was further confused because, in southern Europe about 30,000 years ago, there was an abrupt improvement in the sophistication of tools and cave paintings. A new type of human, dubbed "Cro-Magnon," appeared on the scene. There was puzzlement about what it all meant.

Finally, in the 1960s, the anthropologists Louis and Mary Leakey (and later their son, Richard) began uncovering extremely old, humanlike bones in tropical East Africa (Kenya and Tanzania). Some of these bones were several million years old. Two famous skeletons are "Turkana boy" and "Lucy." Once again, it was looking as though humans had their origins in Africa after all.

Remarkable Insights From DNA

During the 1990s, from the most unexpected direction, came dramatic confirmation of our origins from an extremely powerful tool: DNA (deoxyribonucleic acid) analysis. It just so happens that our genes contain the key to the whole history of the human race. Our genetic material tells us that, with the exception of the Cro-Magnon, all these human-like creatures that inhabited Europe and Asia for over a million years, including the Neanderthals, are not our ancestors at all. They are a different species. Neanderthals and *Homo sapiens* were closely related species, granted. They were almost as close as the donkey is to the horse, but they did not successfully interbreed; there are no Neanderthal genes in *Homo sapiens.*

Allan Wilson and Rebecca Cann are Berkeley genetic microbiologists who have used sophisticated DNA analysis techniques to trace the ancestry of humans back to their origins.[1] They and other pioneering researchers, such as the geneticist L. Luca Cavalli-Sforza,[2] have built up a remarkably precise picture of our ancient genealogy. The molecular evidence indicates that *Homo sapiens* arose around 250,000 years ago. The population of *Homo sapiens* was small—no more than about 10,000 of them—and the population remained at around this level for a very long time. Furthermore, studies of the genes of different peoples from all over the world show that all their ancestral lines lead back to a single location for our homeland. This key information tells us that our mother country is an area bounded by Kenya, Tanzania, and Ethiopia.

Indeed, these studies show that our ancestors remained in their homeland until about 60,000 years ago. According to the eminent Anglo-American anthropologist Ian Tattersall, we now know that everyone on this planet is descended from a group of people who lived in the savannas of East Africa until just 60,000 years ago.[3] This is a highly significant piece of information—it tells us that our origins are tropical African and *recent* in evolutionary terms.

We can now piece together what happened. Over a period of a million years, successive waves of humanlike creatures overflowed out of Africa to populate most of the Old World. They had brains about half the size of ours, but walked upright and had many humanlike traits. They have been broadly called *Homo erectus*, of which the Neanderthals were just one branch. Then, about 250,000 years ago, a radical thing happened: a new breed of *Homo erectus* arose in East Africa, our own ancestor, *Homo sapiens*.

Homo sapiens were brainier, more agile, more inventive, but more lightly built than *Homo erectus*. They were successful in their ability to survive and to multiply. However, to feed themselves, they needed around 100 square miles of living space per band of 50 people. So, in their turn, about 60,000 years ago, they overflowed out of Africa into Asia.

How Humans Migrated Around the World

Homo sapiens spread further than *Homo erectus*. They migrated along the coastlines of India and Indonesia and got to Australia approximately 50,000 years ago. That continent was empty of humans at that time. Within 2,000 years, they occupied every corner of it, from the harsh Central Desert to the lush tropical rainforests. These are the ancestors of the Australian Aboriginals.

The Human Timeline

We have our humanlike beginnings with East African *Homo erectus* over 1,000,000 years ago. Out of that population, *Homo sapiens* arose and existed for 190,000 years before leaving Africa about 60,000 years ago. This period, from over 1,000,000 years ago to 60,000 years ago is critical—it is our *formative era*. It is the time when the African environment forged the bodies that we possess today and when the "Owner's Manual" was written.

I will refer to this formative era frequently throughout the book, so I will give it a specific name. Geologists have a convenient, often-used epoch for this approximate time period—the Pleistocene, which runs from 1,600,000 years ago to 10,000 years ago. However, I want to conclude the formative era earlier, at about 60,000 years ago. Since our ancestors spent this time entirely in Africa, I will call this critical formative era the "*African Pleistocene.*"

On the one hand, those areas that are rich in game and vegetation could support a relatively dense population of up to 50 people per 25 square miles. On the other hand, the early European settlers thought, wrongly, that the deserts and 'outback' were empty. Even they were populated, but at lower densities—down as far as 50 people per 300 square miles.

The total Aboriginal population of the Australian continent (about the same area as the continental United States) stabilized at around 800,000 people. The population density is said to have reached "saturation." These densities are, of course, much lower than we are used to seeing in the industrialized West today. The U.S. supports 280 million people, an average density of 50 people on only 480 acres, or three-quarters of a square mile.

About 35,000 years ago, *Homo sapiens* was knocking at the doors of Europe. Here they found themselves in stiff competition with the Neanderthals. John Kappelman, an anthropologist who has written about the biology of ancient, humanlike creatures, reports that the Neanderthals were massive, at least 30% larger than the ordinary human today.[4] They had the heavily muscled body and stature of an Olympic wrestler and weighed up to 200 pounds (91 kg). On the other hand, their brains were somewhat smaller than modern man's is today.

We will never know exactly what happened to the Neanderthals. However, every human male was a potent "Jack-the-Giant-Killer:" he was smarter, wilier, and more organized than the more powerful, yet dim-witted, giant of the forest. Over several thousand years, it is probable that he killed them all off. That is what happens when too-similar species compete for the same living space.

By 30,000 years ago, the Neanderthals had gone and the *Homo sapiens* newcomers had introduced their own, developing culture. This explains the quantum leap in art and technology of the time. These new people were the Cro-Magnons, the ancestors of Europeans. Meanwhile, in the Middle East, India, China, and Siberia, other *Homo sapiens* similar to the Cro-Magnons drove all the other branches of *Homo erectus* into extinction. By 20,000 years ago, humans had fanned out over the whole of the Old World.

About 15,000 years ago, toward the end of the last ice age, sea levels were still low and it was possible to canoe or walk from Siberia, across the Bering Strait to what is now Alaska. Finally, the first few humans broke out of the Old World and penetrated into the Americas. There they found a New World rich in plants and game, empty of humans, and free of competition, and they prospered well.

As they multiplied, their frontier advanced south. The swelling population spread, at an average rate of 8 miles per year, through territories that now include Canada, the United States, Mexico, and Central and South America, right down to Patagonia. By about 10,000 years ago, the Americas were peopled 'to saturation' for their ancestral lifestyle. We must remember that 'saturation' is still a very low density by modern standards: an average of 100 square miles of living space per band of 50 people. These first, pioneering peoples became the indigenous Indian tribes or "Amerindians."

The essential idea to retain about our past is this: that we are all still tropical creatures who only left our homeland 2,000 generations (60,000 years) ago.

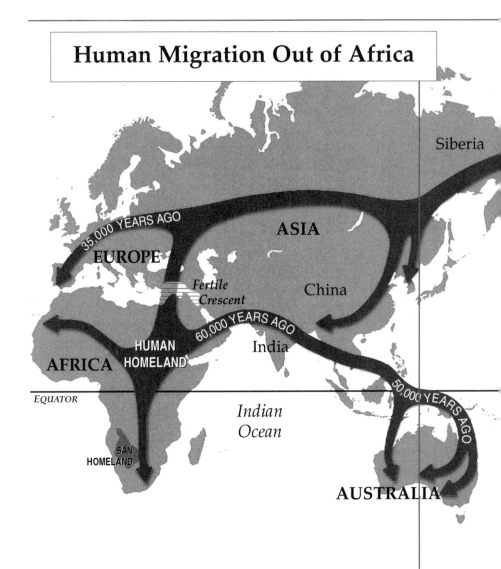

Human Migration Out of Africa

This map of the world shows the broad migration pattern of our human ancestors as they overflowed out of their "Human Homeland" in east Africa. Note that we are just showing the overall pattern and timings, not the detailed wanderings and itineraries. The earliest wave of migrants, 60,000 years ago, went via India and Indonesia to Australia. Later migrations arrived in Asia and in Europe. Finally

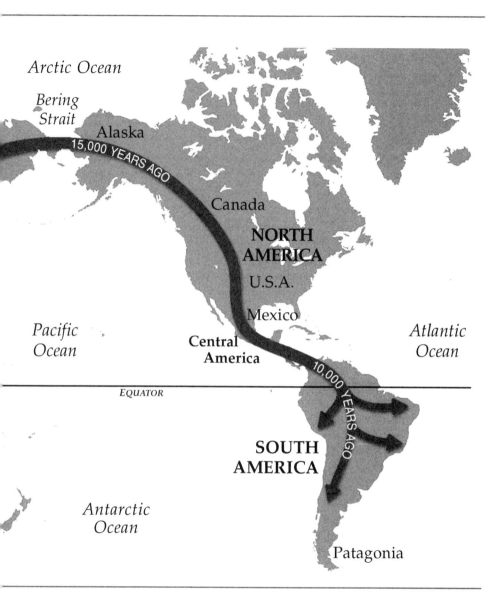

humans crossed from Asia into North America and penetrated all the way down
to the southern tip of South America. Meanwhile, other groups had already spread
into the other parts of Africa itself. We show the location of one of these groups,
the San Bushman, whom we talk about in some detail later in this chapter. We also
show an area known as the Fertile Crescent, which we discuss in Chapter 2.

While 2,000 generations might seem like a lot, it is just an eye-blink in evolutionary terms. The bacteria in our guts go through that many generations in the space of two months. We do not expect a species to change much, if at all, in such a short space of time. We know that our bodies are still the same, we have the same biochemistry, and we have the same digestive arrangements.

We look a little different on the outside, of course. Over the last 2,000 generations, superficial racial differences have evolved, but underneath we are all still the same. We all have a common recent origin. In other words, everyone on this planet still inhabits a body designed for life in our ancestral homeland, the tropical, east African savanna. The DNA evidence is a ringing endorsement of the Leakeys' fossil evidence. The cradle of mankind is in the African Rift Valley stretching from Olduvai in northern Tanzania, all the way through Kenya to Lake Turkana in southern Ethiopia.

What was Our Homeland Like?

What was this overflowing pot, our homeland or Garden of Eden, like? This environment and lifestyle shaped our natures, our bodies, and our biology. Let us look at a snapshot of this place.

If we conjure up a picture of the African savanna landscape, it is the classic image of open, rolling grassland with the occasional tree, bush, and shrub. In the wetter areas, there are thickets and groves of beautiful flowering shrubs and trees. In parts, termite mounds stand up to 25 feet (8 meters) high. The floor of the African Rift Valley is not very high above sea level, but there are nearby plateaus; some mountains rise to over 10,000 feet (3,000 meters). There are several large, and many small, lakes, many waterholes, and some streams and rivers. Many of the watercourses are dry for most of the year, but flood during the rains.

How Long is a Human Generation?

A human generation can only be approximated and we have to work with averages. Conventionally, many scientists "assume" that a generation is 25 years, which is a suspiciously round and convenient number. As we shall see, in our hunter gatherer past, women bore children from about 20 years old to about 46 years old. The mid-point is therefore around 33 years. If we allow for some tapering of fecundity with age, it is likely that the *average* age of a generation for most of human history is around 30 years. This is the figure we have used.

The weather fluctuates between mild and hot for most parts of the year, about 55°F to 90°F (13°C to 32°C). There are rainy and dry seasons. Annual rainfall is moderate: between 35 inches (900 mm) and 60 inches (1,500 mm), and the rain comes in unpredictable storms and showers.

Our ancestors were not alone in the savanna. They shared the land with a wide variety of creatures: giraffe, lion, elephant, warthog, rhinoceros, hyena, antelope, gazelle, zebra, baboons, chimpanzees, vultures, eagles, flamingos, and many more. In addition, there were snakes, porcupines, crocodiles, lizards, tortoises, snails, grasshoppers, and a myriad of small mammals, reptiles, and insects. The lakes, streams, and waterholes teemed with many species of freshwater fish, shellfish, frogs, toads, ducks, geese, and other aquatic creatures.

Our ancient ancestors lived for countless generations in these circumstances. This environment fashioned our bodies, our naturally adapted lifestyle, and our mentality. With this sketch of it in mind, we can discover how nature designed us to live in this environment. In particular, we will focus on the kind of eating pattern that is right for us.

THE SAN BUSHMEN

How did our human ancestors make use of this environment? We can learn a great deal by examining how primal tribes live today. However, there are allowances to be made: such tribes have been pushed into more marginal lands, and sometimes modern materials filter in from the outside world. Nevertheless, working from studies carried out over the past 150 years, we can piece together a good, solid picture of our anscestors. As our main illustration, we will look at the San Bushmen who live in southern Africa (see *Human Migration Out of Africa*, pp. 10-11).

The San Bushmen (more correctly called by their own name, the !Kung) at one time occupied a large part of southern Africa. Negroid Bantu herders (Zulus and Xhosa) migrating from West Africa have pushed them into a smaller, remote area—the Kalahari—over the past 600 years. The Kalahari is a sandy wilderness, well covered with trees, scrub, vines, creepers, and grasses. The sand drains the rainfall fast, so there is little surface water, just scattered waterholes. Animal life is varied, and many species such as antelope, lion, giraffe, zebra, and elephant thrive there. It is very like our ancestral homeland, but without the streams and lakes.

The San are short, slender, and fine-featured with a reddish-yellow skin. Laurens van der Post describes the color as "Provençal apricot."[5] The San have tightly coiled, peppercorn colored, and woolly hair. Their noses are broad, and they have pointy ears with no lobes. They have high cheekbones and somewhat Mongoloid eyes.

The Italian geneticist Ornella Semino and others have shown that the San are southern Africa's most ancient inhabitants.[6] In 60,000 years, they have migrated only 1,500 miles from humanity's homeland in the African Rift Valley. Anthropologists have studied the San extensively since the 1950s and found the San living the same way that our ancestors have since the dawn of time.

The San live in groups of 40 to 60 people (about 6 to 10 families). A typical group (or band) has about 15–20 men, 15–20 women, and a further 15–20 dependent children. The group "owns" their territory of some 125 square miles (320 km²) within which they roam. They camp for a few days in a place and then move on. In the space of six months, one band was recorded by the ethnic archaeologist John Yellen, as having moved 37 times, an average of once every five days.[7] When they have exhausted the food supply of the area, they travel to the next site, which can be up to 20 miles away.

The San wear no clothes. They do not have any possessions beyond what is easily portable and can be carried long distances. Babes-in-arms are carried by their mothers, but everyone else has to walk. They carefully choose the next campsite for the availability of plant and animal food. Sometimes the whole group will move to the place where the men have killed a large animal and then stay until the meat is all gone. Game animals that come to waterholes are a rich source of food. To avoid frightening them away, and in spite of the inconvenience, they camp at least a quarter mile away from a waterhole.

How the San Feed Themselves

What use do the San make of their feeding environment? The Japanese anthropologist Jiro Tanaka and others have lived among the San and monitored their lifestyle for years at a time.[8] The only "work" to be done by the band is the daily quest for food. The roles adopted by each member of the band are natural and instinctive.

Women's Work

Almost every day a large proportion of the women set off, in a group, on a food-collecting expedition. Nursing mothers carry their babies in a leather sling. Older women, old men, and the men not hunting that day stay at the camp with some of the children. The American anthropologist Richard Lee, an untiring researcher of hunter-gatherer societies, reports that during the expedition, the women walk 2 to 12 miles (3 to 20 km).[9] They gradually separate but always stay within hailing distance of one another. On the return leg, a woman will be carrying 7 to 15 kg (15–33 pounds) of collected food. Her family will receive a share of most of it.

The Digging Stick and New Food Resources

The women's digging stick gives humans a big advantage over their competitors in the same ecological niche. Baboons, for example, often get to a fruiting tree and strip it before the humans arrive, but baboons are incapable of digging down to underground foods.

The women have two types of activity: picking and digging. From above ground, the women pick fruits, nuts, berries, flowers, gums, stalks, pods, leaves, and all kinds of edible plant parts. From below ground, they poke out, with their digging sticks, a whole variety of stems, bulbs, corms, and roots.

It is estimated that the San use over 100 species of plant as food, although many of them are tiresome to collect and not always agreeable to eat. Given the chance, they tend to concentrate on just 15 to 20 species that are reliable to find, tasty, and easy to gather. The most consumed species is the fruit and nutlike kernel of the mongongo tree. Groves of these trees are found all over San territory, and their edible parts are available for large parts of the year. The baobab fruit is another staple. It is delectable, rich in vitamin C, calcium, and magnesium. It too has a kernel that is nutlike. Raw, the tsin bean is slimy and inedible, but once roasted is an enjoyable delicacy.[10]

John Yellen and Richard Lee record the San as eating peanuts on a regular basis.[11] This demonstrates some of the difficulties of reconstructing the ancestral diet. The peanut is native to tropical South America and was introduced to Africa by European explorers only around 400 years ago. Since then, it has spread so rapidly that hunter-gatherers in the Kalahari desert can think of it as a normal native food. However, we can be sure that our African Pleistocene ancestors never ate peanuts.

Green salad vegetables, such as scilla and talinum (a kind of purslane), appear at the start of the rainy season. Fruits, such as the !igwa, ochna, and grewia berries and the ivory fruit, yield hundreds of pounds during their seasons. None of these fruits is sweet and many are bitter. Most foods are highly fibrous. Jiro Tanaka estimates that the San eat on average 2 pounds (900 g) of plant food per person per day.

Plant foods are an important, even critical, source of water. One of the most important is the bitter-juiced tsama melon, from which our familiar (but sweet) watermelon is descended.[12] Indeed, the San obtain more than 90% of their water needs from plants. This is not typical for our African Pleistocene ancestors, who would have had access to waterholes, ponds, and streams year round. It is fascinating to realize that the human body can survive without free water at all, provided there is access to enough plant food of the right type.

The women also collect eggs of all kinds and capture small animals such as locusts, caterpillars, grubs, toads, tortoises, and snakes. Ostrich eggs are particularly valued. The contents supply a good portion of food, the shells make containers for water, and bits of shell are carved into beads.

On their gathering trips, the women will note and report to the men any signs of game that might be good to hunt. Both men and women live in an intimate relationship with the natural world around them. They are incredible botanists and can identify all the plants and know exactly which ones are good to eat and what else each plant might be good for. They are amazing naturalists—they live in close contact with animal life and seem to know what it is like to be in the mind of the larger mammals, such as elephants, lions, or antelopes.

Men's Work

The men concentrate almost exclusively on hunting. This is sporadic and depends entirely on their reading of the opportunities. Hunting parties are small: usually just one or two men in a party; more if it is a big animal. Hunting trips are made an average of three times a week. The men are away for several hours, sometimes up to 10 hours. Frequently, the hunters return empty-handed.

Most of the hunting is unspectacular. The men go after small creatures using snares, traps, and guile. Commonly, the San hunt for springhare, a type of large rodent that sleeps in its deep burrow during the day. The hunter pokes a flexible, barb-tipped 20-foot pole down the burrow until he has hooked the animal. He then digs the creature out. Porcupines and 150-pound 'antbears' are smoked out, dug out, or even speared by crawling down the burrow. Warthogs are run to death with hunting dogs. A fire is lit at the entrance to the tunnel and then they are speared as they try to escape. The warthog is highly prized for its fatty flesh, a rarity in the San diet.

Game birds like guinea fowl, francolin, and bustard are captured in cunning snares. Ostrich is hunted on occasion. As mentioned earlier, the San do not have much access to water, but when they get the chance, they spear fish, trap toads, and collect shellfish.

Big game, such as eland (a huge, ox-like antelope weighing up to one ton), gemsbok, and wildebeest, are hunted as the occasion presents itself. However, the effort required is enormous and the outcome uncertain. In one incident, the San tracked a herd of eland for eight days and finally shot one of them with poison arrows. They followed the wounded eland for another three days before it collapsed and could be killed and butchered. Giraffe are occasionally hunted, but not with much success.

How Important is Hunted Food?

Hunted food does not actually provide a large percentage of the diet. Jiro Tanaka measured the number of game animals caught by one San band. The hunters brought in just 140 animals in six months—about three for each member of the band. About one-third of the weight of an animal (consisting of bones, horns, hooves, and so on) is inedible waste. Tanaka estimates that the weight of game animals actually consumed per person averages about 5 ounces (150 g) per person per day.[13]

When the kill is made, the hunters are allowed to eat the liver immediately and they will eat more of the meat as necessary to satisfy their hunger. If they are far from base, they will eat the parts that spoil fast first. The animal is butchered on the spot. Only the gallbladder and the testicles are discarded.

Everything else is taken back to base and will be eaten. Blood is carried in bags made from the stomach or bladder. The hunters wring out the half-digested grasses in the paunch and drink the fluid to save precious water.

Back at the camp, they dry surplus strips of the meat to a kind of pemmican. Even the hide is pounded up and eaten, or parts are kept to make leather artifacts as needed. Soft parts such as udders, fetus, heart, lung, brains, and blood are given to old people with worn down teeth. The intestines are emptied of their excrement, cleaned, and are much prized as a delicacy.

Hooves and trotters are picked clean; gristle is dried and pounded. Sinews are used to make string. The major bones are eagerly cracked open for their fatty marrow; marrow fat is mainly of the monounsaturated kind. The conventional muscle meat is, of course, much desired. Nothing is wasted.

Children eat what the adults eat. Babies and toddlers are breast-fed until they are about four years old. The mother introduces easily chewed, solid foods after the first teeth have broken through.

The search for honey occupies an inordinate amount of effort, guile, and time. The reason is simple: it is just about the only source of sweetness in the San diet. When they find a bees' nest (usually in a hole in a tree), they waft smoke from a smoldering bunch of specially selected herbs toward the bees. The bees think a forest fire is coming, gorge themselves on honey, and then flee the hive. In this state, they are both absent and docile. This is just as well: these insects are the fearsome African killer bees that make mass attacks and kill anything that gets in the way.

When the coast is clear, the San puts his hand into the nest and scoops up a handful of comb, dripping with honey and flecked with half-developed grubs. This is shared out and eaten on the spot, wax, grubs, and all. The San try to leave enough intact comb so that the bees are not driven away permanently. That way they can come back from time to time and harvest more honey. The San are so possessive about this resource that ownership of the nest is passed on from father to son. From a nutritional point of view, the amount of honey is insignificant; they only get the equivalent of a candy bar three or four times a year. However, from a psychological point of view, this is a high point in the San life.

The San Food Supply

Total animal matter consumption (that is, game animals plus eggs and all the gathered and fished animals) is no more than around 8 ounces (225 g) per person per day. Plant food is about 2 pounds (900 g) per day. This weight of food is rather less than even the San would like to be eating and we will see how this relates to the way we eat today. Nevertheless, the proportions are worth noting: about 20% animal food to 80% plant food measured by weight. Measured by calories, Richard Lee estimated the ratio to be 33% animal food to 67% plant food.[14] The reason for the difference is that there are more calories per pound in animal foods than plant foods.

The San can survive very well without hunted food at all. However, it is certain that they could not survive without the women's gathered animal and plant food. The men's work—hunting—is an optional extra. In spite of that, hunting preoccupies the thoughts of both men and women. It inspires songs, dances, storytelling, and interminable plotting and cogitation. Why this might be so, and why men are necessary, especially husbands, is discussed in Chapter 8.

Richard Lee estimates that an adult San spends about 12 to 19 hours per week getting food.[15] That is the only "work" there is; after that, it is just lazing around, chatting, singing, dancing, making the odd piece of body adornment, and preparing hunting equipment. It is a very easy-going lifestyle. Compared to today's average 40-hour work week, which does not include food shopping and preparation time, the San lifestyle was very leisurely. This is all very agreeable, but what is the effect of this lifestyle on the health of the San?

The State of the San's Health

Austrian biologist Sylvia Kirchengast reports that the San are, above all, slim and they stay slim throughout their lives.[16] Their average body mass index (BMI) is around 19. That corresponds to a weight of 110 pounds (50 kg) for a height of 5'4" (163 cm).

Body Mass Index

The body mass index (BMI) is a useful rule of thumb to test whether you are a healthy weight for your height. Conventional medical wisdom considers a "healthy" BMI to lie between 18 and 25; "overweight" is 26 to 30; "obese" is 31 and over.

Stuart Truswell and John Hansen are medical doctors who conducted nutritional and medical research on the San in the 1960s. They found that, predictably, the San do not suffer from diseases associated with obesity.[17] Diabetes is unknown. They have one of the lowest cholesterol levels in the world: total cholesterol levels for all age groups are around 120 mg/100 ml; phospholipids and triglycerides are low too.

The diet is very low in fats of all kinds, and the types of fats are healthier. They are mainly polyunsaturated fats with very little saturated fat. It is interesting to compare the fats in the San's blood with those in the average European's blood. The San has a much higher percentage of the polyunsaturated omega-3 fat (26% to 9%) and a lower percentage of the polyunsaturated omega-6 fat (34% to 40%). This is not surprising: in contrast to Westerners, the San are eating a diet

The Australian Aborigine

Another example of a primal tribe, very remote from the San Bushman, is the Australian Aborigine, who lived a completely primal existence until European settlers first arrived in Australia 200 years ago. The continent of Australia has a wide variety of climates, ranging from tropical in the north to temperate in the south. The vast interior of Australia is very dry and much of it is desert.

Remarkably, in spite of the wide variation of climate and geography, the Aboriginal living arrangements hardly differed from the Bushman. They lived in bands of 30 to 50 people, men, women, and children included.[24] Each group circulated in its territory, which could have an area of up to 300 square miles in barren regions. They were constantly on the move, camping for a few days and then moving on 10 to 15 miles to the next campsite.

How the Aborigines Feed Themselves

The basic food collecting patterns were similar to the San's, especially in the savanna areas that mirror our African homeland.[25] The women gathered and the men hunted. The women used digging sticks and collected plants, insects, and small animals, providing the base load of food on a daily basis. The kinds of plants collected were quite different species to those of the Kalahari, but had very similar characteristics: young leaves and shoots, roots, tubers, bulbs, fibrous fruits, nuts, gums, flowers, water lily roots, and berries.

The animal food collected would be eggs, turtles, snakes, shellfish, crabs, caterpillars (e.g., the witchety grub and the bogong moth), land snails, and the goanna (a giant lizard). Sweet foods were very rare but much prized. Disproportionate amounts of time were spent on finding a bees' nest to smoke out. Other sweetmeats were the honey ant, gorged with nectar, and "lerp," a sweet insect secretion on eucalyptus leaves. In times of scarcity, grass seeds were collected, winnowed, and ground between two handheld stones.[26] The drudgery of this task was viewed with such distaste that it was only done very rarely.

The men would spend a lot of thought, ingenuity, and time on the hunt, which was often unsuccessful. Stories about the hunts, past, present, and future dominated their conversations. Unlike the San, the Aboriginal did not have the bow and arrow—they still used spears, traps, snares, boomerangs, and fire. They hunted and trapped wallaby, kangaroo, freshwater fish, snakes, platypus, possums, birds, ducks, and emu.

The Aboriginal Food Supply

The Aboriginal food supply was similar to the San in the proportion of food coming from animals and plants. About 35% of calories came from animal sources and 65% from plant sources. In traditional aboriginal diets, the animal matter was very low in fat (less than 3%).[27] It was mainly polyunsaturated fat, and there was little saturated fat. The polyunsaturated fat was composed of equal percentages from the omega-3 and omega-6 families. As with the Bushman, fat was much sought after: fatty parts of the carcass were prized, distributed with ceremony, and eaten with relish. The witchety grub was rich in monounsaturated fat, similar to olive oil.

The Aborigine ate most plant food raw, but if it tasted better roasted, some was tossed into the embers of a fire. Animal food was mostly cooked. Small game, snakes, lizards, and grubs would be baked in the embers. Larger animals would be gutted and the variety meats (offal) cooked and eaten separately; the carcass would be baked whole.

The State of the Aborigine's Health

At the time of European settlement 200 years ago, the Aboriginal was described as being in good health and of athletic physique. In the 1960s, researchers studied Aboriginals still living the traditional way and found that they were incredibly lean by our standards, with body mass indexes ranging from 16 to 20.[28] They also had low blood pressure, low cholesterol, and no atherosclerosis or diabetes. Their blood samples showed high levels of hemoglobin, vitamins C and B_{12}, folate, and a good sodium/potassium ratio. However, the Aborigines' health disintegrates when they adopt a European lifestyle.

that contains roughly equal amounts of omega-3 and omega-6 fats. The main sources of fats for the San are nuts and wild creatures, both of which have very different fatty acid profiles to the foods habitually consumed in the West. In addition, their bodies are not fabricating fats out of the kinds of food that are making Westerners fat.

There is no sign of coronary heart disease, atherosclerosis, or thrombosis. Researchers have found no case of varicose veins, piles, or hernias. No cases of cancer or osteoporosis were seen either. Average blood pressure is a low 120/75 and it does not increase with age; not a single case was found of high blood pressure.

In 1966, the South African ear, nose, and throat specialists John Jarvis and H.G. van Heerden made hearing tests on 10 old Bushmen and found that they had perfect hearing.[18] There was little or no earwax and the drum could be easily seen. Teeth were also free of caries (cavities). In old age, eyesight still remained excellent for distance, but, in a few, the lens has lost some transparency.

Other researchers found that the San received healthy levels of vitamins A, B_{12}, C, and D, folate, thiamine, riboflavin, niacin, iron, calcium, iodine, zinc, copper, and other trace elements.[19] The human body is designed to manufacture vitamin D from sunlight. The San, like our African Pleistocene ancestors, lived in a sunny place and spent all day outdoors, with no clothes on. Their bodies manufactured all the vitamin D they needed. Nobody suffered from anemia or protein deficiency. The kidneys were functioning normally on the low-salt diet and were excreting very little salt in the urine. Levels of phosphorus in the urine were very low.

Lactose is a type of sugar found uniquely in milk. It is an aggressive allergen for most adults, although some Caucasians can put up with it. The San, in common with most peoples of the world, are uniformly intolerant of lactose. In glucose tolerance tests, the San had responses that are within the normal, nondiabetic range. Insulin response was slow, as is normal for humans who have virtually no sugars in the diet.

The San are in excellent health by any terms, let alone under the arduous conditions in which they live. Their old people live to a venerable yet healthy old age, in good shape right to the end. The "end" comes when they are too old to walk the 10 or so miles to the next campsite. The aged San makes contact with the spirits of his waiting ancestors. He is propped up under a bush with a supply of water, food, and weapons; he is surrounded with a thicket of thorny branches to keep the predators away. Sorrowful goodbyes are said and the band moves on. That is how it has always been, and there is nothing else to be done. After a day or two, the carnivores will snout the thorns aside and close in.

A Potent Lesson

For most of us, this lifestyle seems remote and outlandish, yet that is how our ancestors lived for endlessly cycling seasons in harmony with our African Pleistocene environment. Time is now out of joint and we have to make a mental leap to accept that the San's present is a potent lesson about the past that shaped us. We have spent some time on the San for a very good reason: their lifestyle gives a very good picture of how our African Pleistocene ancestors lived for eons. It is the way of life for which our bodies are designed. Our studies of tribes like the San give a good picture of the kinds of foods that fueled the machine of our ancestral bodies. We are starting to get an idea of the composition of these foods and the proportions in which they were consumed.

FOSSIL EVIDENCE

We have looked at what primal tribes do today; but what can we learn directly about our ancestors who lived in African Pleistocene times? Ancient bones are a rich source of a surprising amount of information. Rutgers University anthropologist Robert Blumenschine and others have discovered that Stone Age humans were scavengers.[20] He and other researchers excavated the fossilized bones of butchered carcasses. By clever analysis, they found that the marks from the stone chopping tools came *after* the marks from the predator that did the killing. In other words, the lion killed his prey and took his fill, then the humans rushed in to fight the hyenas for the leftovers. As anthropologist Pat Shipman observed, "Meat-eaters scavenge when they can and hunt when they must."[21]

However, there is more to bones than just the marks on them. A person builds bones from the foods that he or she eats, so it is possible to analyze the chemical composition of a bone to find out the foods eaten to make that bone. Michael Richards, a specialist in prehistoric diets from the University of Bradford, finds that, 30,000 years ago, the Cro-Magnons of Europe ate fish, turtles, shellfish, and birds.[22] Meanwhile the Neanderthals, who lived alongside them, ate reindeer, mammoth, and other large herbivores.

Ancient teeth are another rich source of information. Have you ever wondered why your back teeth have those difficult-to-clean biting surfaces? Dental researchers like Peter Lucas and W. Maier studied what is so special about these shapes. They find that they are best for grinding up plant food; on the other hand, they are not very good for meat or seeds.[23] Other researchers have examined the tooth enamel and find that the thickness and strength of human enamel is designed for a plant food diet that is halfway between that of a chimpanzee and a gorilla.[29] A chimpanzee eats mostly soft plant foods like fruits and tender leaves, while a gorilla eats tough leaves and even twigs and branches.

Yet other researchers look at the scratches and wear on ancient teeth. The Spanish biologist Carles Lalueza and others find that Neanderthals have tooth wear typical of a meat diet.[30] In contrast, the teeth of African Pleistocene humans show that they were eating an abrasive, high plant food diet.

Remarkably, fossilized excrement, known as coprolite, has been discovered and is a good source of information. Michael Kliks, a specialist in intestinal health, has studied ancient coprolites and reports that, until quite recently, human populations took in impressive amounts of plant fiber—around 130 grams per day.[31] Fascinatingly, also in the fossilized excrement, he found undigested residues of bones, teeth, hair, feathers, fish scales, and insect shells.

CIRCUMSTANTIAL OR INDIRECT EVIDENCE

Up to this point, we have been examining direct evidence—data that we can measure directly and is fundamental to understanding our ancestral nutritional heritage. It paints a picture of human beings as a species and gives strong guidance to our naturally adapted feeding patterns. But we must also take into account other fields of scientific research which have an *indirect* bearing. This is a demonstration of our approach set out at the beginning—to break across barriers between scientific compartments and bring a satisfying harmony to the totality of knowledge. Understanding this circumstantial evidence brings unexpected insights on a whole range of perplexing health mysteries. Here, we look at some of this intriguing indirect, or circumstantial, evidence.

The Path of Least Work

The review of foraging tribes such as the San and Aborigine sets the scene for understanding the kind of lifestyle led by our ancestors for eons. One factor that emerges very strongly is that humans are *economical* with their energy. They seem to have a calculator in their heads, whirring away, working out what is the best return for the effort they spend. This is known as finding "the path of least work" to get what they want. (No surprises there!) In terms of finding food, this is known as "optimal foraging" strategy. Very simply, how does a human being efficiently find food in the African savanna with only bare hands, a pointed stick, and loads of ingenuity?

Several studies have examined the effort compared to the benefit for various feeding patterns. Not surprisingly, they find that, overall, it requires the least effort to collect foodstuffs that stay still or only move very slowly. Therefore, plants of all kinds, eggs, and slow-moving animals provide the vast bulk of the diet. In addition, foods that require little or no *processing* are given top priority. As we saw, the Aboriginal only ate grass seed as a last resort; it was just too time-consuming and tedious.

These optimal foraging analyses all reinforce our picture of the true eating pattern practiced by the San and Aboriginal. However, it begs the question why humans bothered with *hunting* at all: it is dangerous, it requires lots of energy, and the results are uncertain. Worse, the hunter, instead of finding dinner, could *become* dinner! The answer to this fascinating question is explored in Chapter 8.

What Kind of Food is Our Digestive System Designed For?

Another piece of indirect evidence comes from answering the question, "What kind of food is the human digestive system designed to operate on?" After all, we know that a canary eats birdseed but a cat eats canaries—and they each have a digestive system and enzymes to suit their particular natural diets. One illuminating approach is to take a critical look at creatures that are most similar to us in biological terms.

The closest relatives to humans in the evolutionary tree are the chimpanzee and the gorilla. Since we share the same lineage, we can expect to share similar, if not identical, eating habits too. At the very least, our digestive systems will share a common heritage, even if they have been pressed into slightly different uses since our ancestral lines diverged. Several groundbreaking studies, including those by the geneticists Charles Sibley,[32] Jeffrey Rogers,[33] and Morris Goodman[34] show that the chimpanzee and the gorilla share over 98% of their DNA with human DNA. Their body plan is almost the same as each other's and ours.

The gorilla is what is known as a vegan, a creature that consumes no food of animal origin whatever. A male gorilla is a gentle giant weighing 450 pounds of solid bone and muscle. He can climb trees with ease and swing his great weight through the branches. Even so, to keep his body supplied, he needs to eat 50 pounds of vegetation per day. His diet is chiefly leaves, fruit, and even small twigs and bark. He can spend up to eight hours eating. Vegetation is not rich in calories, so the gorilla has to economize energy expenditure—he is a slow, deliberate mover.

Chimpanzees are rather smaller than the average human and they are much more active than the gorilla. They, too, have a diet that is focused on plant food, but more oriented to ripe fruit and young leaves. In addition, they kill and eat small creatures, particularly monkeys and small wild pigs. Some chimpanzees even poke a stick into a termite nest and eat the termites that crawl out. It is estimated that around 6% of the chimpanzee's calories are of animal origin.

Humans, gorillas, and chimpanzees share an ancestral line that goes back to fruit-eating creatures. Over the millennia, their eating pattern has diverged somewhat, but the same digestive system is pressed into service. All humanlike creatures share the same basic pattern. As anthropologist Katharine Milton observes, they have a simple stomach, a lengthy small intestine, a modest-sized cecum, and a corrugated colon.[35]

The cecum is the first region of the colon. It has a deep layer of muscle that kneads the contents and propels them forward. In contrast to the human cecum, the *carnivore* cecum is much smaller. There are other differences too: in the cat and dog, muscle contractions of the cecum are much more vigorous and they can reverse direction, sending the contents back up into the intestine.

Humanlike creatures also have an appendix. This is an unusual structure and contrary to popular belief, it serves a useful purpose. It secretes digestive helpers such as mucin, eripsin, and amylase; the appendix is also a powerful producer of antibodies for the immune system. The only other type of creature that has an appendix is leaf-eating animals (folivores), notably the rabbit and the capybara (a large, vegetarian, South American, semi-aquatic creature related to the guinea pig).

Surprisingly, it is difficult to be precise about the true dimensions of a digestive system. The various components are particularly elastic and the proportions can vary significantly from one individual to another. According to an individual's eating habits, the stomach is contracted or bloated; the colon longer or shorter. Indeed, a baby's colon has proportions similar to those of other apes. As humans mature, their colon, relatively speaking, shortens.[36] But this may only happen to Westerners on a low-fiber diet. It is suggestive that in other apes, the opposite happens—their colons get longer with age. It would be surprising if ours were not intended to do the same. Gorillas have long colons anyway compared to humans. This is where they digest their large intake of plant material.

However, we can learn even more from the curious fact that our digestive system is even closer in design to that of the capuchin monkey. Capuchins are little, stocky, nimble creatures that live in Central America. Like humans, capuchins have a small intestine that is lengthy compared to the colon. The overall length of gut (small intestine plus colon) compared to body size is also small compared to other apes and monkeys. This indicates that humans are designed for a similar *type* of food supply. Capuchins eat a high-quality diet made up of unusually rich wild foods, both fruits and oil-rich nuts. They also spend a disproportionate amount of time seeking out animal matter, including grubs, grasshoppers, and small animals.

Similarly, savanna baboons painstakingly seek out small nutritious food items—up to 3,000 in a day, including gums, flowers, fruits, and small animals and insects. Neither the baboon nor the capuchin monkey is as close to us genetically as the great apes. However, they have feeding environments that are more similar to the human one and they evolved digestive systems that have a similar design to ours.

What Kinds of Foods are Our Bodies Designed to Capture?

Just like the gorilla and chimpanzee, our jaws and molars are designed for chewing and grinding. Like the great apes, we have front teeth in the shape of a chisel—good for taking a bite out of an apple. As we saw earlier, we have back teeth made for grinding. Unlike carnivores, our jaws can move from side to side for better chewing. Our teeth are closely spaced, unlike those of a carnivore, who has needle-shaped teeth with wide gaps. Our saliva contains the enzyme ptyalin, which powerfully pre-digests plant carbohydrate.

Chimpanzees and baboons use their hands a great deal to prepare their food. It is no coincidence that the same hand, with its ability to grasp an object, is also one that is good for grasping a branch. Like us, these creatures show great dexterity: they will pick out the choice part of a plant or unwrap a leaf to find a grub inside.

LIVING THE WAY NATURE INTENDED

In this chapter, we have set the scene, noting many facts and describing the remarkable advances in knowledge about our human origins. It is a story that could not have been written even ten years ago. We can now properly understand how human beings are a part of nature—it is liberating to know how to live the way nature intended.

We have built up a picture of the lifestyle experienced by our ancestors for hundreds of thousands of years. We have identified the kinds of feeding opportunities they had and described the use that they made of their environment, including their behavior within it. We know that even today, our digestive systems, biochemistry, brains, psychology, and bodies are still those designed for life in the savanna of East Africa. I call this lifestyle the "Savanna Model."

We have not yet done any interpreting or drawn any conclusions, which will come later as we piece together yet more evidence. However, already we can discern the major outlines of our Owner's Manual. Our African Pleistocene ancestors had a food supply in which plant material was a major component and animal matter was a moderate component. We have seen that the *types* of plants and animal matter were quite different from what we consume today. We will discover that these differences are of capital importance. Their diet contained certain types of fat but not others. What they did *not* eat is of equal importance: we eat many groups of food today that did not form part of our ancestral diet.

Contrary to modern myth, those far-off ancestors lived long, healthy lives. In so many fundamental ways, our modern lives have diverged from the lifestyle that Nature intended. It is estimated that the average Westerner loses 10 to 15 years of life thanks to dysfunctional eating habits. Furthermore, those extra years would be lived in great physical shape to the end.

This ancestral lifestyle seems exotic—far removed from how we live today—and few would like to return to it. Indeed, population densities are now so high that there just is not enough space to go around. So, we are stuck with what we have got; there is no going back. However, the good news is that we can work intelligently to get the best of both worlds, ancient and modern.

In the next chapter, we look at the distortions that have occurred in human dietary patterns worldwide since that far-off time. We will see what impact these distortions have on our health and well-being, and we will use these insights to write more segments of the Owner's Manual.

2. The Farming Revolution and Its Consequences

I n the last chapter, we explored the lifestyle of our ancient ancestors in our East African homeland and dubbed it the "Savanna Model." Remarkably, our bodies have not changed significantly since then and, ideally, we would still live and feed ourselves the same way, even today. However, as history will show, things changed. We will now continue our human story by exploring how and why human lifestyles drifted away from this ideal.

Just before the dawn of recorded history, so-called advancements took place that set most of humanity on a path that led firmly away from our naturally adapted lifestyle. This process repeated itself throughout the world. As we will see, most humans were no longer nourishing their bodies to the best advantage.

This chapter puts the spotlight on the major departures from the ideal diet, departures which happened, for the most part, quite unwittingly. As the centuries rolled by, new techniques and new foods came along that led us ever further from our ancestral feeding patterns. From the 19th century, it became obvious that our food supply was not always nourishing populations properly. It also became apparent that the food supply was increasingly vulnerable to dubious practices. We review how government agencies tried to correct both these matters and why we cannot rely on them to protect the public interest. This will give us a perspective on how we ended up with the food supply that we have.

THE MAJOR UPSET IN HUMAN NUTRITION

By about 11,000 years ago, the human race had occupied the majority of the world's land and there was nowhere else to go. The wandering bands of foragers still needed 100 to 200 square miles for each group of 50 people. Nevertheless, as their numbers were still multiplying, these groups came into conflict with one another over territory. More and more they would fight each other with increasing ferocity to protect their living space. The archeological evidence is clear: there are traces of Stone Age battlegrounds from Australia to Europe.

Then, a group of foragers stumbled on a solution to the problem. They discovered how to feed themselves on a much smaller area of land. Instead of wandering their territory in search of their next meal, they took control of their food supply. They had figured out a way to survive on 4 square miles instead of 200 square miles. This was a huge innovation for the human race: for the first time, humans stayed in one place and planted. It would not only change the social behavior of these bands forever, it would also cause a dramatic shift in the human diet, not always with positive results.

The place where it all started was the grasslands of what is now Kurdistan in northern Iraq. Historians call this lifestyle upheaval the "Farming Revolution." It was important enough to mark the end of the Paleolithic Age and the beginning of the "Neolithic" or New Stone Age. The start of agriculture marked the beginning of this period. It would take man's use of metals several thousand years later to create the next important period—the Bronze Age. However, for us, it is this agricultural revolution that still influences our life and health today.

The New Stone Age ushered in unforeseen consequences. Because those pioneer farmers were not able to cultivate their usual diet of foraged plants, they found themselves compelled to grow those items that it was possible to grow. For this reason, completely new food groups entered the diet. For the first time in the history of the human race, people started to eat grass seeds. Put plainly like that, it sounds faintly ridiculous, but today we eat grass seeds on a huge scale. Of course, we know them by another name: grains. Those first farmers took the grasses that surrounded their living space and learned to plant, grow, harvest, winnow, and mill their seeds. These grasses were the ancestors of today's wheat and barley. This dietary change marked a massive upheaval in human nutrition. It was the first step—but a major one—away from our ancestral diet. We are only now beginning to understand the severity of the consequences.

Cereal and Legume Defined

Cereal is just another word for grain. They are all varieties of grasses. *Legume*, also known as "pulse," is the collective term for lentils, chickpea (garbanzo) beans, peas, soybeans, peanuts, and similar seeds. Some authorities, such as the United States Department of Agriculture (USDA), use the term *dry beans*. They are part of a very large family called Fabaceae, the pea family.

About the same time, the first farmers also discovered how to grow lentils and garbanzo beans (chickpeas). In this way, 11,000 years ago, and for the first time, we humans started to consume two completely new food categories: grains and legumes. It was the first demonstration that humans could harness nature. However, as we shall see, nature can play tricks on us. Just because we can consume something without an immediate negative reaction, it does not always mean that we *should* consume it. Indeed, humans can train themselves to eat almost anything. It is one of the lessons that we shall learn: contrary to what most of us fondly imagine, we cannot trust our instincts to tell us what to eat.

A TECHNOLOGICAL REVOLUTION AND A SHIFT IN SOCIETY

The implementation of basic farming skills meant that other inventions had to follow. Farmers had to devise baskets, fences, hoes, and sickles; they had to build storage silos and houses. Humans found themselves on an exciting, yet demanding, treadmill of creation, manufacture, and construction.

All these pressures made for a huge change in human activity. Humans had exchanged the mobile, instinctive, and day-to-day existence of the forager for the responsibilities of the structured, disciplined, and productive life of one who farms and processes food. A remarkable adjustment had to be made: evolution had equipped humans with a mentality for survival in the savanna environment. Fortunately, some of the same qualities, such as ingenuity, fortitude, and persistence, could be pressed into service to make a success of this new existence. On the other hand, humans are not by nature tidy or given to planning for the future or to organizing large groups. These first farmers had to learn, the hard way, the skills to manage themselves on a larger scale and to make provision for the future.

Farming fixed people in one place, so they created the first permanent villages. This marked one of man's most important shifts from animal clan-like life. The density of their populations increased vastly. As foragers, an individual would rarely see a group of more than 50 people; in a whole lifetime, he or she might encounter no more than 400 strangers. Today, we come across just as many on a single visit to the shopping mall.

There was a second, quite unexpected consequence that changed forever the way human society is organized. As foragers, humans lived day-to-day and hand-to-mouth. They gathered what they needed for the day and consumed it, then they repeated the process the next day. Everybody took part in the procurement of food—if not, they starved. With the advent of farming came a radical change: farmers had to produce food in advance of requirements and store it. This enabled the production of food surpluses. In a very short time, these surpluses were used to support artisans whose skills only indirectly helped food production. Here was the start of the "division of labor," where individuals specialized in just one activity, such as the making of tools, baskets, or bricks.

The farming life was in many ways more insecure than the foraging one. The stores required protection from pilferers and bandits, so warrior castes arose. The total dependence on a successful harvest required the gods to be placated, so priestly castes came into being. As intermediaries between the people and the gods, the priesthoods in turn developed ever more complex rituals, sacrifices, taboos, and superstitions.

In forager societies, the barter system is well developed. Humans are very good at keeping a record in their heads of who owes what and to whom: they keep score and make sure that they leave no obligation unreturned and that nobody cheats or gets a free ride. It is easier to police this in a forager society. They know everybody with whom they are dealing and many of them are direct relatives. There is a high degree of trust. However, in these new, densely populated farming societies, this delicate balance breaks down. With the division of labor, the number of transactions multiplies. Farmers, tradesmen, artisans, and all the different occupations have to make deals with each other all the time—just to stay fed, get raw materials, and trade finished product. Furthermore, they were less likely to know each other or have mutual kinship ties.

There was an urgent need to keep records of who does what—and owes what—to whom. This led to another revolution in human society: the invention of writing and numbering. In this way, an intellectual class of scribes and book-keepers came into being. It is from this time that we have the first written records, or "history." (Everything that happened before this time is known as "prehistory.") Barter of goods is an unwieldy and inflexible way of trading on this scale, so money was invented. With that came special classes of financiers, money lenders, and accountants. With the multiplication of transactions between people who did not know each other, lawyers and judges were needed to draw up contracts and resolve conflicts. To manage these complex societies, a class of bureaucrats came into being. All these specialized groups were fed from the food surpluses.

The food reserves were a fabulous source of wealth quite unknown to hunter-gatherers. With concentration of knowledge in just a few hands, some people were able to commandeer an unequal share of these resources for themselves and their relatives. In this way, potentates, priests, and merchants accumulated vast amounts of power and wealth.

Dating the Earliest Farming Sites

The dates we give for the start of farming are the best estimates available. Exploration of ancient sites is ongoing and new sites could yet be discovered that push the earliest dates back in time. In addition, it is possible that improved dating technology will cause minor revisions to currently accepted dates. However, for our purposes, we are only interested in seeing the general pattern of when farming came about. It does not really matter exactly when it happened or, indeed, which farmers were the first. The essential points are that, in the grand sweep of human history, it is a recent occurrence and that farming started in certain localities and not in others.

In due course, many villages grew into cities; some cities became the centers of great empires such as Sumer, Babylon, and Egypt. With this evolution came a completely new way of organizing society. By necessity, and in a great many ways, the new society was at variance with our naturally adapted Savanna Model society. This dislocation affects us even more today, leading to all kinds of unwarranted stress and psychological disturbances.

The people who adopted farming had, unknowingly, grasped a tiger by the tail. Their population densities had grown well beyond the point where they could return to a simple forager existence. So, all peoples who depend on farming (and that includes us) have to put up with its inherent drawbacks. However, until now, we had not even realized the extent to which our lives are affected by this lack of harmony with our savanna-bred natures.

THE SPREAD OF FARMING

As biologist-historian Jared Diamond points out, only a few varieties of plants in the world lend themselves to being farmed and the farmer had little choice but to focus his efforts on those few.[1] This practical reality greatly reduces the *variety* of foods eaten. So, it was for our first planters in Kurdistan. Instead of consuming plants from the hundreds of wild, foraged species, the farmers' diet was now limited mostly to just four farmed species—wheat, barley, lentils, and beans. As the centuries rolled by, farmers gradually domesticated some fruits (such as apricot and apple) and vegetables (such as onion and leeks), but they remained a tiny part of the diet.

The farming techniques developed in Kurdistan spread rapidly to neighboring areas. Within 1,000 years, farming was practiced in the plains between the Tigris and Euphrates (in present-day Iraq) and eastwards to western Persia (Iran). Farming spread westward into areas of present-day Syria, Turkey, Lebanon, Jordan, Israel, and finally the Nile valley of Egypt. It was the scene of the struggles and migrations of some of the earliest known peoples, including Sumerians, Assyrians, Akkadians, Semites, Babylonians, and Phoenicians. On a map, the area traced out looks rather like a French croissant (a crescent shape). In 1916, an American Egyptologist at the University of Chicago, James Henry Breasted, coined the term the *Fertile Crescent*, which became the byword for the cradle of farming (see map on pp. 10-11). Farming was also quickly taken up even further to the west, in Cyprus, Crete, and Greece, and in India to the east.

As time went by, other groups of people, quite independently, discovered how to farm grains using whatever resources were locally available. The Chinese began with millet about 7500 B.C. and moved on to rice about 1,000 years later. From there, rice cultivation spread to Burma, Indo-China, and India. Rye, which grows well in cold climates, was first harvested 3,000 years ago when agriculture spread to northern Europe. Oats came along only 1,000 years ago, also in northern Europe.

Recent Origins of Breakfast Cereals

The modern commercial concept of corn as a breakfast food originated in the vegetarian beliefs of the American Seventh-Day Adventists. In 1906, a Seventh-Day Adventist named Will Kellogg founded a company to make "Corn Flakes" for this niche market. Then, in the late 1950s, came a remarkable example of how smart advertising can dramatically change a nation's eating habits. A new marketing campaign promoted "breakfast cereals" so persuasively that consumption skyrocketed. In just a generation, they became the chief food of choice at breakfast for an entire nation. Progressively, governments have required the cereals to be fortified (or, as the cereal companies prefer, "enriched") with an ever-lengthening list of vitamins and minerals.

The Indians of Mexico were the first to cultivate corn (maize) 7,000 years ago. By ingenious selection of the best varieties, they gradually bred it from a normal grass seed into the much larger and plump cob that we know today. Columbus brought corn back to Spain and it spread to similar climates in the Old World.

In the United States, the main communities cultivating corn were those living close to their Mexican counterparts in the Southwest. It was not until 200 A.D. that corn spread out from that area and then only to the Indians on the eastern seaboard, such as the Iroquois. Even so, it was regarded as a minor crop. Most of the other Indians of the United States—the Apache, Comanche, Sioux, Cheyenne, the Cahuilla in the south, and the Chinooks in the north—were hunter-gatherers. After the arrival of European farmers to America, wheat, not corn, was the main crop planted for human consumption. It may come as a surprise to learn that in the United States corn did not become a big item of human consumption until the 1950s. Until then, Americans only consumed corn in a minor way in the form of popcorn, corn on the cob, and hominy; corn's main use was to fatten cows and hogs.

We have so far focused on grains because they were the storm troopers of the farming revolution. As the centuries rolled by, many more foods were brought into production (and others abandoned). In the next chapter, we will look at how these new foods were introduced and the consequences (for better or for worse) of human consumption. In the meantime, let us note that it took a long time for farmed products to become common around the world.

The peoples of ancient Kurdistan (northern Iraq) happened to be the first to develop farming, but as we have seen, later and quite independently, cereal farming was invented in China and Mexico. However, not all farming started with cereals: the Incas of Peru began with potatoes (5,500 years ago) and moved on to a grass seed called "quinoa" only later. The Indians of the eastern United

States first cultivated the sunflower for its seeds 4,500 years ago. The root of the sunflower (we know it as Jerusalem artichoke) was also eaten.

THE INDUSTRIALIZATION OF FARMING

Over the centuries, farmers gradually improved their techniques. Irrigation was an early innovation practiced by Sumerians and Egyptians alike: it improved yields and removed much of the uncertainty of unpredictable rainfall. Farmers learned to maintain soil fertility in several ways. They would plant a field with a different crop each year and in one of the years, the farmer would leave the field unplanted and allow nature to replenish soil nutrients, a process known as "lying fallow." The Romans knew that alternating a leguminous crop with a cereal crop improved the quality of the latter, but without knowing why. We now understand that legumes put an important nutrient back into the soil—nitrogen.

Sometimes, farming percolated outwards from these centers, often by conquest, to neighboring territories, but the process was not always rapid. For example, the Celts, Germans, Anglo-Saxons, and Scandinavians did not farm until 2,500 years ago, a mere 100 generations past. Indeed, up to the present day, there are still a few non-farming populations: isolated forager bands of San Bushmen (Southern Africa), Aborigines (Australia), Hadza (Tanzania), the fierce Sentinales (Nicobar Islands), and Aché (Peru) have escaped efforts to corral them into fixed hamlets and farms.

Farming always began with plants. However, where suitable animals existed, their domestication quickly followed. In the Fertile Crescent, sheep and goats were soon farmed. The same happened in China (pigs), Mexico (turkeys), and Peru (llamas and guinea pigs). The types of plants cultivated and breeds of animals raised were specific to the locality. But the plants and animals of the Fertile Crescent are the ones that spread to Europe and came to dominate the Western food supply until the late Middle Ages (around 1300 to 1500).

Farmers learned that spreading farmyard manure on the land improved the quality of the crop. Farmers were great naturalists: they watched out for the best growing plants and selected their seeds for the next planting. In this way, they developed varieties that possessed more desirable qualities: for example, they resisted disease better, had better yields, or were easier to harvest.

Yield

The term *yield* simply means the amount of crop that is produced by a given area of land. It is often measured as bushels per acre. (A bushel is about 9.3 gallons.) A good yield for wheat is 50 bushels per acre; for corn, it is 130 bushels per acre.

The earliest farmers used hoes to till the ground. But as soon as they had domesticated cattle, oxen were available as a source of power. So, some ingenious person invented the first plows. They were already in use 5,000 years ago in present-day southern Iraq. The technique quickly spread to everywhere in the Fertile Crescent, including Israel and Egypt. The earliest known use in China is more recent, about 2,500 years ago. This basic plowing technique hardly changed for several thousand years although there were gradual improvements: more efficient plows were devised and draft animals became bigger and more powerful. Most farming centers followed this pattern, but in the Americas, no suitable animals were available, so the Aztecs and Incas continued to cultivate by hand.

The first farmers had to grind their cereal grains into flour. They did this with a device called a quern, which consisted of a flat stone with a rounded stone on top. A few grains were put between the two stones and someone pushed the rounded stone backwards and forwards to pulverize the grains into coarse flour. By Roman times, the quern had become a much bigger, rotary device operated by slaves or donkeys. About this time, there was an important advance: nature, in the form of flowing water, was harnessed to turn the millstones. These early "watermills" were built of wood including all the mechanism. In some areas where free flowing water was not readily available (for example, Holland), the watermill technology was adapted to harness wind power; thus the windmill was born. The technology improved steadily over the ensuing centuries. It took steam power during the Industrial Revolution to replace these mills during the 19th century.

The late Middle Ages in northern Europe saw two big leaps in farming practices. In England and Germany, it was discovered how to get three crops every two years instead of just two crops. This is known as the three-field system: one-third was planted in the fall for harvesting early summer, one-third in the spring for harvesting in late summer, and one-third remained fallow. This increased production by 50%. Mediterranean countries like Italy, Greece, and Spain could not benefit from this innovation: unlike northern Europe, they do not have summer rain, which is essential for the system to work.

Secondly, the problem of feeding livestock during the hard winters held back northern Europe. The practice was to slaughter a large part of the herd in autumn and start again in the spring. The three-field system generated a surplus of fodder that farmers could feed to the beasts through the winter. But this could only work if there was a good way of preserving the fodder for several months. This led to a second major development—silage, a way of conserving fodder in deep pits and allowing it to ferment. This stops it from going rotten and preserves its nutrients. These two developments marked the rise in economic power of northern Europe during the Middle Ages to the detriment of the countries of southern Europe.

So, farming techniques improved, at least in the sense that farmers obtained higher production for the same effort. Farming had evolved in a slow and steady way from its early roots and most of the basic principles would have been familiar to a Sumerian from 5,000 years earlier. During all this time, no one knew what was happening to the nutrients in the plants and animals, but no one really thought about it either. They were being kept alive in an uncertain world and survival was the goal.

Plant Chemicals

In spite of 5,000 years of gradual improvement, there was one big area that remained a problem: the loss of crops to diseases and pests of all kinds. It was not until the 19th century that a pest was successfully controlled on a large scale. This was an infestation of vines in the 1840s by a kind of mildew and it was cleared up by dusting with sulfur. However, advances on this front were slow. It took another century before the agricultural world was turned upside down by a discovery by Paul Müller, a Swiss chemist. In 1942, he developed the highly effective and long-lasting insecticide DDT. DDT's ability to kill just about every insect, yet leave plants and warm-blooded animals apparently unharmed, was so successful that Müller received the Nobel Prize in 1948.

Research on poison gas in Germany during World War II led to the discovery of another group of yet more powerful insecticides—the most common being a compound called parathion. Some of these compounds were "systemic"—that is, the plant absorbed them into its tissues and became itself toxic to insects. Though low in cost, these compounds were toxic to humans and other warm-blooded animals.

These chemicals were designed to kill insects. However, there are other nuisances that harm crop yields: funguses, weeds, worms and viruses. Attention was turned to developing fungicides, herbicides (to kill weeds), and vermicides (to kill worms), with almost equal success. Viruses cannot be attacked by chemicals, but they are transmitted from plant to plant by insects, worms, and other bugs; by killing the bugs, virus damage was controlled too. It seemed that almost any pest, disease, or weed problem could be mastered by suitable chemical treatment. Farmers foresaw a pest-free millennium. Crop losses were cut sharply, locust attack was reduced to a manageable problem, and the new chemicals, by dramatically improving food production, saved the lives of millions of people.

But problems began surfacing in the early 1950s. In many crops, standard doses of DDT, parathion, and similar pesticides were found ineffective and had to be doubled or trebled. Resistant breeds of insects had developed. In addition, the powerful insecticides often destroyed helpful insects too. Resistant survivors soon produced worse outbreaks of pests than there had been before the treatment.

Soon, concern was expressed about pesticide residues. It was found that many birds and wild mammals retained considerable quantities of DDT in their bodies. Rachel Carson, in her 1962 book *Silent Spring*, sounded the alarm. Since that time, agriculturalists have tried to find a middle way between the well-tried traditional methods and the use of chemicals. Even so, chemicals have become ever more sophisticated and widespread, and they are not just restricted to controlling pests either. Fruit trees are sprayed to heighten the color of the fruit; they are even treated with hormones to get all the fruit ready for harvesting on a programmed day. Residues in foods are strictly controlled, but there are always some left on our plates. No one really knows the consequences of consuming them over a lifetime or the effect they have when they are added to each other.

Plant Fertilizers

The ancient techniques of enriching the ground with manure had been known for a very long time. However, it was not until the 18th century that a chemical found naturally in India, saltpeter, was used to fertilize fields in England. Ground-up bones, especially if treated with sulfuric acid, were found to be useful too. All kinds of other materials were tried, such as powdered gypsum and blast furnace slag, but one of the most successful was guano. Guano is a massive thick deposit of bird droppings accumulated over the centuries in the Peruvian Lobos Islands.

It took a while for anyone to work out why these materials had their effect. Then, the brilliant English chemist Sir Humphry Davy, in an 1820 treatise, explained just what these fertilizers were doing. They were adding three bulk elements essential for plant growth: nitrogen, potassium, and phosphorus. Deposits of phosphorus and potassium were discovered in many parts of the world and their availability, even up to the present day, is not a problem. Sources of nitrogen (as in saltpeter) were scarce and its supply was not assured until, in 1909, the German chemist Fritz Haber discovered how to make nitrogen fertilizer from the nitrogen in the air. These three chemicals—nitrogen, potassium and phosphorus—still form the basis of all bulk fertilizers.

Plants grow in soil that contains a vast range of chemicals and they absorb them, even if they don't need them. Over the years, scientists have identified those other elements that are essential to a healthy plant. They are needed in much smaller quantities (so they are known as "trace elements") and there are only about 14 of them. They include chemicals like copper, zinc, manganese, and sulfur. With this discovery, it was possible to grow plants without soil altogether, just dangling their roots in nutrient-rich water. This system is known variously as "hydroponics," "nutriculture," and "soil-less culture." A variant is used extensively in desert areas where plants can be grown, under suitable cover, with their roots in gravel or sand. Beautiful vegetables and fruit can be grown this way by just using these basic nutrients. However, what makes a plant grow is not always sufficient for animals and humans. We need those other trace elements that plants normally absorb when they grow in soil, such as iron, chromium, and selenium, even if the plants themselves do not need them.

Animal Husbandry

In parallel with the developments in pest control since World War II, animal husbandry was under examination. It is expensive allowing cattle, hogs, and chickens to roam freely, feeding as they choose. Much better to restrict their movements and give them feed that is designed to make them grow faster, fatter, and with less waste. Proteins, fats, and carbohydrates are the basic elements of animal nutrition, so does it matter where they come from? Yes, indeed it does. For example, cows' natural food is found by browsing in trees and bushes. This might come as a surprise, because we think of cows sitting in a grassy meadow chewing the cud. It was only at the end of the Middle Ages when herdsmen discovered that, by feeding cows on "high energy" grass pastures, they would grow more quickly. We now know that this restricted, single-food diet changes the nutritional quality of the meat.

But cattlemen have gone one step further: corn is plentiful and easily made into a concentrated feed, and it fattens cows fast. But corn is not normal cow food at all—they cannot digest it properly and it disrupts the working of their intestines. Their colons become overgrown with bacteria, which in turn produce nasty toxins that get into the carcass. Cattlemen even have a name for this phenomenon: "bloody gut." Ever cheaper sources of fodder were sought, however outlandish. Even the last swillings from the slaughterhouse floor were collected, dried, and pressed into cake as animal feed. In this way, we were treated to the ultimate spectacle of dead cows being fed to live cows. This practice allowed the incurable sickness bovine spongiform encephalopathy (BSE; familiarly known as "mad cow disease") to spread in British herds and to fatally sicken many humans who ate the beef.

But that is only the start. Chickens would normally lay only about 170 eggs per year. With clever feeding, suitable lighting, and other stimulation, they now average 240 eggs per year. The ambition is to increase this to 700 eggs per year by the addition of sex hormones to speed up the chicken's egg-production cycle. They are fed dyes to make their yolks bright yellow, they are dusted with insecticides against parasites, and fed antibiotics to stop them from getting sick in the crowded conditions.

Since 1993, dairy cows have been injected with the hormone known as rbST to increase milk production by up to 25%. Antibiotics have routinely been added to animal feed since the 1950s to increase growth rate. All these measures are sanctioned by government authorities, chief among them the U.S. Food and Drug Administration (FDA). But even this is not enough for some: the competitive pressures to produce cheap meat are so great that unscrupulous cattlemen inject their herds with illegal substances, such as muscle-building steroids.

Mechanization

Meanwhile, in the 19th century, another major development was taking place—mechanization. Early steam "traction engines" were developed for plowing. These were cumbersome but were a great improvement on the horse-drawn methods. Soon, they were supplanted by the internal combustion engine in the form of tractors. The first successful gasoline tractor was built in the United States in 1892. The number of tractors increased dramatically in America from 600 in 1907 to almost 3,400,000 by 1950. Thus, mechanization was a tremendous force for increasing productivity and reducing the need for farm labor.

Through all these changes, the *nature* of the plants was changed by selective breeding. Combine harvesters, tomato reapers, or cotton pickers need plants that grow in specific ways to work efficiently, so the plants were bred to be more suitable for mechanical harvesting. In this way, mechanization drove a trend to change plants for convenient handling. Many plants do not lend themselves to mechanized production, so they were no longer farmed.

"A chicken in every pot and a car in every garage"—that was the slogan used by Herbert Hoover in his 1928 presidential campaign. It is hard to imagine that, for the average American in those times, it was as rare to eat chicken as it was to own a car. Mechanization changed all that for both chickens and cars. Animals such as hogs and chickens could be kept in large sheds and reared in much more densely packed conditions. Their products became much cheaper. By the 1930s, farming had become so mechanized that this marked a major change: agriculture flipped from being a labor-intensive industry to one that used few farmhands but invested heavily in machines.

Plant Genetics

We have seen how ancient farmers selected the best plants for cultivation. This was a continuous process down through the centuries. Indeed, many plants that we know today are unrecognizably different from their wild ancestors. However, the process accelerated as commercial pressures of farming intensified. There have been some major successes. Millions more could be fed after the "green revolution" that occurred during the 1960s in Asian countries, when new, highly productive strains of rice were planted. However, often plants are modified for seemingly trivial reasons. Take, for example, wheat flakes: different varieties of wheat respond differently to milk. One of the major producers of breakfast cereal, General Mills, has a brand called "Wheaties." They wanted a flake that curled on contact with milk and reduced sogginess in the breakfast bowl. General Mills undertook a development program to breed such a wheat and then contracted with farmers to supply only this variety.[2] What happened to the nutritional quality? Perhaps nothing changed, but no one cared to find out either.

This kind of plant breeding has a long history, but this does not automatically make it an acceptable thing to do. The whole point is that plants have been changed for a variety of reasons, but none of them has to do with nutritiousness. We just do not know what has been lost or gained in the process. However, with plant breeding, at least scientists were working with combinations of genes that could have occurred in nature.

Carrot Color Frivolity

The ancestral wild carrot came from western Asia (the region of Turkey, Lebanon, and Syria). It was a deep purple color and it was skinnier and had a hard yellow core. As long ago as the 16th century, Dutch farmers thought it amusing to breed a carrot in the Dutch national color: bright orange. For us in the West, this is the "proper" carrot color; however, for the people of western Asia the carrot has remained purple. Now, growers want to jazz up their product and make it more appealing. Plant breeders are experimenting to make carrots with all kinds of hues, from white through primrose and bright red to black.

Since the 1970s, scientists have been artificially manipulating plant genes to achieve desired characteristics. Sometimes genes from a quite different species, or even an animal, are introduced to modify the plant genes. Their goals have been to make farming easier and cheaper by improving yields, and by producing crops resistant to pests, drought, salt, and weedkillers. A second objective is to make foods that transport well, are easily packaged, and have a long shelf life. It is an incredibly powerful technique that has few boundaries. A Supreme Court decision in 1980 made genetically modified organisms (GMOs) patentable, so there is a strong incentive for agri-business to focus on GMO plants and to ignore conventional breeds. The momentum is so great that it is like a runaway train hurtling into the darkness. No one knows what will come of it, but one thing is clear—the train is rushing us on an enforced journey away from our human origins.

FOOD PROCESSING, TRANSPORT, AND STORAGE

With the Industrial Revolution going full-swing during the 19th century, cities grew to sizes never before seen in history. Chicago's population increased 17-fold from 30,000 in 1850 to 500,000 in 1870. New York City grew 25 times bigger, from 60,000 in 1800 to 1.5 million in 1870. In contrast, Babylon at the time of the Biblical exodus (1447 B.C.) was only about 60,000 total.[3] Feeding populations in these enormous agglomerations required novel methods. It was quite impossible to get most fresh foods to them in the normal way. Food had to be "preserved,"—that is, processed in a way that stopped it from going bad. Meat and fish were a particular problem but there were tried-and-true methods to conserve it: salting and smoking. Salt beef, bacon, cured ham, kippered herring, and bologna were just a few examples that took over the diet of city dwellers, replacing their fresh equivalent.

Wheat quickly goes rancid when made into flour. For this reason, since time immemorial, bakers only milled their flour when they were ready to use it. However, ingenious industrialists found that the problem lay in the wheat germ. By the simple expedient of removing the wheat germ as the grain was milled, flour would keep almost indefinitely. Mechanization was brought to traditional processes of grinding cereal grains into flour. For 10,000 years, this had been achieved by grinding the grains between two stones. In the 19th century, that process changed. Steel had arrived and the quirky millstones were replaced by banks of steel cylinders rotating at high speed. These progressively ground the grain down to ever finer particle sizes.[4] At every stage, there were sieves to separate the bits of outer husk (bran) from the flour itself. The whole lot was driven by steam-powered machinery—it was a tremendous advance in productivity. This procedure has been continued right to the present day.

The Importance of Micronutrients

We know that there are many active compounds in the foods we eat, particularly fruits and vegetables. We are familiar with the "classic" micronutrients that have been identified over the past 100 years: vitamins A, B, C, and so on, and minerals like iron, selenium, zinc, and iodine. However, we now know that there are thousands of other micronutrient compounds that play a part in the smooth functioning of the body. In this book, we call them "background" micronutrients. For example, there is the family of carotenoids, of which there are over 600. They give the color to carrots, oranges, tomatoes, and melons. There is the phenol family with over 5,000 members. They too are present in all fruits and vegetables, and strongly present in tea, coffee, and wine. And there are the 7,000 terpene compounds, which are omnipresent in all plant foods, particularly in spices and aromatic herbs. We must not forget the thousands of bioflavonoids, yet another vast range of compounds that are essential to health.

We know that all these micronutrients, both classic and background, are important to optimum health. We can't define exactly how all these compounds work, but we ignore their importance at our peril.

The industrialization of milling and baking also changed the nature of bread. The bakers like the new "refined" flour. It was uniform in size and free of bran and wheat germ, so bread-making became much more predictable. It did not need human skill to ensure that the bread baked properly every time, so this meant that bread could be made on a production line too. But both the bran and the wheat germ had been stripped out of the bread. It was not until much later when scientists discovered that wheat germ is a powerhouse of important nutrients, including omega-3 oil, vitamin E, and choline (a B vitamin). It was the precious and fragile omega-3 oil that went rancid so quickly. In one stroke, this processing deprived city populations of vital nutrients. As we shall see, this had surprising and unexpected negative consequences for the consumer.

The first patents for canning food were issued as early as 1810 in England; the United States soon followed. The technique involves sealing the food in the can and then heating it to over 200°F. Most animal foods can be preserved this way and a good many plant foods as well. Always the pressure is on to select variations of the food that withstand this treatment best. Some foods, like milk and fruit juices, are "pasteurized"—the food is heated very briefly to an elevated temperature and then sealed into bottles. No one thought particularly hard about what was happening. Heat, it was known, killed the harmful bacteria that cause food to rot, so that was good. It was less understood that heating also destroyed natural enzymes and many other micronutrients.

Systems of food transport became quicker and more reliable, so many more food products were grown for export to the burgeoning cities. Thus, varieties of plant were chosen that survived transportation well. Bulk storage systems improved with the development of refrigeration in the 1920s and of scientific techniques of "conditioning," which sought to slow or prevent spoilage by careful control of moisture and gases in the silo. Plant varieties that stored well were favored.

THE FAST-FOOD INDUSTRY

In just the last 50 years, there has been a tremendous shift in the way families get their meals. In the year 1950, the average American spent $2,625 for food eaten at home and a further $724 on food eaten out.[5] (All money is expressed in year 2000 dollars.) In other words, about 20% of the food budget was spent on food eaten away from home. In contrast, in the year 2000, the average American slashed nearly in half the dollars spent on food eaten at home to $1,500. Meanwhile, consumption of meals eaten out jumped by almost 50% to $1,125. In other words, over 40% of the food budget is spent on eating out.

An industry had sprung up to fulfill a need. Americans were earning more money but they had less free time, and more and more women were working. This "fast-food" industry, as it came to be known, provided attractive, tasty, and cheap food—and you did not even have to stop the car engine while collecting your order at the "drive-thru" window. It is hard to imagine that in 1950, McDonald's had just one outlet (in San Bernardino, California). Today, they have over 11,000. They were quickly followed by imitators such as Burger King (now over 6,000 outlets) and Wendy's (now over 3,500 outlets). These establishments specialized in a new type of food, the hamburger. However, other enterprising food suppliers introduced different but new foods to the scene: pizza and tacos, for example. Others reworked traditional ideas: fried chicken and sub-sandwiches.

Almost always, the accompaniment was french fries and a soft drink. The soft drink industry had gotten going earlier, partly encouraged by Prohibition in the 1920s. Even so, in 1940, the average American consumed only about 6 ounces per week. By 2000, that had jumped by 20 times to a gallon a week (128 ounces). These changes are radical. At the 1950s family meal, hamburger, pizza, and tacos were either unknown or rarely served. Potatoes were not often served in the form of french fries; soft drinks were absent. All these changes have occurred just in living memory and we will later look at the consequences of this dramatic shift in feeding habits.

FOOD SAFETY

Like any traded item, food is vulnerable to cheating. The Code of Hammurabi, in 1750 B.C., laid out penalties for brewers who sold short weight. The Greeks and Romans struggled with vintners who dyed and flavored their wine. In 1202, King John of England proclaimed the first English food law, "the Assize of Bread," which prohibited adulteration of bread with such ingredients as ground peas or beans.

As the food supply was industrialized during the 19th century, more and more foods were processed and packaged for sale. Unscrupulous merchants adulterated their products with cheaper and sometimes harmful substances, labels were deliberately misleading, inferior food was fancied up with dyes and artificial flavors, and food was preserved with noxious chemicals. In the United States, Abraham Lincoln set up the U.S. Department of Agriculture (USDA) with a division called the Bureau of Chemistry to look into such matters.

Following his investigation of food adulteration, in 1880 the chief chemist Peter Collier recommended a national food and drug law. The bill was defeated, and this was a portent of battles ahead. Why would Congress refuse to legislate for food purity? Only if there were powerful forces opposed to these measures— the nation's food supply is the subject of a titanic battle between the food industry and governments that try to regulate it for the public good.

In 1883, Dr. Harvey Wiley became chief chemist and took up the battle. He expanded the Bureau of Chemistry's food adulteration studies and campaigned for a federal law. He was so vigorous and forthright that was called the "Crusading Chemist." Finally, a law was passed in 1906. The pure food regulations were scientifically sound, thorough, and gave strong powers to the Bureau of Chemistry to enforce them. Had these regulations been allowed to remain in place, they would have made America one of the healthiest places in the world to eat, but trouble was already on the horizon.

On signing the regulations, the Secretary to the Treasury complained that they were too severe on the food industries. The fishermen of Massachusetts wanted to keep borax; the dried fruit industry of California wanted to use sulfur dioxide; ketchup interests begged for benzoic acid. Very quickly, industry forces set about undermining the Bureau of Chemistry. The Secretary of Agriculture, James Wilson, was persuaded to set up a board, under chairman Ira Remsen, to protect the manufacturers. This "Remsen Board" started making its own recommendations to Wilson, who often upheld them, over the head of the Bureau of Chemistry. The Crusading Chemist's success was short-lived. In Dr. Wiley's words, "The food and drugs law became a hopeless paralytic."

In spite of the restrictions and difficulties, Dr. Wiley battled on. He tried to stop the bleaching of flour, which often uses chlorine dioxide, a chemical akin to household bleach. In a test case, the Bureau of Chemistry sued the Lexington Mill and Elevator Company for contaminating flour with nitrogen peroxide, another bleaching chemical. The case took almost 10 years to complete as it went all the way to the United States Supreme Court. The Supreme Court finally ruled against bleached flour in 1919. But mysteriously, the USDA wrote the application guidelines in such a way as to make the ruling easily circumvented. Bleached flour has never been removed from commerce in the U.S. to this day. On the other hand, bleached flour has been banned in many European countries.

Dr. Wiley took on the Coca-Cola company for dispensing its wares without disclosing the ingredients. The two sides fought to a standstill. Coca-Cola made a concession: it removed cocaine from the formula. On the other hand, it retained the right to keep some of the ingredients secret from the public. In 1912, Dr. Wiley resigned in disgust and wrote: "The makers of unfit foods have taken possession of Food and Drug enforcement, and have reversed the effect of the law, protecting the criminals that adulterate food, instead of protecting the public health."[6]

The Bureau of Chemistry nevertheless continued with its work. By chipping away at its task, Congress passed a series of piecemeal laws. For example, requiring that food packages be "plainly and conspicuously marked on the outside of the package in terms of weight, measure, or numerical count" and banning labels that "may mislead or deceive." In 1930, the Bureau of Chemistry was restructured into the Food and Drug Administration (FDA). Little by little, the law was clarified on a number of fronts. In 1958, manufacturers of new food additives were required to establish safety, and in 1960 the manufacturers of new color additives were required to do likewise. Even these gains are not quite what Dr. Wiley had in mind—he wanted food to be free of additives altogether.

That is the situation today. Manufacturers can make up a confection of anything they like, so long as no one ingredient is "harmful." In all these matters, there is a further weakness: the FDA relies on the manufacturer's own laboratory tests to prove safety. The confection can be totally without food value. Indeed, food can now officially be adulterated so long as it is declared on the label! In this way, hot chocolate, for example, has a poor cocoa content but a high level of cheap fillers, artificial colors, and flavors. Still, manufacturers have to be careful about health claims and they must declare somewhere on a label what is in the food.

Both from its founding as the Bureau of Chemistry and under its present banner, the FDA is supposed to be a guardian of the public interest. However, in many respects it gives the impression of being a watchdog that is conspiring with the burglars. This may be a somewhat unfair characterization, but the reality is that the FDA has to work in a highly political environment. The general public cannot therefore rely on the FDA's protection from many of the dubious practices carried out by the food industry. We have to do that for ourselves.

GOVERNMENT EATING GUIDELINES

The story of this evolution of our diet is crucial to understanding why foods are having such a powerful impact on our health today. It took a very long time before it was recognized that many common diseases were linked to nutrition. One of the first was scurvy. The British navy used to lose more sailors to scurvy than to warfare until the 1790s. Then, a discovery of naval surgeon James Lind was put into practice. Sailors were fed lemon juice on long voyages and scurvy disappeared "as though by magic." We now know that scurvy is caused by a deficiency of vitamin C.

Scurvy

Scurvy is a disease that has been known from ancient times, although it was rare. It became common among early Europeans who had to endure long winters in places like central Canada and among sailors on long sea voyages. Scurvy's symptoms are swollen and bleeding gums, loosened teeth, sore joints, bleeding under the skin, slow wound healing, and anemia. If not treated, it results in death.

Also in the 18th century, it was found that rickets, a bone disease common in poor parts of cities, could be cured by the consumption of cod liver oil. We now know that rickets is caused by a deficiency of vitamin D. Pellagra is a disease that used to be common in the southern states of the U.S. where poorer people lived almost entirely on corn. In 1937, it was discovered that pellagra is caused by a deficiency of tryptophan, an essential protein that is unavailable in corn. It can easily be cured by eating small amounts of protein-rich foods.

The Japanese Navy used to lose 50% of its seamen to beriberi. They were eating a diet of polished white rice and not much else. In the 1870s, the Japanese reported that they could cure beriberi by feeding their sailors with some extra rations of vegetables and fish. We now know that beriberi is a disease caused by a deficiency of vitamin B_1 (thiamine).

The list goes on, but the message is simple: for the last 250 years, more and more diseases have been linked to nutritional deficiencies. Governmental authorities have learned the lesson from this and, in a bid to improve the health of their populations, started to advise them how to eat. One can imagine the early messages: "eat citrus fruit to avoid scurvy" and "eat beans (which are protein-rich) with your corn to avoid pellagra." There were early attempts to smuggle essential nutrients into the food supply by "enriching" some foods: vitamin D was added to butter and calcium was added to flour.

Magic Bullet Mirage

An unfortunate side effect of these discoveries was the encouragement of the notion of a "magic bullet"—that is, one simple cure for one simple disease. As we shall see, this is too simplistic. Most of our modern diseases are due to a complex interaction of many factors that are going wrong at the same time.

For over a century, the U.S. government has been interested in helping Americans to choose a healthy diet. The agency charged with this responsibility is the USDA. As early as 1894, the USDA developed the first food composition tables and dietary recommendations. However, they found quite quickly that, to communicate the ideas to ordinary folk, they needed to group the various foods into categories. Then, they could give recommendations for each category. This gave rise to the concept of "food groups." These food groups have become entrenched, in various forms, in the way we think about our diets. For this reason, and because we will be using this concept as we move through the book, we will look at the story of food groups and how to interpret them.

The History of Food Groups

In 1917, the USDA established its first food groups: milk and meat, cereals, vegetables and fruits, fats and fat foods, and sugars and sugary foods. The government released their publication called "How to Select Foods" using these categories and called them "food groups" for the first time. These early recommendations used a breakdown of five food groups for the American food supply. However, when it was put into practice, dieticians and doctors found that it was too broad-brush and was easily circumvented. It was necessary to be more detailed, so, after due consultation and reflection, in 1933 the USDA published family food plans using 12 food groups. These subdivided the earlier large groups into more meaningful categories.

It might be thought that this was very clear. However, in 1942, the USDA issued a new food guide that reduced the number of food groups to what they called the "Basic Seven." These were: green and yellow vegetables; oranges, tomatoes, and grapefruit; potatoes and other vegetables and fruit; milk and milk products; meat, poultry, fish, eggs, and dried peas and beans; bread, flour, and cereals; and butter and fortified margarine.

Twelve Food Groups
(USDA Categorization of 1933)

Milk	Butter
Eggs	Sugars
Lean Meat, Poultry, and Fish	Other Fats
Dry Beans, Peas, and Nuts	Flours and Cereals
Tomatoes and Citrus Fruits	Other Vegetables and Fruits
Leafy Green and Yellow Vegetables	Potatoes and Sweet Potatoes

It is interesting to see what has changed. "Potatoes and sweet potatoes" have been lumped in with "other vegetables and fruit." "Eggs" and "dry beans, peas, and nuts" are lumped in with "meat, poultry, and fish." The "butter" group has been expanded to "butter and fortified margarine." The word *lean* has been dropped from the category "lean meat." The "other fats" group and the "sugars" group have disappeared entirely.

This does not look like a move in the right direction, but worse is to come. In 1956, the "Basic Seven" groups were condensed to the "Basic Four": milk and milk products; meat, fish, poultry, eggs, dry beans, and nuts; fruits and vegetables; and grains. This time the "green and yellow vegetables" group has disappeared. "Butter and fortified margarine" has been dropped. "Oranges, tomatoes, and grapefruit" are lumped into the catch-all category "fruits and vegetables."

This took the simplification too far. In 1979, the USDA issued the "Hassle Free Guide to a Better Diet." This added a fifth group—"fats, sweets, and alcohol"—to the Basic Four. The guide recommended moderation in the use of the fifth group and also mentioned calories and dietary fiber for the first time.

Finally, in 1980, the USDA released the first Dietary Guidelines for Americans. The only change was to split the "fruit and vegetable" group into separate groups. So, now we are up to six groups. The USDA, for ease of reference, condensed their designations to: the Grains group, the Vegetables group, the Fruit group, the Milk (Dairy) group, the Meat and Beans group, and the Fats, Oils, and Sweets group.

Six Food Groups
(USDA Categorization of 1980–2004)

Grains	Milk (Dairy)
Vegetables	Meat and Beans
Fruit	Fats, Oils, and Sweets

Since that time, the USDA has issued revisions to its Dietary Guidelines every five years, but the food group classification has remained broadly the same. More recently, the USDA mentioned the use of "salt and sodium" and recommends moderation. Finally in 2005, the USDA issued the following redefinition of the food groups:

Six Food Groups	
(USDA Categorization 2005)	
Grains	Milk (Dairy)
Vegetables	Meat and Beans
Fruit	Oils

The only food group that the USDA changed is the "Fats, Oils, and Sweets" group—it is now just the "Oils" group. Where have fat and sugar gone? The USDA has created a new concept: that of optional treats. If your daily intake of calories on the conventional food groups leaves a shortfall, you can top-up with sugars and fats. By removing sugar and fat from food groups altogether, the USDA is placating the sugar, snack-food, soft drink, and confectionary lobbies, and it is also an attempt to feed consumers' weakness for pleasurable and comfort foods.

In 1992, to give a pictorial presentation to the Dietary Guidelines, the USDA introduced the Food Guide Pyramid. This is a neat way of showing the *priority* to be given to each group as well as depicting the food groups themselves. However, as we shall see later, there are serious flaws both in the groupings and the priorities.

So, there is nothing special about the way our food supply is categorized today. Other categorizations have been used in the past and every few years the USDA reviews and makes changes to them. Most Americans will be familiar from their school days with the idea of food groups. However, depending on just what year they went to school, the food groups were different. No wonder people are confused.

Why are the contents of the food groups shuffled around so much? One of the reasons has to do with pressure groups. The sugar lobby did not like being singled out, so they got sugar dropped entirely in 1942. Only in 1980, and against bitter opposition, did the USDA get sugar mentioned again, but only as an afterthought in the "Fats, Oils, and Sweets" group. Likewise, butter and margarine were quietly merged into the same group. For similar reasons, the potato lobby got their product dropped as a food group in 1942; the potato and its french fry variant have remained submerged in the "Vegetable" group ever since. For this reason, in the minds of most Americans, a french fry has just the same value as a tomato. As for "lean meat" and "green and yellow vegetables," they were leveled down and airbrushed out of special mention.

The Bond Effect Food Groups

When we look at the history of our food supply in the next chapter, we will follow the USDA's broad food group categorizations because most people are familiar with them. However, there is an arbitrary nature to some of the groupings that has more to do with political expediency than scientific rigor. So, we will subdivide some of the groups in a way that allows us to make important distinctions between the types of foods within the group. We will also add groups that do not exist at the moment, namely a "Sugars and Sweeteners" group, "Salt and Sodium" group, and a "Beverages" group. We will also add fats back into the oils group.

By the term *vegetable*, the USDA means any plant food that is not a fruit, grain, nut, or legume. Even after excluding these categories of plant food, the term *vegetable* covers a wide range of plant types. For reasons that will become clear later, we will divide the "Vegetable" group in two: "Vegetables (Starchy)" and "Vegetables (Non-Starchy)."

One USDA group, "Meat, Fish, Poultry, Dry Beans, Nuts and Eggs," seems to have been lumped together because they are, on the whole, protein-rich foods. However, not all protein-rich foods (for example, cheese) are included and some protein-poor foods (for example, chestnuts) make the list. This USDA food group is just too incoherent for our purposes. There are significant differences among these items, so we will break down this group into three major classes. One is protein-rich foods of animal origin: "Meat, Poultry, Eggs, and Fish." The other two are protein-rich foods of plant origin: "Dry Beans and Peas (or Legumes)" and "Nuts."

By making these adjustments to the familiar USDA food groups, we will be able to highlight in a more precise way how foods conform to, or diverge from, the Savannah Model. As we proceed through the book, it will be necessary to make even more subtle distinctions, but for now, this breakdown will serve our purposes. Our modified groupings then are: Grains; Vegetables (Starchy); Vegetables (Non-Starchy); Fruits; Milk and Dairy; Meat, Fish, Eggs, and Poultry; Dry Beans; Nuts; Fats and Oils; Sugars and Sweeteners; Salt and Sodium; and Beverages. Table 2.1 (shown on page 49) shows how the modified groups can be compared to the current USDA groups.

Dietary Guidelines for Americans

The categorization of the nation's food supply into food groups is the first of a two-stage process. The second, and more important, stage is then recommending to Americans how many servings of each food group they should be consuming every day. These recommendations are embodied in the impressive-sounding "Dietary Guidelines for Americans." First instituted in 1980, they are revised every five years, on the decade and on the half decade.

TABLE 2.1 COMPARISON OF FOOD GROUPS	
USDA 2005 FOOD GROUPS	**BOND EFFECT FOOD GROUPS**
Grains (Bread, cereals, rice, and pasta)	Grains (Bread, cereals, rice, and pasta)
Vegetables	Vegetables (Starchy)
	Vegetables (Non-Starchy)
Fruit	Fruit
Milk and Dairy (Milk, Yogurt, and Cheese)	Milk, Yogurt, and Cheese
Meat and Beans (Meat, fish, poultry, dry beans, nuts, and eggs)	Meat, Poultry, Eggs, and Fish
	Dry Beans, Peas
	Nuts
Oils	Fats and Oils
	Sugars and Sweeteners
	Beverages
	Salt and Sodium

However, these recommendations do not consist of the best advice given by impartial scientists. We have already had a glimpse of some of the political pressures at work. The USDA's Dietary Guidelines are drawn up only after negotiation with all interested parties. These interested parties are powerful and include agro-industrialists, farmers, food lobbies, trade associations, labor unions, politicians, and financiers.

Every five years, we are treated to the spectacle of a new round of negotiations for an agreed text to put in the Dietary Guidelines. It is not edifying: each interest group brings the maximum of financial and political pressure to bear. Regrettably, in the mêlée, the scientists' impartial advice is mostly watered down or abandoned. In other words, the USDA's Dietary Guidelines are not a gold standard—on the contrary, they are a weak and deceitful compromise between all the competing interests.

This is a major cause for concern. In spite of their debased nature, these recommendations are then taught to our children in schools and used to design meals in hospitals, schools, prisons, and retirement homes. Worse, these recommendations become the dogma in which professional dieticians and nutritionists are trained. The conventional platitudes for healthy eating have become as sincere as a harlot's kiss. Integrity has abandoned the field, leaving it wide open to all kinds of alternative dietary nostrums. Most of them are questionable, some are plausible, but none of them gets to the fundamentals. They cannot, for they do not know the truth about our human heritage. The whole point of this book is to provide those fundamentals and to do so in an honest, and coherent way.

ADRIFT FROM THE IDEAL

In this chapter, we have reviewed all the various ways in which diets have changed not just in the last 50 or even 500 years, but in *50,000* years. We catalogued the Farming Revolution's upheaval of our eating pattern 11,000 years ago with the introduction of grains and legumes into the human diet for the first time. We recounted the major changes in farm practices and technology since that time. And we traced where today's diet comes from and pinpointed when and how we drifted away from the ideal.

In the 1940s and 1950s, the Americans led the way in intensifying agriculture. Now, we have found scientific ways of altering foods for all kinds of reasons. When the supply of untouched fertile soils run out, we find ways of pressing exhausted soils back into service using fertilizers, pesticides, and other chemicals. We are capable of producing what look like real plants but which simply do not contain the same nutrients. We can mass-produce animals on a production line system and their flesh finds its way onto our plates—injected with hormones, fed with antibiotics, and dusted with insecticide. Foods are processed and refined in ever more sophisticated ways. Artificial dyes, fillers, preservatives, colorings, flavors, and odors are routinely used in manufactured foods. Foods are routinely adulterated with cheap, nutrition-free fillers and extenders. We have seen how government agencies try to hold the line, but their efforts are subverted by political and financial pressures. They cannot be relied upon to protect the public interest.

All this sounds alarming, but which factors are of primary importance and which of secondary importance? In this chapter, we have reviewed familiar territory concerning the intensification of agriculture; but the main theme has focused on the idea that many of these foods are new to the human diet anyway. Perhaps *in themselves* these foods are posing problems: just maybe, no matter how pure or sullied they are, they need to be treated with caution. In the next chapter, we will look more closely at the origins of the foods commonly available today and examine the consequences of consuming them.

3. How We Eat and Its Consequences

In this chapter, we will examine the history of the current food supply using the new food groups defined in Chapter 2. We will indicate in general terms the consequences of accepting these foods into the diet. There are some surprises: many foods that we think of as being traditional and acceptable are in fact recent and sometimes harmful. Many foods, although newcomers to the human diet, are perfectly acceptable and in conformity with the Savanna Model. To improve our health, we have to confront some incorrect yet ingrained ideas about how we should be feeding ourselves.

GRAINS GROUP: BREAD, RICE, AND PASTA

Wherever we look, we find that farming was initially based on the cultivation of grains of some sort. The reason was simple: it was *possible* to grow, harvest, and store grains. Grains were the first major new food to enter the food supply since the origins of the human species. None of the world's major civilizations could have gotten started without them. It is not surprising, therefore, that we think of grains as a normal, even essential part of our food supply. We are taught by our parents and teachers at an early age that eating grains helps build our bodies. This accepted belief has led most government authorities to give farmers incentives to grow this crop and to recommend grains as the staple (principle component) of their population's nutrition. But such advice is mistaken, even for unrefined grains.

Nature has equipped many creatures to eat grains. For example, the chicken has a hard, ridged palate to husk the seed and a powerful, muscular gizzard to grind the grain into flour. It even swallows gravel to help the grinding process. However, nature did not so equip humans. Let us look at the processing required to turn grains into something that will feed us. The hard, outer husk of the grain is inedible and difficult to remove just by chewing, so the first farmers had to think up new mechanical techniques to achieve what nature alone could not provide. First, they had to split the edible part of the grain ("wheat") from the inedible husk ("chaff") by a process known as threshing. They did this with a flail (two long rods joined by a leather thong) and beat the wheat until the grains were separated from the chaff. It took a man one day to thresh the amount of wheat that grows on about 100 square yards. Second, the wheat is "winnowed" (separated from the chaff) by tossing the mixture of wheat and chaff into the air; the wind then blows away the lighter chaff.

Even then, the food processing is not finished: humans do not have teeth designed to chew the grain, so the farmers had to find mechanical ways to break down the seeds into something the body can handle. The solution is grindstones: with a lot of physical effort, they could mill the grain into a coarse or fine powder called flour. Finally, nature did not equip the human body to digest flour in its raw state. Real grain eaters, like chickens, have special enzymes for the digestion of raw flour. Their pancreas, the chief organ for secreting starch-digesting enzymes, has several ducts,[1] while the human pancreas has only one. The only way the human digestive system can handle flour is by cooking it first. Those first farmers had to take the flour, make it into patties, and roast them in the embers of a fire. In this way, humans were already moving from a natural diet to one based on a rudimentary technology. Rudimentary, yet quite impractical for the average hunter-gatherer. In making these changes, those first farmers were smart enough to grow foods that tasted good and provided a level of nourishment. However, although these new foods filled their stomachs, they were not necessarily helpful to their general health.

Those early farmers were eating flour cooked without yeast—in other words, unleavened bread. It took another 5,000 years before someone in the Egyptian civilization discovered the use of yeast to "raise" bread and give it a more agreeable texture. Modern breads still owe their basic recipe to an inventive Egyptian baker who lived around 4500 B.C.

The Problems with Eating Grains

Grains, as a class of food, were never part of our ancestral diet. We are speaking of all types of grains—wheat, rye, rice, barley, oats, quinoa, and so on—and all forms of these grains, including bread, pastry, breakfast cereals, pasta, pizza, oatmeal, and cookies. Consumption of all these grains is linked to a range of

Hormones

Hormones are potent chemical messengers. Thousands of them are in continual movement, whizzing around the body, instructing organs to do something or other. Tiny amounts of hormone have powerful effects: for example, they turn caterpillars into butterflies. In humans, they regulate every function of the body, including the immune system, sexual functions, pregnancy, digestion, blood clotting, fat control, kidney function, bone building, growth, blood pressure, and even mood and behavior.

conditions such as heart disease, high cholesterol, cancers, osteoporosis, obesi-ty, depressed immune system, premature aging, and diabetes. There is a com-mon thread to some of these conditions: they are, in part, provoked by abnormal surges in blood sugar. These surges in turn disrupt hormones that control other processes, such as bone building, immune function, cell renewal, and cholesterol control.

Grain consumption leads to micronutrient deficiency. Even whole grains have poor concentrations of the multitude of these vital substances that are essential to human health: vitamins, minerals, carotenes, flavonoids, and many more. Grains are basically bulk fillers that displace more nutritious foods from the diet. The situation is even worse with refined grains, because with mecha-nization, the millers strip out the most nutritious part of the grain. Now we know why governments try to compensate for this shortfall by insisting on the "fortification" of breakfast cereals and many other grain products. Of course, these efforts are only a crude and inadequate substitute for the real thing—the marvelous cocktail of thousands of compounds working together as a team, which are provided by plants conforming to the Savanna Model.

From anthropological evidence, we know that the earliest farmers suffered a sharply reduced quality of life: reduction of stature,[2] increase in infant deaths,[3] reduction of life span,[4] increase in infectious diseases,[5] increase in ane-mia,[6] diseased bones,[7] and tooth decay.[8] Today, we can also link grain con-sumption to many other conditions that cannot be preserved in the archaeological record, including brain disorders, such as autism,[9] schizophre-nia,[10] and epilepsy,[11] and immune system disorders, such as multiple sclero-sis,[12] rheumatoid arthritis,[13] eczema,[14] and allergies. There is even a common occupational ailment in the baking industry, "baker's asthma," a debilitating allergic reaction to cereal flours. We are only recently beginning to discover a host of microscopic substances, known as antinutrients, that are common in grains and are secretly gnawing at the foundations of our health in many unsuspected ways.

Antinutrients

Antinutrients are undesirable substances in food that work against the good nutri-ents and often disrupt the inner workings of the body. They are usually secreted by plants to kill predators such as germs, fungi, and insects. In other words, anti-nutrients are often naturally occurring germicides, fungicides, and insecticides.

Grains are also linked to colon disorders, including irritable bowel, colitis, colon cancer, and celiac disease. Full-blown celiac disease has symptoms of diar-rhea, depression, vitamin deficiency, mineral deficiency, epilepsy, stunted growth, and osteoporosis. These conditions had been observed for centuries. It is astounding to think that it was only in the 1960s that a substance in grains known as gluten was found to be the cause.

Gluten is more properly called "the gluten complex," because it is not a single compound but a cocktail of many similar proteins. The human system is particularly irritated by the cocktail found in wheat, followed by rye, barley, and oats. However, in Asia, sensitivity to the gluten cocktail found in rice is also known. Indeed, all grains contain gluten in some form or another and all of them cause trouble in the human system.

VEGETABLES AND SALADS

"Plant food" or vegetation has been the major component of the human food supply since our origins. Some creatures, like our cousin the gorilla, are designed to eat tough vegetation like twigs, bark, stringy leaves, and fibrous stalks. However, humans are not able to digest these plant parts. Moreover, our ancestors did not cook their plant food either, so they focused on the young and succulent plant parts. When we think of vegetables, we do not think of them as a botanist does, as distinct parts of a plant with different functions. However, each part has its own nutritional profile and a role to play in our diet. Even today, we eat from a wide variety of plant parts, sometimes raw in salads and sometimes cooked.

Above ground, the edible part can be the stem, bud, leafstalk, leaf, bean pod, or the immature flower. In addition, there are some fruits, such as the avocado and tomato, which are included in the vegetable category. Indeed, most people think of them and use them as vegetables, so they are surprised to hear that, botanically, avocado and tomato are fruits. A large percentage of our ancestors' food supply came from vegetation that was levered out of the ground with a digging stick. Today, we still eat many foods that grow underground—roots, tubers, bulbs, and corms (solid bulbs).

Most of the vegetables we use today have been known since ancient times. Merchants, traders, and empire builders spread them around the Old World. The Romans in particular moved plants around their territories wherever they would flourish. Later, the Spanish, Portuguese, Dutch, and British spread vegetables that they found with the Inca, Aztec, and Maya, to the rest of the world. During all this time, gardeners were hybridizing and "improving" the species, so that it is often uncertain just what the original, wild species was like.

The U.S. Department of Agriculture (USDA) does not subdivide its Vegetable Group: they classify french fries and ketchup as vegetables just like lettuce and broccoli. As this example shows, it does indeed make a difference just what kind of vegetable we are eating—not all "vegetables" conform to the type of plant food to which we are naturally adapted. It is also true that our Pleistocene ancestors in East Africa would not be familiar with a single vegetable species in our present food supply. For reasons that will become clear later, we divided vegetables into two new groups, "starchy" vegetables and non-starchy vegetables.

Starchy Vegetables

Certain plants have evolved the ability to store food during times of plenty to see them through times of hardship. Some of them store the food in the form of starch. In most cases, the roots are pressed into service as storage organs. Examples are Old World vegetables such as beets from southern Europe, parsnips from temperate Europe, and carrots from Afghanistan. An aboveground example is the chestnut. This might come as a surprise, for the chestnut is usually lumped in with all the other tree-nuts. However tree-nuts typically are rich in oil (around 50%), rich in protein (up to 25%), and low in starch. The chestnut is very starchy and very low in protein and oils (both around 1.5%). Its nutrient profile is like other starchy vegetables and we therefore class it as such.

However, it is a tuber from the New World that has relegated all Old World starchy root vegetables to minor players—the potato. The Spanish conquistadors first brought it back to Europe from Incan Peru in the 16th century. A relative of the tomato plant, it was a small, wrinkled tuber, rather like a walnut. For a long time, Europeans did not know what to do with it; some farmers grew it to fatten their pigs. Then, in the 1800s, the British blockaded France during its war against Napoleon. With their regular foods in short supply, the French developed ways to incorporate potatoes into their daily diet.

Potatoes are not even edible in their raw state, as the human digestive system can only cope with them if they are cooked—they require processing. So, it is only in the last 200 years that the potato entered the diet. But its success was immediate, widespread, and rapid. It has relegated every other root vegetable to the sidelines. However, this has not been a beneficial development.

We all love the potato: it is the most commonly consumed vegetable, served up in dozens of tasty and imaginative ways. Unfortunately for us, its consumption is linked to readily observed conditions, such as obesity, diabetes, high cholesterol, heart disease, and cancers, because of abnormal surges in blood sugar. There are potential difficulties as well with some of the other "starchy" root vegetables, such as the aforementioned parsnip, beets, and carrots.

We think of the potato as a safe food to eat—even if it might be fattening—but very few people are aware that the potato is also mildly toxic. Potato consumption is directly linked to allergies, bowel disorders, confusion, and depression. Every year, dozens of people are hospitalized with potato poisoning, and many more cases go undiagnosed. These problems are directly linked to antinutrients in the potato that our bodies can't cope with. We will deal with the science behind these startling assertions in Chapter 4.

Non-Starchy Vegetables

Not all underground vegetables are starchy. For example, turnip and radish, which both originated in Asia, are non-starchy, as are bulbs such as onion and garlic from Asia and the leek from the Middle East. Corms such as Chinese water chestnut are also non-starchy. Unlike the starchy roots, they mostly get their bulk from another compound called "inulin." We will reveal the significance of this in Chapter 4 when we look at the science behind our food supply.

The vegetables from above ground cover a huge range of plant parts: stems, such as asparagus from the Mediterranean and kohlrabi from Europe; buds, such as Brussels sprouts from Belgium; leafstalks, such as celery from the Mediterranean and rhubarb from Asia; leaves, such as Europe's cabbage, lettuce, and spinach; immature flowers, such as cauliflower from Europe, broccoli from Turkey, and artichoke from the western Mediterranean; immature fruits, such as eggplant from southern Asia and cucumber from northern India; mature "vegetable-fruits," such as tomato from Peru, avocado from Central America, and bell pepper from the Andes; edible bean pods, such as runner beans from tropical America; and edible fungi (mushrooms) from just about everywhere. Of course, today, these plants are grown all over the world, wherever farmers can produce them economically.

The tomato is an unusual case. First known to the Incas, 500 years ago the Spanish conquistadors brought samples back to their homeland from Peru. The tomato comes from the same family as deadly nightshade, so for a long time, Europeans, warned off by the bright red color, thought the tomato was drop-dead poisonous. Finally, some brave souls tried it and survived the experience without any ill-effects. About 200 years ago, the tomato made it into the food supply. Like the potato, it has now eclipsed all other Old World vegetables and conquered cuisines around the world. It is not without its drawbacks: it does indeed contain low levels of plant poisons[15] and some people react to them, with arthritic symptoms, for example.[16]

It is hard to believe, but true, that the tomato was unknown to Italian cuisine just 200 years ago. The chili pepper, which gives Asian cooking and curries their fiery properties, was unknown before the Spanish introduced it (from Mexico) to India and Malaya 400 years ago.

We have seen just how many new non-starchy vegetable foods have been introduced into the human diet all around the world relatively recently. Remarkably, with the exception of chili pepper, they are all beneficial entries to the diet—none of them seems to have a major adverse effect on human health. The chili pepper, however, irritates the lining of every part of the digestive tract: it causes the colon to become more porous, allowing germs, fungi, and food particles to enter the bloodstream. This can lead to a whole range of conditions from allergies to migraines to a depressed immune system.

FRUIT GROUP

Imagine that you are one of our ancient ancestors rummaging for food on the African savanna 60,000 years ago. You see a familiar ripe fruit and pounce on it— you know it is going to taste good! Fruit and humans have evolved together over eons to help each other. The fruit wants its seeds dispersed, while humans want nutritional gratification. The fruit immediately rewards you with its gratifying, jazzy, sweetish taste, which is known as the "sugar reward." Moreover, since fruit was a rare commodity on the African savanna, our brains are programmed to continue eating that sweetish thing until the supply runs out.

Our early ancestors of the African savannas would not recognize the fruits available in our modern supermarkets. First, our fruit selections are vastly different: apples, cherries, and plums originated in the Middle East, pears in Europe, grapes in the Caucasus, strawberries in America, oranges in China, and bananas in Malaya. Second, gardeners, through selective planting techniques, have heavily modified these different species from their original state since the farming revolution. One has to admire the persistence and foresight of those early New Stone Age farmers. They took the sour-sweet, woody crab apple of the region and patiently bred it over many generations so that it became a tasty apple. They did the same with many other fruits that are familiar to us today, such as the plum, pear, and cherry. However, in the last century, the process has accelerated: agro-industrialists have selectively bred modern fruits to have an attractive appearance, long shelf life, few seeds, less fiber, and a powerfully sweet taste.

Ancient farmers developed most of these fruits in temperate regions. More recently, with the immense growth in global shipping during the age of European exploration, many tropical fruits became popular. The most common is the banana, originally from the jungles of Malaya, along with the pineapple from the Caribbean, the mango from India, and the papaya from Central America. The watermelon is from tropical Africa and it is just about the only plant food that our Pleistocene ancestors would have recognized. The one we eat today is a sweet-tasting descendant of the bitter-juiced tsama melon, still used by the San as a water source. Just in the 1970s, enterprising New Zealanders provided the most recent addition to mass-market fruits, the kiwi fruit. They bred it from the Chinese gooseberry, whose origins lie in subtropical parts of China.

So, today's common fruits are, in many respects, not like the fruits in our Savanna Model. There are potential snags related to the massive increase in sweetness from various kinds of natural sugars, some of which are relatively harmless and others may pose problems. Fruits rich in the wrong sugars can aggravate pre-existing ailments such as diabetes, allergies, high cholesterol, and cancers. There is a massive rise in indigestion in the U.S. and one major reason is eating fruits at the wrong point in a meal: our bodies were not built to handle the mixing up of unfamiliar foods. Different fruits have different proportions of each kind of sugar. Later in the book, we will discuss what fruits to choose and how much and when to eat them.

PROTEIN-RICH FOODS OF ANIMAL ORIGIN

At the U.S. Department of Agriculture (USDA), *meat* is the term applied to the flesh of domesticated mammals, such as cattle, pig, and sheep. More conventionally, this is known as "red meat," which is the designation used here. Similarly, "game" refers to the flesh of any wild land animal, such as wild boar or pheasant. "White meat" refers to flesh taken from domesticated birds, such as chickens, and "seafood" refers to fish and shellfish. We will look at both wild and domesticated sources of animal products. The USDA does not include certain classes of animal foods that were common in our ancestors' diet—the "exotic" categories of reptiles, worms, insects, and gastropods (snails and slugs). This is fair enough as these foods are not commonly eaten in developed countries, although there are many societies around the world that still make use of them.

Red Meat and Game Mammals

We saw with the San how mammals such as springhare (a kind of rodent), porcupine, and warthog were part of our ancestral diet. Less commonly, there would be big game such as antelope and, occasionally, giraffe and even leopard. We now look in detail at sources of meat in our food supply, starting first with farmed meat and then wild meat.

Within about 1,000 years of learning to farm plants, the first cultivators turned their attention to farming animals. They were fortunate that, still in the same location of the Fertile Crescent, there were several species of animal that were *capable* of being tamed and raised in captivity (a process known as "domestication"). This is an important point: as biologist and historian Jared Diamond shows, the absence of farmable plants and suitable animals in their locality held back many other societies around the world in the development of farming.

These early farmers, about 8000 B.C., found three creatures that lent themselves to taming and breeding in captivity: the "mouflon," the "pasang," and the wild boar. In 6000 B.C., this same ingenious people domesticated the massive aurochs, an ox-like creature that stood six feet high at the shoulder. All four species of animal had body compositions very similar to the wild game eaten by our ancestors of the Savanna Model. So far, so good.

Ever inventive, these New Stone Age farmers bred these animals to improve their value and usefulness. However, in doing so over the past 10,000 years they, and all farmers since, changed the breed. The mouflon has been transformed into the sheep, the wild boar's descendant is the pig, the aurochs became the smaller cow, and the pasang became today's goat. As we shall see, with the exception of the goat, the changes were not beneficial.

In discussing meat, we tend to think of the muscle flesh—beef steaks, lamb chops, and pork spareribs. However, our ancestors would eat just about every part of the animal, from the brains, heart, and liver to the guts and the trotters. A few regional cuisines still make use of these so-called variety meats or offal. However, most of us get to eat them in another form. Ever since antiquity, these animal parts have been processed into sausages, pâtés, hamburgers, luncheon meats, and meat pies. The manufacturers of these products mostly have free license to mix-and-match all the animal parts as they see fit and add fat to "extend" them, bulk them up with low-cost ingredients. In no way can these products be compared favorably to the offal eaten by our ancient ancestors: they are from the wrong kind of creature and they are adulterated in many unknown ways. Worse, unlike our ancestral diet, we eat these processed meats in vast quantities on a daily basis rather than when there is the occasional kill. In addition, many meats, both generic and manufactured, are preserved by drying, salting, or smoking, such as bacon, salami, and bologna.

These processes certainly avoid sudden death from some nasty disease contracted from decaying meat. However, they do some necessary things in order to preserve the meat. For example, some (like bacon and salami) are soaked in salt. That keeps harmful bacteria under control, but the salt is detrimental to the human body. Most are fatty (which is not good in itself) and the fats and oils have to be converted into more stable varieties that do not go rancid—saturated fats. These are heart harmful and disrupt many other workings of the body.

The amount of wild meat that the average person in the developed world consumes in a year is close to zero. However, both in North America and in parts of Europe, the hunting of wild animals is still possible on a controlled, recreational basis. In this way, the meat of bear, moose, caribou, deer, wild boar, elk, and similar creatures enters the diets of some hunters' families and the diners at specialist restaurants. This meat corresponds quite closely to the hunted big game of the Savanna Model. The same applies to small game such as the squirrel, hare, and rabbit.

We are beginning to see the introduction of some "managed" wild animals on the market, such as venison (from deer), kangaroo, antelope, and bison (Plains buffalo). These creatures are not strictly speaking domesticated—they breed according to their own inclinations and are allowed to roam relatively freely on a range that closely resembles their natural habitat. Their numbers are culled in a sustainable way and their meat is introduced into the food chain. The American researcher Loren Cordain considers that the meat from these animals is similar to the Savanna Model, with the proviso that they browse the naturally occurring vegetation and are not given commercial feed.[17]

White Meat and Game Birds (Fowl)

We saw how the San would catch various wild birds in traps and snares and even hunt the ostrich. Our lakeshore-inhabiting ancestors would have caught waterfowl too. Not surprisingly, fowl (by definition any wild bird) are relatively hard to catch and so they did not form a huge part of our ancestral diet. On the other hand, the USDA applies the term *poultry* to birds that are farmed.

Chicken, Turkey, Duck, Goose (Farmed)

It took quite a while before any farming community discovered how to tame and raise birds in captivity. The first was the chicken, which was domesticated from the red jungle fowl by the civilization in India around 4,000 years ago. Since then, chickens have become a familiar sight, ranging freely in farmyards all over the Old World.

Chicken. After the World War I, intense efforts were made to industrialize the process of raising chickens. It was found that the chicken could survive being cooped up in batteries of tiny cages under controlled conditions of nutrition, light, heat, and humidity. Britain developed the first "battery farms" in the 1920s. In the United States, mass production of chicken meat took off after World War II. American consumption quadrupled from 14 pounds (boneless) per person annually in 1946 to 59 pounds annually in 2004.[18] Today, the vast proportion of chicken eaten in the developed world is from intensively reared, caged birds; only a tiny proportion comes from a "free range" farmyard lifestyle.

Turkey. Turkeys are native to large parts of North America. The Aztec of Mexico and the Zuni Indians of the American Southwest were the first to domesticate them. In 1519, the Spanish brought the Mexican species back to Europe. In 1621, the Pilgrims were able to put hunted wild turkey on the Thanksgiving table in New England. It was not until after World War II that turkeys were raised for meat on a wide scale. They, like chickens, are raised intensively in large covered sheds where they are crammed in so closely that they hardly have room to fall over. Their meat is now almost as cheap as chicken and American turkey consumption has quadrupled too, going from 3.5 pounds (boneless) per person annually in 1946 to 14 pounds annually in 2004.[19]

Duck and Goose. Duck and goose consumption is minimal compared to chicken and turkey. Domestic ducks are descended from a hybrid of the Muscovy duck domesticated by Incas in Peru and the mallard duck domesticated by the Chinese some 2,000 years ago. Duck raising is practiced on a limited scale in most countries, usually as a small-farm enterprise, although large flocks of duck are bred in some areas of England, The Netherlands, and the United States. Geese are described as domesticated in the Egyptian and biblical writings of 3,000 years ago, but modern breeds are descended from the greylag, a wild goose of northern Eurasia. Geese have not attracted the attention of intensive farmers on the same scale as chickens and turkeys. Goose raising is a minor farm enterprise in practically all countries, but in central Europe and parts of France there is important commercial goose production. Notably in France, these birds are raised specially to make the fatty delicacy "pâté de foie gras," made from the diseased livers of force-fed geese.

Game Fowl (Wild)

The early civilizations carried on the old traditions of hunting, trapping, and snaring fowl. The ancient Egyptians caught and ate ostrich, bustard, crane, dove, pigeon, duck, quail, partridge, pheasant, and goose. Birds associated with the gods were taboo, notably the falcon, the ibis (a kind of heron), and the vulture. The Greeks and Romans did not eat much fowl, although at feasts peacock, thrushes, and ring-dove might be served. However, we must remember that the food of the ordinary citizen was extremely frugal; banquets and feasts were for the few, the wealthy gentry.

Managed Game Birds. Wild bird flesh corresponds closely to the Savanna Model. In addition, there is a large production of "managed" game to provide sport for shooting parties. These are predominantly pheasant, grouse, pigeon, partridge, and quail. (The partridge is related to the francolin hunted by the San.) However, often the managing techniques involve intensive feeding and the production of slow-flying birds. Their meat might well be closer to battery chicken quality than their wild counterparts.

Ostrich and Emu. We are beginning to see some ranching of large flightless birds, notably ostrich and emu. The ostrich is the same species as the ostrich of our African homeland and hunted by the San; it can stand up to 8 feet high. The emu, from the savannas of Australia, is a slightly smaller bird, but still stands up to 6 feet high; it has flesh similar to the ostrich. Provided the farming of these creatures does not intensify (like it has for the chicken), their meat is in conformity with the Savanna Model.

Eggs

Eggs formed a regular part of our ancestors' diet whenever they could find them. Of course, they were not restricted in the species of bird—anything from guinea fowl eggs to ostrich eggs would do just fine. Being in the tropics, the seasons did not vary much throughout the year, so there was usually the egg of some bird or another available most of the time for the San.

Farmed. The first farmers had to go looking for wild eggs. The Fertile Crescent is outside the tropics (it is about the same latitude as Washington, D.C.) and mostly eggs only came along in spring. It was not until chickens were domesticated that eggs were "farmed": wherever the chicken arrived, the hen's egg arrived too. In due course, as duck, goose, and turkey were domesticated, these creatures were bred for their eggs as well. Today, with the enormous advantage of price and the massive volume of battery-hen production, it is the hen's egg that totally dominates the food supply. Does this matter? Are there significant differences between battery-farmed hen's eggs and wild eggs from a variety of birds? We will see later that there are differences, but not necessarily the ones we think.

Wild. The gathering of wild eggs today is greatly restricted by government regulation in most developed countries. However, the eggs of many species are available in small quantities as a by-product of the management of game birds. In this way, eggs from quail, pigeons, gulls, lapwings, plovers, pheasants, and ostriches are available to culinary enthusiasts. We must also mention eggs from reptiles: eggs from crocodiles and turtles would have been quite common in the diet of our African Pleistocene ancestors. Turtles lay eggs in prodigious numbers in sandy shorelines, and collecting and commercializing them has become a major industry in Malaysia. Wild eggs in general form a tiny part of consumption in the developed world and, with the possible exception of quail eggs, most people have never even seen one.

Seafood (Fish and Shellfish)

Our ancient ancestors certainly consumed fish and shellfish on a modest scale—up to 12% of calories according to Michael Crawford, professor of nutrition at London Metropolitan University.[20] As we saw in Chapter 1, fish were speared and trapped as the occasion presented itself. Pleistocene man (or more likely women) easily collected shellfish along the shoreline of African lakes and rivers.

Farmed. Early civilizations took a long time to learn to farm fish. Carp originated in China and have been raised in ponds and rice paddies there for 3,000 years. From about 500 B.C., the ancient Egyptians raised fish in specially built ponds. The main species was Nile perch, a variety of tilapia, which is still commonly available today. Carp cultivation has spread all over the world, notably central Europe, but it was always on the scale of the village pond or its equivalent. It was not until the 1960s that fish farming or "aquaculture" came of age. Since then, salmon, trout, catfish, and tilapia have been farmed on an industrial scale. They have almost completely displaced their wild counterparts from our tables. Less commonly farmed are carp, mullet, redfish, and sea bass. Efforts are already under way to farm tuna, cod, sea bream, and turbot in vast enclosed offshore pens.

The farming of shellfish, mainly mussels, oysters, shrimps, and prawns, has been carried out on a minor scale for centuries in Europe and Japan. Again, since the 1970s, rapid advances in technology have allowed the farm production of shrimp and prawns to explode. They have elbowed out the wild variety. The farming of clams, crayfish, oysters, and mussels is also growing fast.

The fish and shellfish consumed in our ancestral diet were entirely of freshwater varieties. On the other hand, modern fish farming is concentrated mostly on seafood. It appears that this is not an important distinction—if there is a problem with aquaculture, it is with the way the creatures are often fed and the pollutants that get into their bodies.

Wild. Up until the 1970s, virtually the only fish on our plates were ones caught in the wild. Now, we have seen the huge volume of fish, notably salmon and trout, that are produced by fish farms. Even so, most other species that we find in our supermarkets (fresh, frozen, or canned) are still wild. Cod, halibut, tuna, sardine, plaice, mackerel, pollock, herring, and many others, for the time being at least, are all caught in the wild. We can say that many of them conform to the Savanna Model while the others, if not conforming, are certainly not harmful.

Exotic Animal Foods

Reptile foods, including crocodile, alligator, and turtle, although uncommon in the Western diet, are still readily available to the enthusiast. In addition, many societies make use of snakes, such as python and boa constrictor, and the French have made a delicacy of frog's legs. All of these foods, as they are currently available, readily fit the Savanna Model.

There are many gatherer societies around the world, such as the Yanomamo Indians of the Amazon and the Cahuilla Indians of California, that eat (or used to eat) worms of all kinds. Curiously, there is little evidence that the San ate worms and we can only surmise if they were a common component of the Pleistocene diet. It is likely that they were—worms are easy to unearth at certain times of the year by wetting the ground and drumming to bring them to the surface. Italian biologist Dr. Maurizio Paoletti, from Padua University, has made a study of "mini-livestock" eaten by forager tribes today and finds that earthworms are an excellent food source,[21] which we authenticate as conforming to the Savanna Model.

Hunter-gatherers around the world still eat insects of all kinds and anything is fair game. They collect the immature and adult forms of grasshoppers and crickets; the caterpillars of silk moths; and the larvae and pupae of beetles, bees, ants, flies and hornets. Dr. Paoletti has found that the larvae of palm weevils, as raised by certain Amazonian tribes, have an excellent nutritional profile and no drawbacks.[22] The Australian Aborigines prize the witchety grub, a kind of large caterpillar up to 3" long and $1/_2$" in diameter. It is relatively fatty (19%) and, when toasted in the embers of a fire, tastes a bit like roasted sweet-corn.

Many primitive societies eat snails and their shell-less cousins, the slug. The idea to some minds seems grotesque, yet they are a valuable, easily collected source of food. In fact snails have been commonly raised and eaten in the Middle East and Europe for thousands of years. The French, of course, have made a national dish out of snails: "escargots" cooked in garlic and butter are even considered a delicacy. Snail and slug flesh conforms to the Savanna Model, although the French recipe is not ideal nutritionally.

The Consequences of Eating Animal Foods

We have seen how the New Stone Age farmers "improved" the breed of the pig, cow, and sheep. Quite inadvertently, these improvements changed the nutritional qualities. The flesh became much fatter, increasing from just 4% fat to 25% fat. Also, the type of fat changed from certain kinds of polyunsaturated fat to various types of saturated fat. We now associate the consumption of beef, pork, and lamb with cancers, heart disease, high cholesterol, and cardiovascular diseases. In the next chapter we will examine this link. The goat, which has remained popular with many simpler farming cultures, has not been subjected to the same processes of intensive breeding and has largely escaped this unhealthy transformation. Its meat is low in fat (just 2%), half of which is harmless monounsaturated fat. Most meats of wild origin have a similar fatty acid composition, in conformity with the Savanna Model.

Similarly, wildfowl and wild fish are just fine. Poultry, particularly chicken and turkey, tend to be fattier and contain more of the unhealthy fats. The breast (white meat) of the bird is the best, when it has the skin and fat removed, and free-range chickens tend to be leaner and healthier. Duck and goose are also fatty birds, but their fats are semi-liquid at room temperature, indicating a low saturated fat content. Eggs have more "good" fats if they come from chickens who have ranged freely and eaten a diet natural to their species. Fish have more "good" oils if they are wild or have at least been fed correctly on the fish farms.

PROTEIN-RICH FOODS OF PLANT ORIGIN

Protein-rich plant foods fall into two broad classes, nuts and legumes. Their protein content is comparable to that of lean beef steak—20% to 25% and sometimes more. In contrast, an egg is only around 13% protein. Nuts are often called "tree-nuts" to distinguish them from the peanut, which grows underground and is a legume.

The Coconut

The coconut is native to Malaya, but the first European to see one was the Venetian adventurer, Marco Polo, in his travels to China in the 13th century. Conventionally, the U.S. Department of Agriculture classifies the coconut as a tree-nut. However the nutritional profile of coconut meat is nothing like other nuts: its predominant constituent is in fact water, around 45%; the rest is oil (35%) and a high percentage of dietary fiber (9%). There is some sugar (5%) and very little protein (3%). The oil content is the determining nutritional characteristic of coconut meat and for this reason we group coconuts with fats and oils.

Nuts

In Chapter 1, we saw how the mongongo nut was a great standby for the San. There were many other nuts too, including those of the baobab tree, the ochna, and the soapberry tree. However, the nuts that we know today have come from all over the world. Almonds, walnuts, pistachios, and chestnuts are all native to the Fertile Crescent and were domesticated early during the farming revolution. The Brazil nut and the cashew nut are native to South America, the pecan to North America, and the macadamia to Queensland in Australia, and all of these nuts have become familiar to us in the West. They are often processed in various ways, notably by roasting and salting, which improves shelf life and taste, but it is not a nutritional improvement.

Legumes

We saw too that the San consumed foods called "beans," notably the tsin bean. These are podded seeds that belong to the pea family, similar to the legumes. However, the class of legumes known as "dry beans" first entered the food supply of humans only 11,000 years ago with the Farming Revolution. Lentils and chickpeas are indigenous to the Kurdistan area and their cultivation spread rapidly to other civilizations in Egypt, India, and China. Those peoples then developed local varieties—for example, the soybean in China, the fava (or broad) bean in Egypt, and mung bean in India. Across the Pacific, the new civilizations in Central and South America were developing the native kidney bean, pinto bean, haricot bean, and lima bean. These beans, together with the fava bean and mung bean, all come from the genus (a grouping of species) *Phaseolus* and form the class of legumes that we think of as "beans." Unlike the case with grains, consumers in the developed world have not taken up the use of beans (*Phaseolus*) with enthusiasm: in the U.S., consumption is around 7 pounds per person annually; in Europe, it is 5 pounds annually. We will see that this is not a bad thing.

Soy comes from a different genus of legumes called *Glycine*. Even though soy originated in China, consumption there was minimal. According to K. C. Chang, editor of *Food in Chinese Culture,* the total soy protein intake in 1930s China was no more than 5 grams per person weekly. In Japan, consumption has increased slowly since those days, but even now soy protein intake is still only a modest 8 grams per day, according to Chisato Nagata, a researcher at Gifu University School of Medicine, in Japan.[23] In America, soy was unknown until about 80 years ago, when it was introduced to feed cows. Then, in a promotional campaign reminiscent of Kellogg's breakfast cereal marketing wonder (see Chapter 2), just since 1970 Americans have been taught to eat soy. Consumption has been doubling every 12 years. The publicity touted soy as a meat substitute with supposed health benefits and vegetarians and vegans have enthusiastically adopted soy in all its forms—tofu, soy burgers, soy yogurt, soy milk, soy cheeses, and so on. Their consumption can reach a massive 70 grams per person daily. Even the average consumer is unwittingly consuming soy as soy flour is added to all kinds of processed foods.

When we buy a pack of dried beans or lentils, the label warns that the contents must be thoroughly boiled. This tells us that, in their raw natural state, legumes are poisonous. Our savanna ancestors could not even boil water, let alone cook legumes, so humans never developed resistance to the poisons in them. However, even after boiling, legumes still contain harmful substances, slow-acting poisons that disrupt the harmonious working of the body. According to their variety, beans and lentils can provoke immune depression, malignant tumors, red blood cell disruption, pancreatic problems, intestinal disease, and allergies. Soy contains at least 15 allergens, of which three are considered "major" by researcher Hideaki Tsuji of Okayama Prefectoral University, in Japan.[24] Soy is also strongly linked to cancers,[25] senile dementia,[26] thyroid disorders,[27] pancreatic problems,[28] and disrupted hormone function.

MILK GROUP

The San tribe hunter would track an antelope for several days to get close enough to shoot it with poisonous arrows. We can be certain that neither the San, nor our Pleistocene ancestors, ever got close enough to a mother antelope to suckle its teats. Such a feat only became possible after the farming revolution with the domestication of farm animals. Even so, not many societies made much use of this unusual idea.

It took the special circumstances encountered by the nomads of the Russian Steppes to change that. They were early Europeans who lived in the treeless plains of what is now the eastern Ukraine. By 4000 B.C., these people had learned to keep herds of horses, cattle, sheep, and goats. However, under the sparse conditions of the steppe, a migratory way of life became necessary. The animals consumed the grass faster than it could grow, so the herders had to keep their animals moving in search of new pastures and, as a consequence, abandon planting. This was the first time that human beings learned to live largely from their animals. In practice, this meant consuming the only renewable resource: milk, cheese, and other dairy products. To do that, they had to tame mother animals that had just given birth to a calf to allow milking by human hand. By about 2000 B.C., the herders had mastered their techniques and, constantly in search of new pastures, these nomads infiltrated much of northwest Europe, carrying the practice of dairy farming with them.

In this way, Slavs, Germans, Scandinavians, and Anglo-Saxons became dairy farmers too, focusing on the cow. Some parts of southern Europe adopted, in a minor way, sheep's milk and goat's milk. Roquefort cheese is made from sheep's milk in Toulouse, France, and the Greeks use goat's milk to make feta cheese. To the east, the Mongols took up the practice of dairying with the yak (a kind of massive ox).

Other nomadic tribes stumbled upon the use of milk too. About the time the Ukrainians were carrying dairy farming to Europe (4,000 years ago), another herder, Abraham, was setting out from present-day Iraq for his "land of milk and honey" in Palestine. However, neither the Israelites nor for that matter the Egyptians, Greeks, or Romans made an industry out of dairying.

Just 500 years ago, Mongol invaders (the descendants of Genghis Khan) brought dairying to the fringes of their empire in northern India and Persia. A little later, the English, Germans, and Scandinavians brought dairy farming to North America, Australia, and New Zealand. Nevertheless, it comes as a surprise to us in the West to discover that, as dairy consumers, we are in a small minority. A large majority of the world's population (some 5 billion out of 6 billion people) had no idea about dairy until the last 50 years. These non-milk drinkers lived in vast swathes of territory, from Africa to southern India, from China to Japan, and from Latin America to Polynesia. The regular consumption of dairy foods, even today, only applies to a minority of people on the planet—those mostly living in the industrialized West.

Interestingly, when in recent years Western dairymen entered these untapped markets, they hit upon an unexpected difficulty. The new, potential consumers thought that dairy consumption was a strange practice and found that it often disagreed with them. We now understand that dairy products can be a problem. For example, the San are uniformly intolerant of the lactose in milk and this applies in some degree to everyone on the planet. Lactose intolerance gives rise to allergies, headaches, bloating, colon diseases, and many other disorders.

The unhealthy properties of milk fat are now mostly accepted. We are told that fat-free milk is good for us and it is even better to stay away from cream, butter, and ice cream. For many years now, the connection between these foods and high cholesterol, heart disease, strokes, and hardening of the arteries has been well known. Scientific findings show that dairy consumption from any source (cow, goat, sheep) and in any form (including skimmed milk, cheese, and yogurt) is associated with a number of serious, slow-acting diseases, including osteoporosis, high cholesterol, cancers, allergies, heart disease, and obesity. The notion that dairy products *cause* osteoporosis is so contrary to conventional nutritional dogma that it needs solid justification. In Chapter 4, we will look at the scientific background to these assertions.

It has been noted that the Germanic peoples, the ones who adopted dairy farming early, seem to tolerate milk quite well in their early years. We find, however, that childhood tolerance to milk wears off. Germanic senior citizens are just as vulnerable to milk intolerance as everybody else. This is one of the few instances that we know of where a human tribe has evolved an adaptation to a new food. We now suspect that early dairy herders must have suffered a very high percentage of weanlings dying from a bad reaction to milk. The ones that survived had a genetic makeup that allowed them to live through the experience and pass their genes on to their descendants. Even so, such people still suffer, like the rest of the population, from the slower-acting diseases caused by dairy foods.

FATS AND OILS

The term *fat* and the term *oil* mean essentially the same thing. A fat is simply an oil that is solid at room temperature. Fats (oils) fall into three classes: saturated, polyunsaturated, and monounsaturated. In nature, any particular fat (oil) is a cocktail of all three classes. As a rule of thumb, if it is solid (fat) at room temperature, then the chief component is saturated fat.

We have seen that the food supply of the African savanna was very low in fat. It was never available on its own and the foods themselves did not contain much. The San really loved to eat the warthog, which had a relatively high fat content of around 10% (but still a lot lower than red meat's 25%). The other major source of fat was the mongongo nut. The situation remained much the same throughout history until well after the farming revolution. It was not until a few thousand years ago that domesticated animals, notably the pig, were bred porky enough to yield a fat that could be separated out. This kind of fat is lard, whereas fat from cows and sheep is known as tallow. Even so, it was only in certain places and certain levels of prosperity that farming peoples had the luxury of free animal fat in cooking. Traditionally, Chinese, Indian, and Japanese cooking is done with water, not fat.

Butter is also an animal fat, so the first dairy farmers were among the first to have fat as a separate entity. Several thousand years later, it was the same people (mostly northern Europeans) who, in the Middle Ages, discovered more efficient ways to raise livestock. This was the first time that a large group of humans had an abundance of meat and fat throughout the year. Fatty cuisine, utilizing cream, lard, and butter became the norm in Germany, Central Europe, and England. These same peoples then brought the animal fat habit to North America, Australia, and New Zealand. Animal fat consumption in U.S. was already strong in 1909 at 34 pounds per person per year; by 2000, consumption had accelerated to 42 pounds annually.

Meanwhile, in the southern parts of Europe and in the Near East, early farmers had domesticated the olive. The earliest recorded occurrence is from the Greek island of Crete around 3500 B.C.[29] Its cultivation was important to the ancient Greeks and Romans and they spread it to all the countries bordering the Mediterranean. Fresh olives are extremely bitter and must be treated with lye (a strong alkali leached from wood ash) before they can be eaten. Today, olives are grown primarily for olive oil. The Greeks first extracted the oil simply by heaping the olives on the ground in the sunshine and collecting the oil as it dribbled out of the ripe fruit. Now it is pressed out, but in the first pressing not a lot of pressure is used so that the bitterness stays behind; this is known as "extra virgin oil." Greece remains the biggest consumer at about 42 pounds per person per year, while the tiny consumption in the U.S. has risen from 10 ounces to 1.5 pounds per person annually. Similar figures are seen in England, France, and Germany.

It is difficult to imagine, but just 100 years ago corn oil, peanut oil, sunflower oil, rapeseed oil (Canola oil), safflower oil, cottonseed oil, and other "vegetable" oils were virtually unknown to the ordinary consumer. They existed, of course, but only as an unwanted by-product of agricultural processes. The U.S. cooked with solid animal fats as did northern Europe, including Britain and Germany. Then, in 1910, the first process was developed by the food giant Procter and Gamble, in Cincinnati, Ohio, for turning these waste vegetable oils into something useful—cooking fat. The process was "hydrogenation." Thus, Crisco[r] vegetable shortening was born and swiftly commercialized as a replacement for lard. It was cheaper, more convenient, and the quality more predictable than the animal fat alternatives.

Gradually, vegetable fat became popular until, by World War II, farmers grew plants specifically to supply oil to the new vegetable fat industry. Beginning in the 1950s, the budding fast food industry discovered and liked these fats: they had a long shelf life and could be reheated and reused repeatedly without producing "off" flavors. Similar qualities endeared vegetable fats to the rapidly expanding snack food industry. It is remarkable to think that fast foods and snack foods have only been commonplace since the mid 1960s.

However, in the 1970s researchers made the connection between saturated fat and heart disease and the spotlight was put on the practice of hydrogenation—yes, it was turning a relatively harmless plant oil into a health-threatening saturated fat. The solution was straightforward: just use the oil in its original, unhydrogenated state. Supermarket shelves filled with a wide range of vegetable cooking oils. By this time, the extraction technology had become more sophisticated. Today, high temperatures and pressures double the yield and petroleum solvents, such as hexane, extract the last drop out of the crushed oil seed. The raw oil is then bleached, deodorized, de-gummed, de-waxed, and refined with caustic soda. This produces vegetable oils that are clear, heat stable, bland, and odorless (some varieties can be used as engine oil).

Meanwhile, the fast food industry, expanding rapidly, continued using solid hydrogenated vegetable fat (commonly known as "shortening") for its french fries until the 1990s. Recently, the concerns about hydrogenation encouraged them to convert to the original, liquid, unhydrogenated vegetable oil. This is a step in the right direction, but not the whole story, as we shall see.

The net result of the enthusiastic adoption of vegetable oils is a dramatic, 24-fold increase in U.S. consumption, from 1.5 pounds per person per year in 1909 to 36 pounds per person annually in 2000. Overall consumption of all fats and oils combined has more than doubled from 35 pounds per person per year in 1909 to 77 pounds annually in 2000.

We saw in Chapter 1 that humans are not designed to consume much fat and oil, and what little they *do* consume has to be of a certain kind. Today, we are consuming very high quantities of oils and fats—40% of calories for the average American—and these fats and oils are different from those found in our ancestral homeland. We can trace a range of diseases to this departure from the Savanna Model: artery plaque, thrombosis, osteoporosis, high blood pressure, arthritis, allergies, cancers, obesity, diabetes, asthma, menstrual cramps, and many more. What is going on? We've all heard the slogan "fat makes you fat," but how can fat (oil) possibly be responsible for such a wide range of other illnesses? The answer lies in our hormones: many fats manipulate our hormones, others do nothing, and yet others block hormones altogether. In other words, like bulls in a china shop, we are blundering about, knocking over our hormones, blissfully unaware of how the fats and oils we eat are disrupting the fine balance of our bodies' workings. This is a crucial, but neglected aspect of what we eat: it can affect our body in subtle, unseen, yet harmful ways.

SUGAR GROUP

In Chapter 2, we split the USDA's "sweets" section from the Fats, Oils, and Sweets group and renamed it the "Sugar Group." What the USDA means by "sweets" is sugar and foods with a high sugar content, such as candies, soft drinks, and some desserts. They are mainly thinking of the familiar sugar that we know as "table sugar," although they also mention other sources of sugar, including honey, maple syrup, and corn syrup.

There are, in fact, several types of sugar. Fructose is a sugar that is commonly found concentrated in many fruits (from which it gets its name); another common sugar is glucose. Frequently, the two combine equally to form a new type of sugar called sucrose. Table sugar is 99% sucrose and comes either from sugar cane or sugar beets. As we have seen, sweet foods were a rare commodity in the ancestral diet. The main source was honey, which is composed of several different sugars, with glucose and fructose as the major components.

Honey

Even though most people today do not eat much honey, it has become a byword for innate goodness, sweetness, and even love. Winnie the Pooh said that "eating honey" was his favorite pastime. Shakespeare mentions honey 47 times: as endearments ("honey-love"), as flattery ("honeyed words"), as a sugar-coating for something unpleasant, as a delicacy, as something healing, and, by its association with bees, with industry and chasteness.

Our Pleistocene ancestors gave priority to finding honey, but they would not have found much. Australian anthropologist Betty Meehan lived for a year with the native Anbarra aboriginals of Northern Australia and she recorded an average honey consumption of around 4 pounds per person per year.[30] That contrasts with the current average consumption of sugar in the U.S. of about 160 pounds per person per year—40 times as much.

The situation would have remained much the same up until the first farmers learned how to "farm" bees. The first recorded instance of beekeeping is in Ancient Egypt around 2400 B.C. From that time on, it is clear that, for the ancient Egyptians at least, honey became more available. Even so, it is certain that honey consumption was limited to the affluent classes: in 2100 B.C., the 1,000 manual workers building a monument ate "bread, vegetables, and meat," whereas the king's messenger received in addition "oil, fat, wine, figs, and honey."[31] A marriage contract of around 1200 B.C. provides the bride with "12 jars of honey per year" (around 20 pounds), so honey is still precious and rare enough to form part of a marriage bargain. The boy-Pharaoh, Tutankhamen, had jars of honey buried with him. On the other hand, it seems that the ordinary populace had to make do with other sources of sweetness, which archaeologists have identified as syrups made from the juices of figs, dates, and grapes.[32]

The practice of beekeeping spread to ancient Greece and Rome, while the ancient Chinese imported honey from the Mediterranean area. In A.D. 500, one retired Peking bureaucrat was paid a quart of honey per month as pension. In late Bronze Age Britain (around 1000 B.C.), the production of beeswax was vital for the casting of bronze objects. We can suppose that the Ancient Britons enjoyed eating the honey that came with the wax.

In Europe's Middle Ages, there are many records of honey production. In England, Dame Alice de Bryene recorded in her household accounts for the year 1412 to 1413 a consumption of 6-$\frac{1}{2}$ quarts of honey. In her 40-strong household, this works out at less than half a pound per person per year. By Shakespeare's time, at the turn of the 1600s, just about every smallholder and cottager would have had a hive or two. Honey was commonplace but not available in large quantities, perhaps not even the 4 pounds per person annually that the Australian aboriginal was able to find by foraging. Even today, honey consumption in the U.S. languishes at around 1 pound per person per year, but that is because of the arrival of a powerful competitor—sugar.

Table Sugar

Common sugar (or table sugar) comes chiefly from either sugar cane or sugar beets. Sugar cane is native to New Guinea in Southeast Asia and several thousand years ago, sugar cane cultivation spread throughout tropical Asia, notably to India. Alexander the Great, in his conquest of the Ganges area of India during the 3rd century B.C., was one of the first Europeans to come into contact with sugar cane. He reported the existence of a "stiff grass yielding a kind of honey." Mostly Indians just chewed the cane, but around this time, in 400 B.C., they were trying to develop ways to extract the juice. The methods were rudimentary, but they were the first examples of sugar presses or "mills."

During the Dark Ages (around A.D. 500 to A.D. 1000), all contact with India was lost, so the crusaders in the 11th century became the first Europeans for over a millennium to come into contact with sugar. This was in Arabia and by this time extraction and refining had improved. Sugar came as a solid lump or "loaf" and it was as rare and expensive as spices. The source of sugar was a mystery, one that was closely guarded by the Arab merchants, but the returning crusaders were sufficiently enthusiastic (and entrepreneurial) to start trading sugar with the Arabs. In Europe, as is the way with rare and expensive commodities, wealthy households started to replace "cheap" honey by extravagant sugar. Then, in the 1390s, sugar cane was planted in southern Spain and Portugal by the Arab occupiers. The secret was out and sugar cane was carried to the Canaries, the recently discovered islands off the coast of Africa under Spanish control. In 1493, on his second voyage, Columbus stopped in the Canaries and took the first sugar cane cuttings to the New World.

In the 1550s, the Portuguese already had a strongly developed sugar industry in Brazil, with 2,000 sugar mills along the northeast coast.[33] Even so, until the 1750s, sugar was still worth its weight in gold. Big profits could be made by those who could find new sugar-growing areas and more efficient means to extract the sugar. Speculators, entrepreneurs, and planters hastened to cultivate sugar cane in all suitable parts of the tropics and subtropics. During the 18th century, sugar plantations sprang up all over the Caribbean—in Haiti, Barbados, Cuba, Jamaica, the Virgin Islands, and Guadeloupe. In the century from 1700 to 1800, British consumption trebled from 4 pounds per person per year to 12 pounds annually. By the end of that century, sugar was readily available in rural areas as well as towns and was within the reach of all classes in society. At first, most sugar in Britain was used in tea, but later candies and chocolates became extremely popular. Planting increased during the 19th century, expanding to Fiji, Hawaii, Australia, India, Thailand, and southern Africa. During the 20th century, Florida became a world-scale producer.

An Elizabethan Overindulgence

Sugar was still beyond the means of the common folk, but it seems that the wealthy were already overindulging. Queen Elizabeth I of England in the 16th century received regal presents of loafsugar from the King of Morocco. In 1598, a foreign visitor remarked of Elizabeth that "her teeth were black, a defect to which the English gentry seem subject from their great use of sugar."[34] Perhaps unwittingly, the King of Morocco's generosity was the cause.

That was cane sugar, but in the middle of the 18th century, a German scientist devised a method of extracting sugar from another plant, mangel-wurzel, a type of beet. Fifty years later, another German improved the mangel-wurzel to the plant now known as "sugar beet" and erected the first beet-sugar factory in 1802. In 1811, Napoleon was worried about the British blockade of sugar imports from the West Indies (the same blockade that drove the French to eat potatoes), so he set up sugar-beet schools, factories, and plantations. Sugar-beet grows easily in temperate climates and most European countries quickly set up their own sugar-beet industry. The same techniques were adopted in North America, Russia, China, Japan, and other temperate zones of the world. Now, production of sugar from sugar beets rivals that from sugar cane.

Just in the last century, sugar has moved from being a luxury item to a cheap commodity. Annual consumption in America of sugar from these two sources rose to 61.5 pounds per person in 2004. Even so, supply outstrips demand and competition is intense. Farm prices have been driven down and each country is protecting its sugar industry by holding consumer prices high. This has led to yet another development: the extraction of sugar from corn (maize) starch. It might surprise you to know that sugar can be made from corn, but the marvels of modern technology have performed such a feat. This product is called "high-fructose corn syrup" (HFCS), although the name is a bit misleading, since it has exactly the same quantities of fructose and sucrose as table sugar. It is a lot cheaper than the artificially high price of cane sugar. Particularly in the U.S., HFCS has replaced table sugar in a great many foods. High-fructose corn syrup mixes well in many foods, is cheap to produce, tastes sweet, and is easy to store. It is used in everything from bread and pasta sauces to bacon and beer as well as in "health products" like protein bars. However, by far its greatest use is in carbonated soft drinks—the American soft drinks industry switched from sugar to HFCS in the 1970s. As a result, American annual consumption of HFCS has soared from zero in 1969 to 59.2 pounds per person in 2004.

The Problems with Eating Sugar

When we add all the sugar sources together (including minor sources such as maple syrup, molasses, and so on), annual sugar consumption in U.S. has shot up, just in 300 years, from around 4 pounds per person (as in the Savanna Model) to 141.0 pounds per person.[35] We might suppose that such a dramatic move away from the Savanna Model in sugar consumption has consequences, and indeed it does. As is now commonly accepted, sugar intake is not healthy: it disturbs blood sugar control which, as with grains and potato, is linked to the tremendous increase in heart disease, high cholesterol, diabetes, obesity, cancers, bone disease, allergies, and many more conditions. This constellation of diseases is sometimes called "Syndrome X" or "sugar disease." In addition, sugar is devoid of any other nutrients and it works yet more harm by displacing more nutritious foods from the diet.

SALT

Salt is a compound made up of two elements, sodium and chlorine. As a rule of thumb, 6 grams of salt contain 2.5 grams of sodium and 3.5 grams of chlorine.[36] Put another way, 2.5 grams of sodium make 6 grams of salt. Often nutritionists talk about the "sodium content" of food rather than the "salt content," because the body recognizes sodium in all its forms and sodium, not chlorine, is what has such a decisive effect on our health. Most of the sodium we consume comes in the form of table salt, although some people get additional sodium, for example, from the sodium bicarbonate in antacids.

We saw in Chapter 1 how the San's diet was very low in salt, about 650 mg per day (Americans on average consume ten times this amount). The San have no sources of salt and the only sodium comes from what is naturally present in the plants they eat. Our understanding of this ancestral diet suggests that the situation was identical for the whole of our evolutionary past, as our ancestors lived inland and had no access to naturally occurring salt. The Savanna Model diet is very low in sodium and, significantly, rich in another mineral called potassium.

The USDA, both in its pyramid and dietary guidelines for Americans, subtly but insistently encourages people to reduce salt consumption. They point out that most salt is ingested from prepared and processed foods, so that much of the salt is so disguised that we do not realize it is there. Did you know that cornflakes are saltier than seawater?

But salt was not always so freely available. Homer related in *The Odyssey* that Odysseus should look for a people who had no knowledge of salt—these were the Epeirotes who, even after the capture of Troy, knew nothing of the sea. The Greeks themselves came late to the use of salt and they might have had a taboo against it. Early Indo-Europeans and Sanskrit-speaking peoples (early Hindus) had no word for salt. To the Romans, salt was a scarce commodity and they even paid their soldiers with it (our word *salary* comes from the Latin *salarium* meaning "salt-payment"). The same goes for many other civilizations: salt was a form of money and was treated with respect. Many Central American tribes knew nothing of salt until the Spanish conquest and the same was true of central Africa before European contact.

Of course, many peoples who lived close to the sea had access to salt. They created salt-drying beds along the shoreline and harvested the salt for consumption and trade. Nevertheless, this was a cottage industry until recent times, when salt production was put on an industrialized footing. In some areas, salt beds deep under the Earth were discovered. The Ancient Egyptians, Romans, and Greeks sent unfortunate wretches underground to mine salt by hand. Nowadays, it is either excavated by huge mining machines or extracted through boreholes using high-pressure steam. Suddenly, salt moved from being a rare, tradable product to a freely available, cheap commodity. Salt consumption rocketed in the U.S. from around 1 gram per person per day to 10 grams per day.

Researcher Boyd Eaton estimates that the typical daily consumption of sodium in Pleistocene times was no more than 0.7 gram per person.[37] It was obtained purely from what was intrinsic to the foods they ate. The average American consumes 4 grams of sodium (10 grams of salt) per day, nearly six times as much. This heavy salt load poses a problem for the body: it is linked to problems such as high blood pressure, osteoporosis,[38] and blocked arteries. We tend to think of our arteries as being like inert plastic plumbing, but in reality they are living tissue and high salt levels irritate and scar them. The blood pressure specialist Professor Louis Tobian has shown that salt damages arteries even if your blood pressure is normal.[39] Also, over-consumption of salt drains calcium out of the bones and high salt levels cause our kidneys to malfunction, provoking abnormally high blood pressure.

Nutritionists have demonized salt often enough, so what has been said so far is not a surprise. However, there is another factor that is important—the consumption of the mineral potassium. Sodium and potassium work as a team in tiny, yet vital, quantities in the electrical circuitry of body cells. They need to be consumed in a ratio of about 1 part of sodium to 5 parts potassium. Boyd Eaton finds that this is exactly the ratio consumed, quite naturally and without forethought, by humans in Pleistocene times.[40] Potassium is abundant in fruits, salads, and vegetables. In the average American diet today, the see-saw is unbalanced the other way—1 part potassium to 2.5 parts sodium—and this has repercussions on the efficient working of every cell in our bodies.

BEVERAGES

In Chapter 2, we introduced a new food group, Beverages. The reason is that the USDA in its dietary guidelines for Americans only makes passing reference to alcohol, sodas, fruit juice, and water, and no mention at all is made of tea or coffee. Nevertheless, beverages are an important factor in our food intake and we need to know how they fit into the scheme of things. We therefore make a food group of beverages and single out the ones that dominate our Western consumption pattern.

The main beverage for our Pleistocene ancestors was water, plain and simple. Or perhaps not so plain—often it came from a waterhole used by the other creatures of the savanna, containing all kinds of bugs, germs, and sediment. In addition, fluid was obtained from vegetation such as the tsama melon, roots and tubers, and even from rainwater collected in the hollow trunks of trees. Finally, some liquid was obtained from the mammals that were killed on occasion; the San would drink the blood and stomach contents of antelope, for example.

Alcoholic Beverages

It is an interesting thought that in ancient times, no one had a means of boiling water. It was not until the invention of kiln-fired pottery in Egypt around 6000 B.C.

that water could be heated and infused with herbs to give it flavor. Within a heartbeat of learning how to make pots, these inventive people also discovered how to ferment beverages to make forms of beer and wine. In short order, most civilizations adopted, or discovered for themselves, local variations on these basic beverages. In 2100 B.C., Sumerian doctors prescribed beer for many ailments; Egyptian doctors in 1500 B.C. included beer or wine in 15% of their prescriptions. By 1170 B.C., Hammurabi of Babylon, in his code of laws, regulated drinking houses and pre-biblical Canaanites had a multitude of uses for intoxicating fluids.

Meanwhile, Indians and Chinese made intoxicating beverages from barley and rice. The 3,000-year-old Hindu Ayurvedic medicine teaches both the beneficial uses of alcoholic beverages and the consequences of intoxication and the diseases of alcoholism. Most of the peoples in India, as well as Sri Lanka, the Philippines, China, and Japan, have continued to ferment a portion of their crops. Japanese sake is a well-known drink made from fermented rice.

In Africa, maize, millet, bananas, honey, the saps of the palm and the bamboo, and many fruits have been used to ferment beers and wines, the best known being kaffir beer and palm wines. The Tarahumara of northern Mexico made beers from corn and agave, and the Papago Indians made a cactus wine. Throughout Central and South America, the Indians made alcoholic beverages from maize, tubers, fruits, flowers, and saps. In contrast, the San, the Eskimo, the Australian aboriginal, the North American Indian, and the Polynesian never discovered fermentation.

Today, the choice of fermented drinks has narrowed down to two main types, wine and beer. Wine is made from grapes and can have an alcoholic strength up to 13%. Beer is made from malted barley and has strengths between 4% and 6% alcohol; most varieties of beer are flavored with hops to give it a bitter taste. Consumption of wine in the U.S. has increased from 1.3 gallons per person per year in 1970 to 2.2 gallons annually in 2002. For beer, the figures show an increase from 18.5 gallons per person per year to 22.0 gallons annually. (These are figures covering the whole population, not just those of drinking age.)

Fermentation produces a drink with a maximum alcohol content of only about 13%, but usually it is much less. By about 2,800 years ago, the Chinese had worked out a method to make the alcohol content much stronger—distillation. Around the same time, the Javanese discovered how to distill a potion they call "arrack" from fermented sugar cane and rice. The Greeks and Romans also made crude distilled products. However, it took the Arab alchemists in the 8th century to develop the equipment and techniques to put distillation on a predictable, economic, and palatable footing. By the late Middle Ages, distilled spirits were widespread in Europe. The beverages could now have an alcohol content ranging up to 80%. (Nowadays, most governments restrict the alcohol content to 45% maximum.) In the 19th century, Western entrepreneurs industrialized the production of spirits and actively sold to global markets. In this way, Scottish whisky, Dutch gin, English rum, French brandy, American bourbon, and Russian vodka beat out local brews to become world brands. Consumption of spirits has declined in America from 1.8 gallons per person per year in 1970 to 1.1 gallons annually in 2002. (Again, these figures cover the whole population, not just those of drinking age.)

Back in the Middle Ages, monks were experimenting with making alcoholic "elixirs" designed for medicinal purposes, with closely guarded recipes using fruits, sugar, herbs, and spices. We know these elixirs today as "liqueurs." Benedictine was among the first liqueurs in 1510. Chartreuse came in 1607 and was swiftly followed by Cointreau, Grand Marnier, Curacao, and many more. They have an alcohol content ranging from 25% to 60%.

Tea and Coffee

Earlier, we mentioned heated water and infused herbs—one of them, tea, found by the Chinese around 350 B.C., has come to dominate the market. But tea did not come to Europe until the English East India company, trading with the secretive Chinese in the 1660s, introduced tea leaves to London's coffee houses. This ushered in the picturesque age of the famous sailing clippers: these graceful, high-speed ships raced across the oceans to be the first with their precious cargo in the capitals of Europe. However, for almost two more centuries, no European knew what a tea plant looked like. Then, in 1827, a young Dutch tea taster, J.I.L.L. Jacobson, risked his life to penetrate China's forbidden tea gardens and bring back tea seeds to cultivate the tea plant in the Dutch East Indies. In 1823, coincidentally, a variety of tea had been discovered growing wild in Assam, India. Under British government encouragement, tea plantations were developed using plants from both Assam and China, and India became a major producer and consumer of tea. Most tea in the world today is so-called "black tea": it comes from the same plant as green tea, just the drying and fermentation process is different. Annual tea consumption in U.S. is not as high as in other countries and has been stable since 1970 at around 7 gallons per person.

Coffee rivals tea in worldwide consumption. It is thought to have its birthplace in southern Ethiopia and to take its name from the province of Kaffa. It was as recently as the 15th century that the plant was discovered and transplanted to southern Arabia. From there, it swiftly became popular all over the Arab world. By the early 1600s, major European cities could boast of their coffeehouses, which became centers of political, social, literary, and eventually business influence. By the late 1600s, coffeehouses became popular in North American cities such as Boston, New York, and Philadelphia. Annual consumption of coffee has been falling in the U.S. in recent times, from 33.4 gallons per person in 1970 to 22 gallons in 2002.

Cocoa

Cocoa has its origins in Central America, where the Maya and Aztecs held it in great esteem. At the court of Montezuma, the Spanish conquistador Hernando Cortes was served a bitter cocoa-bean drink. He brought the bean to Europe, where the cocoa drink was sweetened, flavored with cinnamon and vanilla, and served hot. The beverage remained a Spanish secret for almost 100 years. In 1657, a Frenchman opened a shop in London, at which solid chocolate for making the beverage could be purchased at 15 shillings a pound. At this price. only the wealthy could afford to drink it, and fashionable chocolate houses appeared in London, Amsterdam, and other European capitals. It was not until the mid-19th century that cocoa became affordable for all levels of society. Today, "chocolate drink" powders that have only a small percentage of cocoa adulterated with sweetener, fillers, and artificial flavors, dominate the market for cocoa.

Soft Drinks

The first marketed soft drinks appeared in 17th-century France as a mixture of water and lemon juice, sweetened with honey. But the race was on to carbonate water—the idea was to produce cheap versions of naturally occurring health spa mineral waters. In 1772, the English scientist Joseph Priestley demonstrated a small carbonating apparatus to the College of Physicians in London. For this invention, he is nicknamed "the father of the soft drinks industry." Using Priestley's apparatus, Thomas Henry, an apothecary in Manchester, England, produced the first commercial quantities of carbonated water. Jacob Schweppe, a jeweler in Geneva, read Priestley's papers and, by 1794, was selling highly carbonated waters to his friends. He added other mineral salts and flavors, such as ginger, lemon, and quinine (to make tonic water). Schweppe moved to London and built a worldwide soft drinks empire.

In 1886, Dr. John Pemberton, an Atlanta chemist, developed what he called an "esteemed brain tonic and intellectual beverage, a cure for all nervous affections, sick headache, neuralgia, hysteria, and melancholy." Pemberton's product contained carbonated water, sugar syrup, cocaine from coca leaves, caffeine from kola nuts, and other secret flavors. It was later marketed under a telling name, Coca-Cola. Because Pemberton was ill, he sold two-thirds of his business in 1888 to cover expenses. He died later that year, never knowing how successful the product would become. Asa Candler, an Atlanta druggist, bought the entire business in 1891 for $2,300. The Coca-Cola company removed the cocaine by 1929. Even so, consumption has soared. Americans in 1940 consumed an average of one 6.5 ounce bottle per week, or 2.6 gallons per year.[41] This has increased ten times to 25.8 gallons per person for the year 2003. Another carbonated cola beverage has been around almost as long—Pepsi Cola; they sell 22.0 gallons per person annually. Thus, consumption of just these two beverages combined is nearly 48 gallons per person per year, or over a pint a day. Other carbonated soft drinks account for a further 7 gallons per year.

Milk

We examined milk in the Milk Group, but here we look at it as a beverage. Milk in its raw form can be dangerously contaminated with unhealthy microbes. These used to cause a lot of sickness until Victorian times. Then, inspired by the work of Louis Pasteur, it was found that milk could be made safe by heating it to 162°F (72°C) for 15 seconds. This "pasteurized" milk was the form in which milk was commercialized until the 1960s. In those days, milk used to have the cream float to the surface (some may remember bottles of milk with a plug of rich cream at the top). Today, milk is usually "homogenized" as well: the milk is heated and squirted by pressure pumps through nozzles so that the cream stays evenly distributed throughout the milk.

Since the 1960s, there has been an awakening to the dangers of milk fat—nutritionists have been advising the use of skimmed or semi-skimmed milk over whole milk. Skim milk is made in a machine that centrifuges the milk at 6,000 rpm to separate the fat from the skimmed milk. Consumption of whole milk has declined dramatically from 25.5 gallons per person per year in 1970 to 8.0 gallons annually in 2002. Meanwhile, skimmed milk consumption in its various forms has increased from 5.8 gallons to 15.5 gallons annually. Overall, annual milk consumption per person in America has declined from 31.3 gallons in 1970 to 22.2 gallons in 2002.[42] And the unhealthy milk fat? That is recycled back to American consumers as cream, butter, and ice cream.

Juices

From the time when it was learned how to preserve fruit juices in reasonable condition (using pasteurization) in the 19th century, bottlers have canned and packaged various juice products. They pressed the juices from the fruit, strained, clarified, filtered, pectinized, and pasteurized it. They concentrate some juices by evaporation. Today, by far the most popular juice is from oranges; it is followed by apple, pineapple, and so on. Total fruit juice consumption has been rising steadily from 5.7 gallons per person per year in 1970 to 10 gallons annually in 2002.

Water

Our Pleistocene ancestors' water came from rivers, lakes, and waterholes. Often, they had to compete with lions, crocodiles, and hyenas for a sip from a muddy, excrement-infested water source. It is probable that they picked up many nasty parasites and diseases from their water supply. Water supplies in the early civilizations were even worse: the high concentrations of population not only took water out of the river, but put sewage back in. The major cities would be located on a good river, and mostly the population had to get drinking water from it as best they could. There were outbreaks of various waterborne diseases, but usually the gods were blamed rather than unsanitary practices.

This changed dramatically in Victorian times: there were particularly bad outbreaks of cholera, typhoid, and typhus in London and scientists had discovered that sewage-contaminated water was the cause. In reaction, the authorities undertook immense construction projects from 1850 to 1875 to build elaborate networks of pipes and tunnels to collect raw sewage and carry it to treatment works outside the city. In parallel, pumping stations, reservoirs, treatment stations, and pipe networks were constructed to bring safe drinking water to every household. It is said that this new science of public health engineering has done more to prevent and cure disease than any conventional medical treatment. Quickly, public health engineering spread to America and continental Europe. Overseas, the public works department became one of the most important development arms of British and French colonial governments.

Water for municipal supplies comes from two chief sources: surface water from rivers and lakes, and groundwater from water-bearing layers underground. Surface water is usually dirtier and needs several stages of treatment. It is first filtered and then "flocculated," a process whereby certain chemicals are added to the water to make the fine particles clump together and sink to the bottom where they can be strained off. Other chemicals are sometimes added to reduce acidity and to bring hardness to acceptable levels. Both surface water and groundwater need to be disinfected to kill harmful bacteria. Most commonly, this is done by injecting chlorine gas; excess chlorine is removed when it has done its work. The gas ozone is sometimes used instead of chlorine because it leaves less odor, but it is more expensive.

In this way, municipal water contains traces of the chemicals that have been added. They are mostly harmless substances like slaked lime, baking soda, and alum (aluminum sulfate). Chlorine is potentially more aggressive, but the active quantities that remain are usually harmless too, certainly a lot less than in the average swimming pool.

There is some evidence that a chemical called fluoride helps fight tooth decay so, more controversially, some municipalities voluntarily dose their water supply with fluoride. Now it happens that the waters of our African homeland were quite rich in fluoride, certainly no less than the concentrations deliberately put there by some municipal authorities. Nevertheless, many consumers object to being forcibly medicated in this way.

A great many of the water treatment plants and distribution networks were built over 100 years ago. Not only have they reached the end of their useful lives, they suffer a chronic lack of investment. In consequence, they are vulnerable to mistakes in chemical dosage and to contamination through leaky pipework.

Everybody was happy drinking municipal water until the 1980s, when the public became more concerned about the aging equipment, the added chemicals, and the forced fluoridation. The bottled water company Perrier brilliantly exploited this disquiet. They initiated a marketing coup on a scale similar to Kellogg with breakfast cereals (see Chapter 2) and persuaded Americans and Europeans to abandon drinking the water they could get for free out of a tap and buy water in a bottle.

The mineral water companies latched on to another alarm—that we are all dehydrating from lack of water. Remarkably, they persuaded us to not only switch from tap water to bottled water but also to drink much more of it. Such was their success that consumption of bottled water has soared from virtually zero in 1970 to 21.2 gallons per person per year in 2002. Curiously, consumer watchdogs estimate that 60% of the bottled water sold on the market is simply municipal water put into bottles (sometimes with further treatment). Most of the remaining 40% of bottled water does indeed come from natural springs and wells, but it still has to be sterilized, conditioned, and carbonated.

The Health Consequences of Our Beverage Choices

Our species, like most on the planet, are designed to get most of their liquid intake from water. Until recent times, that was still the case for us, even in the West. But we have seen the rise of alternative drinks, which have come along just in the average grandparent's lifetime. Setting aside wine, distilled spirits, and liqueurs, which are not thirst quenchers, what are we now consuming instead of water? When we add up the figures for beer, tea, coffee, cocoa, soft drinks, juices, and

The Problem with Alcohol

Alcohol occurs frequently in nature, especially where ripe fruits ferment of their own accord. There are stories of elephants gorging on overripe, fermenting mangoes and rampaging around in a drunken stupor. The human body handles alcohol perfectly well in these modest, naturally occurring circumstances. However, with our cleverness, we have made alcohol much more readily available and in greater concentrations. Greater consumption interferes with fat metabolism, brain chemistry, and many other bodily functions. The liver, the organ responsible for detoxifying alcohol from the blood, can develop the fatal condition of cirrhosis. Sometimes, the one-way valve into the stomach becomes a two-way valve, leading to acid reflux, when the contents of the stomach rise back up the esophagus and burn the lining. Plus, alcohol is empty calories: at best, it just adds to the waistline, at worst, it displaces more nutritive foods from the diet. Chronic alcoholics frequently suffer vitamin and mineral deficiency diseases and their life span is shortened by 10 to 12 years because of this.

milk, we find that the average American is consuming, in a year, 150 gallons of liquid that is not plain water—that comes to 3.25 pints per day!

The average farm laborer in 1900 consumed a half pint of beer on a Saturday night, and that was it for alcohol for the week. Today, Americans of drinking age are consuming, on average, 5 pints a week, much of it concentrated into one or two binges. Beer drinking on a large scale is linked to obesity (beer gut), heart disease, high blood pressure, high cholesterol, allergies, poor bone health, and cancers. The connection is the same as for sugars: beer contains a hyperactive sugar, maltose, which creates abnormal blood sugar surges. In addition, some people are allergic to the barley gluten in beer. The alcoholic content is also a problem (see inset on page 81), but beer is relatively dilute in alcohol, so this factor is of secondary importance to the sugar diseases.

Tea, whether black or green, seems to be mostly positive in its health effects. It is rich in certain micronutrients that are in short supply in the average Western diet. The body gratefully seizes these and uses them to reinforce the immune system, so that tea drinkers are less likely to suffer certain cancers and infectious diseases. And the caffeine content is moderate: a cup of tea contains about the same as a 12 oz can of cola.

Although consumed by the large mug, the classic American coffee is weakly brewed and relatively benign. The trend now is for coffeehouses to serve much stronger brews but still in large portions, which is getting us into the territory where caffeine overdose (see inset below) may undermine our health. Coffee in these concentrations is associated with raised blood pressure, increased heart rate, strokes, and heart disease. On the other hand, coffee does have some protective effect against some types of cancer, Parkinson's disease, and diabetes. However, the balance of advantage stays with keeping the coffee weak.

Cocoa also contains caffeine at low levels, but it also contains a rich variety of micronutrients that are heart healthy and protective against many cancers. The warning is the same: use the genuine cocoa powder, not the artificial confections that masquerade as "chocolate drinks."

Caffeine Overdose

Caffeine is found to a greater or lesser degree throughout the plant kingdom. The human body is clearly well adapted to handle it. Today, we tend to focus on the plants with a high content, particularly coffee, for its stimulative properties. On the whole, caffeine is quite benign and does not have many drawbacks. However, used consistently and in large doses, it interferes with blood sugar control and with bone health, and it reduces elasticity of the arteries. Caffeine addicts who try to stop often find that they suffer classic drug withdrawal symptoms: headaches, sleeplessness, irritability, tiredness, and so on.

Soft drinks and, by volume, colas dominate the market and have a number of problems. Their sugar content is directly associated with childhood obesity and heart disease. By adulthood, we see diabetes, cancers, raised blood pressure, high cholesterol, and all the usual sugar diseases. Colas, because of certain ingredients, are also associated with poor bone-building in children and osteoporosis in adults.

Fruit juices also have their problems. Fruits lose their fibrous structure in the juicing process. In addition, pasteurization knocks out many micronutrients, dramatically reducing their nutritional value. Finally, juice processing brings out the sugar content, which hits the bloodstream hard—fruit juices too are associated with the sugar diseases and, in particular, obesity and diabetes.

We have dealt with milk at length in the Milk Group and it is associated with all the problems of that group: heart disease, poor bone-building, allergies, obesity, and many more. Milk consumption has been dropping in spite of increasingly desperate promotions by the dairy industry. Studies suggest that they are losing out to carbonated soft drinks, which is simply replacing one problem with another.

Let us now turn to the other alcoholic beverages—wine, spirits, and liqueurs. Wine, particularly red wine, contains a number of micronutrients that appear to be helpful to health, especially cardiovascular conditions and cancers. The proviso is that you should drink no more than a couple of glasses per day. After that, the alcohol content takes over and starts to dominate the consequences. Wine, particularly dry wine, does not have the catastrophic effect on health that beer can have—wine drinkers on the whole suffer less from beer belly and the sugar diseases. Spirits have higher concentrations of alcohol, so the limit is reached more quickly and this is their main danger. But they do not provoke the sugar diseases like beer does. There is some evidence that high alcohol concentrations irritate the mouth, throat, and esophagus linings to the point where cancers develop. Spirits do not have any worthwhile concentrations of nutrients. Liqueurs suffer the same drawbacks and have an additional one—high sugar content. Liqueurs are doubly fattening (sugar and alcohol) and have nothing worthwhile to contribute nutritionally.

Finally, back to water: on the big scale, this is the least of our worries. Municipal water supplies are still far healthier than the fetid, polluted, and disease-ridden waters that our ancient ancestors were obliged to drink. Bottled waters are a harmless diversion. The alarms about dehydration are largely overdone, simply marketing manipulation to get us to drink far more bottled water than we need.

OUR CHANGED FOOD SUPPLY

We have examined how various foods have entered the food supply. Not all newcomers to the diet are unwelcome—many are fine alternatives to the foods our ancestors were adapted to in the Savanna Model. In recent history, new foods have arrived from all over the world. Some of them, such as the potato, have colonized our food supply so thoroughly that we cannot imagine life without them. In a similar vein, most cuisines around the world have accepted that fine addition to our diet, the tomato, which was unknown to Shakespeare just 400 years ago.

However, things are not always what they seem. For example, just in the past few centuries, the carrot has gone from purple to bright orange and now it is going back to purple again. In changing the colors, we keep changing the nutrients. The strawberry used to be just a little fruit about the size of a pea. In this continuous hybridization process, what nutrients have changed? In the industrialized production of the modern world, generic foods can change out of recognition, just in a generation.

Today, we see a host of new diseases afflicting our populations: autism, allergies, asthma, heart disease, cancer, arthritis, bone disease, obesity, diabetes, Alzheimer's, and many more. These diseases have become so pervasive that we think of them as part of the normal human condition. We simply cannot imagine that there is a direct connection between our lifestyle, notably eating habits, and these diseases.

We have catalogued, food group by food group, the major divergences of these foods from our ancestral foods of the African savanna and looked at some of the consequences. We see that there are problems with grains, milk products, potatoes, and dry beans. Less surprisingly, we find that sugar creates havoc with our health. We should never have accepted certain types of vegetable oil in bulk quantities and we have done certain things to red meat that make it unhealthy to humans and non-conforming to the Savanna Model. We come to the startling realization that nature never intended us to eat some very familiar foodstuffs, which are making us sick.

Much of this new knowledge has not yet percolated into the schools, the nutritionist creed, and the medical community. And many of these revelations are daunting—they call into question many of our sincerely held beliefs and make us realize how much our upbringing, our schools, and the health industry have indoctrinated us. In the next chapter, we provide the scientific background to these astonishing conclusions, and then we will pull all the strands together to build the ideal eating plan in modern terms.

4. The Science I— Population Studies and Biochemical Clues

In the last chapter, we thoroughly reviewed how we have arrived at our present food supply. We often focus on the changes that have occurred in living memory and, indeed, the pace of change has accelerated in just the last 50 years. However, our lengthy exploration demonstrates how, over a very long period of time—more than 11,000 years—our food supply has been steadily, subtly, and imperceptibly changing. We can see that the way we eat today is radically different in *nature* from the way humans fed themselves for eons on the savannas of east Africa.

How much does this matter? In Chapter 3, we outlined some of the consequences of these differences but without going into detail. We will now go into justifying these assertions based on scientific evidence. As each piece of the jigsaw slots into place, we will see how this evidence completes the gaps in the "Owner's Manual."

We begin by looking at scientific studies on human populations around the globe and investigate how different diets affect health and life span. Such studies are known as population studies, although scientists often use the term *epidemiological studies.* Then, we will look at the way our biochemistry is supposed to work and what this tells us about the foods we should be eating. In the next chapter, we examine the way nature has designed our digestive system to work. Finally, we will look at what our modern diet is doing to us. Along the way, we will discover insights to thought-provoking conundrums such as how the Eskimo, with a massive calcium intake, suffers from osteoporosis or how the long-lived and healthy Okinawans nevertheless suffer unusually from senile dementia.

POPULATION STUDY CLUES

Humans fanned out from Africa some 60,000 years ago until, by 15,000 years ago, they had ventured to all the major parts of the planet. In this way, this tropical creature, *Homo sapiens,* now lives in places that are not tropical. Moreover, these groups were obliged to live on what was locally available, so humans all over the planet were now consuming new foods in new ways.

Today, the planet is like a huge laboratory with experiments going on in different parts. It is an ideal opportunity to study statistically how different lifestyles affect health and longevity. If a scientific research institution were to propose such an experiment today, the authorities would reject it as being cruel and unusual. However, nature and history have combined to perform the experiment for us, so we can learn from this wonderful resource. Let's look at some examples of interesting populations to see how their diet has changed from the Savanna Model and the effect it has had on their health.

Life Expectancy and "Health Expectancy"

A good starting point is to examine countrywide statistics for death rates and the *reasons* for death. National governments collect these figures and international bodies like the World Health Organization collate them. Life expectancy is the factor that is most often paraded as an indication of how well a country is doing.

The figures most bandied about are for life expectancy at birth. This means, *on average*, for every baby born, the number of years it might be expected to live. In Pleistocene times, or even with the San, 30% of babies would die within the first year. This drags down the averages for life expectancy *at birth*, particularly in the underdeveloped world. For this reason, researchers often look at life expectancy at a later age, often at age 15. This gives the average number of years a 15-year-old is expected to live. This produces some surprising and useful results: we find that once an individual from a poor country has made it safely to 15 years old, he or she can expect to live as long, or even longer, than their counterparts in industrialized societies.

For example, 15-year-old boys can expect to live to the age of 76.5 in Japan, 75.6 in Greece, 75.3 in Hong Kong, but only 72.9 in the United States.[1] Women live longer than men in all countries and the proportions are similar: 15-year-old girls can expect to live to the age of 82.4 in Japan, 80.9 in Hong Kong, 80.5 in Greece, but only 79.6 in the U.S. The Japanese overall have the longest life expectancy in the world, closely followed by people living in Hong Kong. Even

Vanishing Ways of Life

The interesting thing to note about life expectancy is that we do not know how long someone will live until they die. Thus, life expectancies are based on people who were born in the first decades of the 20th century and are now dying. When we look at the life expectancy figures for 1990, those Chinese, Greeks, Hong Kongers, and Americans lived the formative part of their lives through the 1910s, 1920s and 1930s. Those old people have bodies and habits that reflect their traditional ways of life. Nowadays, as international lifestyles converge on the same eating pattern, we are losing this valuable resource.

if we take life expectancy at birth, Chinese boys born in the Shanghai province have a life expectancy of 75.7 years, while American boys at birth have a life expectancy of 71.8.[2] Shanghai baby girls can expect to live for 79.2 years, but American baby girls can only expect 78.6 years of life.

The information gets even more interesting as we drill down to find out what diseases are prevalent in a country and what diseases their populations die of. Deliberately, we go back in time to sample the conditions when people's lifestyles were much more traditional. For example, in 1960, for every 100,000 men, 466 Americans died of heart disease, whereas only 48 Greeks died of it. Greeks were five times more likely to die of a stroke than an Egyptian. Britons were 1.5 times as likely to die of cancer as a Yugoslav.[3] In 1978, Norwegian women were five times more likely to suffer a hip fracture than a Spanish woman.[4] In 1954, Japanese women had a very low incidence of breast cancer— just 4 deaths per 10,000—compared to 18.5 deaths in the U.S.; an American man was 20 times more likely to die of prostate cancer than a Japanese man.[5]

There is little correlation between health and wealth. Japan and the U.S. are both rich countries, but poor countries can be healthy too. In 1978, Albania was the poorest country in Europe with an annual income of only $380 per person. In spite of that, an Albanian man was half as likely to die of coronary heart disease as a British man.[6]

There is another often-used measure of well-being known as "health expectancy"—this is the number of years that a person can expect to live "in full health." Based on this measure, the Japanese have the highest health expectancy of 74.5 years.[7] In comparison, the British come in 14th with 71.7 years and Americans come in 24th with only 70.0 years. In other words, you die earlier and spend more time disabled (on average) if you are an American.

Statistics like this give us plenty to ponder. What is so special about the Greeks, the Japanese, and the Hong Kong Chinese that they live longer (and in better shape) than Americans? Why are some people more vulnerable to cancers, heart disease, strokes, and osteoporosis than others? There is now a mas-

Lifespan in Historical Times

There is a prevalent illusion that we live longer and better than people in historical times. This is perhaps driven by our images of life in the fetid cities so graphically described by Charles Dickens and Victor Hugo. Sure, in those days, and in those places, life for many people was indeed "mean, nasty, brutish and short" (to quote the English enlightenment philosopher Thomas Hobbes). But that is hardly a standard by which we should judge our prosperous and pampered lives today. We have seen that rural Americans have much the same life expectancy at 15 as did their great grandparents 150 years ago.

What about the prosperous and pampered societies further back in time? It is a central thesis of this book that neither the lifestyle of ancient agricultural civilizations nor those of Medieval and Victorian Europe are a good model for us today. Nevertheless, it helps to cast the spotlight on a number of issues. After the farming revolution 10,000 years ago, for the first time in the history of the human race, people were living in close proximity with each other and they were dependent on farming. For the first time, human populations were exposed to the hazards of crop failure, new diseases—particularly new diseases—and disastrous floods and plagues. Babies were born at more frequent intervals, but more babies died in infancy. This drags down the averages. After a natural disaster whole populations would be wiped out. The technology of warfare became ever more murderous. But how are we to put on a statistically sound basis a true estimate of longevity? The answer is that we cannot.

To get another bearing on the question, we can look at what the ancient peoples themselves thought of their life expectancy. First, a quick look at the writings of the ancient Greek, Homer. Based on Homer's directions in the Iliad, the archeologist Schlieman discovered the site of Homer's 3,000 year old Troy in 1870. It was a dramatic vindication of the historical basis of Homer's stories about Odysseus. Homer relates how Odysseus' wife Penelope remained faithful even though he was absent for twenty years. The remarkable, but little commented, feature is that Penelope was besieged by ardent suitors for the twenty years of Odysseus' absence. Some of the suitors were the same age as her son Telemachus. In other words, in ancient Greece, 3,000 years ago, a 40-plus woman was such a marriageable attraction that she was pursued by men half her age. Or we can look at the words of Aristotle living in ancient Greece over 2,300 years ago. He recommended that men wait until they are 35 years old before even getting married. The Greeks in general thought that a man reached his peak at the age of 40. These are hardly the strategies of people expecting a short life or a decrepit old age.

Look again at some of Alexander the Great's generals. Antigonus Monophthalmos was a battling veteran who, encouraging his troops from his warhorse, finally succumbed to a hail of javelins at the Battle of Ipsus. He was 81 years old. His opponent, Lysimichos, was later killed at the Battle of Coropedium at the age of 79. His ally Selfcos Nicator survived all battles only to be assassinated at the age of 78. This is the other side of the coin, old men with a youth's vigor. Old men who could lead their troops into battle, wielding the heavy armament of the period. Of course, this is all just circumstantial evidence. Yet it is surely no coincidence that the ancient Greek diet is still represented, 23 centuries later, by the much studied, and healthful, Cretan diet that we discuss in a later segment.

sive body of research to identify how different populations' lifestyles influence their life and health expectancy. We will look at the knowledge obtained for a few populations to see how the evidence builds up. To get the best contrast, we have chosen some extreme cases.

The Eskimos

As our species spread out around the world, even the most inhospitable regions were settled. The Eskimos were originally Siberians who got pushed across the Bering Strait by population pressures. They arrived in Alaska 6,000 years ago and found the land already occupied by the American Indians, who had migrated there several thousand years earlier. The only available territory was the land that the American Indians had shied away from—the unimaginably difficult Arctic regions of Alaska and Canada.

The Eskimos live in the most extreme of unfavorable environments. It is either cool, cold, or extremely cold most of the time. However, they have no biological special adaptation for these temperatures—the Eskimos are still tropical creatures. They can only live inside the Arctic Circle by insulating themselves from it. This was possible once some Siberian ancestor had worked out how to kill and skin a large furry animal and tailor it into a weather-tight garment. Like astronauts who are obliged to wear spacesuits to work in the vacuum of outer space, so the Eskimos have to cocoon themselves to live in the Arctic cold.

The Eskimos' main activity is hunting and traveling, but they also spend quite a lot of time eating, sleeping, and loafing about.[8] In the depths of winter, just warming up the air they breathe takes 1,000 calories. They eat much of their meat frozen, and that costs their bodies another 300 calories just to thaw it out. Oxford University professor/explorer Hugh MacDonald Sinclair specialized in studying the Eskimo diet, at a time when there were still many Eskimos living the traditional way. In 1953, he estimated that, in winter, the average Eskimo needs to consume about 4,500 calories per day.[9]

In Eskimo society, contrary to the Savanna Model, hunting is not a luxury but a necessity. It is virtually the only source of food—at no time is gathering an option as a mainstay. Men are still the driving force in the hunt, although often the women come along and help. Even so, in complete contrast to the Savanna Model, the women and children are highly dependant on their men to feed them. The women are occupied with the domestic chores of skinning the kill, preparing the food, and making clothes and other artifacts.

The Eskimo Diet

How did the Eskimos feed themselves? Today, the Eskimo has the double-edged "benefit" of modern civilization, so we have to go back to quite old studies, archives, and records. Anne Keenleyside is a Canadian researcher with special interest in paleopathology, the analysis of ancient bones. She found that, with virtually no vegetation in their environment and winter temperatures dropping to below –40°F, the Eskimos had to rely almost entirely on animal sources for their food.[10] Dr. Keenleyside and many other researchers have built up a picture of the traditional Eskimo feeding pattern. Eskimos hunted fish, seal, whale, walrus, musk ox, caribou, polar bears, wolves, birds, rabbits, ducks, and geese. They ate every part of the animal—brains, blood, intestines and even the feces. On occasion, the women would gather eggs, crabs, mollusks, and shellfish.

The Eskimos were particularly fond of the rather sour contents of the caribou paunch. These are the partly digested remains of lichens and mosses. They cut the blubber off the kill for use as lighting oil and other external uses. They ate most animal food raw, sometimes after considerable putrefaction. Other foods, particularly seal meat, were eaten frozen. Some foods were lightly cooked over a seal-oil lamp or boiled or roasted. Because the Eskimo lives above the tree line, a campfire was a rare luxury fed by dried seaweed and other dried plant remains.[11] In times of plenty, the Eskimo could consume prodigious amounts of meat: 9 pounds in a day has been measured as a normal occurrence. They drank prodigious amounts of water too (we will see why later when we discuss acid/alkali balance).

It was only in the short summer that the Eskimo ate any plant food. The treeless plains of the Arctic have a permanently frozen subsoil, known as tundra, and no plants grow more than knee high. The women would forage for berries, roots, stalks, buds, and leaves. They gathered some kinds of algae and seaweed too. It is estimated, however, that plant food represented no more than about 5% of the diet, even during the growing season.

The muscle meat of seal and whale shares similar characteristics with our ancestral wild game—there is little "marbling," or fat permeating the muscle. The small amount of muscle fat and the visible fat (blubber) are particularly rich in essential fatty acids (EFAs), notably one called eicosapentaenoic acid (EPA). Later in this chapter, we'll look at essential fatty acids and their significance to human health.

Dr. George Mann, in a report for the U.S. National Defense Committee in 1962, stated that by eating all the animal parts, the Eskimo obtained enough of the "classic" micronutrients to survive including vitamin C.[12] This might come as a surprise, since we think of vitamin C as only coming from plants. However, the skin and guts of animals like seal and caribou are also rich in this vitamin. On the other hand, the Eskimo diet was very deficient in "background" micronutrients.

Calcium consumption was huge—over 2,000 mg per day.[13] Protein intake was very high and the fat and oil intake was high.[14] However, the types of fat are of key importance: the Eskimo diet was very low in saturated fat, high in omega-3 oils, and quite high in cholesterol; there were virtually no unhealthy trans fatty acids. The Eskimos' intake of fiber, carbohydrates, and sugars was almost nonexistent, although they got some glycogen (a kind of animal carbohydrate) from the meat. Canadian researcher Kang-Jey Ho estimates that 50% of energy came from fat, 35% from protein, and 15% from glycogen.[15] Most notably, there was virtually no plant food, no soluble fiber, nor the myriad of micronutrients that only plant foods can provide.

Eskimo Health

The Eskimos first attracted attention because of an anomaly: in spite of their high-fat, high-meat diet, they had no cardiovascular disease, thromboses, or strokes; they had low blood pressure and good cholesterol levels.[16] In fact, it was too much of a good thing. Their blood was slow to clot when needed (known as a prolonged "bleeding time") and they suffered from difficult-to-stop nosebleeds. These discoveries led researchers to find the vital role of the various fatty acids in manipulating body biochemistry. The Eskimos did not suffer from vitamin C deficiency (scurvy) or from vitamin D deficiency (rickets); nor did they suffer from diabetes, appendicitis, arthritis, cancer, or dental caries (cavities).

On the other hand, the Eskimo aged fast: they became wizened and shriveled so that a 50-year-old looked more like an 80-year-old. It is estimated that the average life span was indeed only about 50 years. We can learn something too from their high calcium intake of up to 2,000 mg per day. In spite of this megadose of calcium, the Eskimos suffered from bone demineralization and osteoporosis.[17] Doesn't this go against all we are told today? This should make us question a major nutritional doctrine—that we have only to swallow calcium by the bucketful to avoid osteoporosis. In fact, good bone health is a very complex matter, easily upset by a myriad of lifestyle factors, of which calcium intake is almost irrelevant. We will see later the chief factor at the root of Eskimo osteoporosis and the lessons it gives us for the Savanna Model.

Today, the Eskimos suffer the same fate as other hunter-gatherers who adopt the Western lifestyle: high rates of obesity, heart disease, diabetes, rotten teeth and high mortality. Life expectancy has dropped even lower. Later, we will refer back to these observations to learn how the Eskimo had remarkably good health in some areas and weakness in others.

The Japanese

We are all familiar with the so-called staple of the Japanese diet, rice. We say "so-called" because there are two misconceptions about rice. First, the Japanese did not eat that much of it—even as recently as 1998, daily consumption of rice was just 6 ounces. And although rice retains a hallowed place in Japanese hearts, it is regarded as a poor man's food to be replaced by plant foods whenever possible.[18]

Traditionally, the Japanese are Buddhists and, as such, they did not eat animals at all. However, they did eat fish, often raw. By Western standards, it was a high consumption, around 90 g (3.15 ounces) per person per day (four times as much as the average American). From this, they got a high consumption of fish oil, notably the essential fatty acid eicosapentaenoic acid (EPA). Even so, their overall consumption of fat was very low—no more than 10% of calories— which is much lower than the U.S. Department of Agriculture recommended (but rarely achieved) maximum of 30%.

The largest percentage of their fat came from rapeseed (canola) oil. East Asians have cultivated rapeseed for millennia, and the Japanese have used rape- seed oil in frugal amounts for at least 2,000 years. To a lesser extent, they used soybean oil. Consumption of saturated fats, hydrogenated fats, and trans-fatty acids was almost zero.

The idea of dairy farming had never reached Japan and dairy products never formed part of their traditional diet. Rice was the staple and other cereals were virtually unknown. The Japanese traditionally did not eat wheat, barley, rye, or oats. And they did not eat potatoes either. So, when we say that Japanese consumption of rice was 6 ounces per day, that is it: no other carbohydrate fillers such as bread, pasta, pizza, or french fries existed in their diet.

The Japanese traditionally had to husband their resources and they ate much more sparingly than is our custom in the West. They had a high consumption of salt (from soy sauce) of 14 g per person per day. This is a great deal worse than government recommendations of 8 g per day maximum. The Japanese also smoke a lot: 70% of men and 45% of women smoke some form of tobacco.

Japanese Longevity and Health

Japanese men have a life expectancy four years greater than Americans and their health expectancy is 4.5 years longer than Americans. But studies show that this only applies as long as the Japanese stay in Japan. When Japanese migrate to America and adopt the American way of life, including its diet, their life expectancy drops to the American norm and they get the same diseases.[19] This suggests that Japanese health and longevity are not about genes but about the way the Japanese live their lives, notably the foods they eat and do not eat.

At home, by a fluke of culture, geography, and luck, the Japanese have hit on a good lifestyle, but even so, it is not perfect. For example, they smoke too much and they consume too much salt. More than in most other countries, the Japanese die of strokes and heart disease. The diet of raw fish means that they absorb the live eggs and larvae of intestinal parasites, so that worm infestations of the gut, virtually unknown in the West, are quite common in Japan.

Within the general statistics for Japan are buried even more startling results. The archipelago of Okinawa is remote from the Japanese mainland and its pop- ulation has an even more enviable record for health and longevity. They have one of the highest proportion of centenarians in the world: their chances of liv- ing to 100 are 12 times those of an American.

A study carried out in the remote and tiny Okinawan island of Kohama found that the inhabitants eat even more fish, 144 g (about 5 ounces), and far less salt, about 6 g, per day.[20] They eat seaweed and herbaceous plants and also sweet potato and tofu (soybean curd). They have adopted some Chinese practices from nearby Taiwan, eating some pork and drinking green tea. And they exercise a lot: 95% of the 80-year-olds studied led active lives, working long hours every day in their fish-farming paddies.

The Okinawans are a poor people, but even the poorest precinct has better longevity—two years more—than the already stellar performance of Japan as a whole.[21] They have the lowest incidence of cardiovascular disease in all of Japan, even though they smoke the same amount. At age 59, only 8% of the population had high blood pressure, 2.3% had heart disease, and 1.2% had diabetes. These figures are two to three times better than mainland Japan. However, the Okinawans had *double* the incidence of senile dementia (later, we will find the explanation for this interesting result). In a study of 80-year-olds, 90% were fully functional human beings without any disability; only three had impaired hearing and only four had fading eyesight.[22]

The remarkable health and longevity of the Okinawans has generated a number of diet programs. However, as we shall see, it is still not ideal. How do we interpret the eating patterns of a poor, agro-fishing Japanese community? Do the types of fish make a difference? Is the green tea significant? Is their "sweet potato" like our sweet potato and does it matter? As we will see later, these matters have a prime importance.

The Cretans

Similar observations have been made with the peoples of the Mediterranean northern rim. The people of the Greek island of Crete had one of the highest life expectancies in the world, in spite of a hard lifestyle. Indeed, although half a world away, there are many similarities with the Okinawan way of life. The Cretans ate frugally; they ate fish but virtually no meat (just the occasional goat's meat, as beef was nonexistent); they ate plenty of plant food (notably an unusual salad-green called purslane); and they consumed very little dairy, pastries, or sugars. Unlike the Okinawans, they ate bread—a rough-ground, whole-wheat variety—and they had a moderate fat consumption through the sparing use of olive oil in the kitchen. They also had an extraordinary custom: for the Cretan, traditional breakfast often consisted of a jigger of olive oil downed in one gulp, and that was it until lunchtime. Wine was also commonly drunk but in moderation.

These people were poor and complained that they felt hungry most of the time. They were obliged to be physically active on their land until an advanced age. Yet, the Cretans had the longest life span in Europe and their incidence of heart disease, colon cancer, high blood pressure, osteoporosis, and diabetes are all much lower than the peoples of northern Europe and North America.

American researcher Ancel Keys, who first investigated the fabled Cretan longevity and health in the 1950s, wrote a book about his findings which became popular as the so-called Mediterranean diet.[23] But this Mediterranean diet has nothing in common with the kind of meal you will find in an Italian, Spanish, or French restaurant. It contains no spaghetti, paella, pizza, or blanquette de veau; even less does it contain their rich cheeses and cream sauces.

With the advance of prosperity and the crumbling of old traditions, the Cretans are now adopting Western eating habits, and their deterioration in health is being documented.

Testing the Cretan Diet

In the meantime, the baton has passed to researchers who investigated the Mediterranean diet with well-controlled clinical trials. These trials are studies where large groups of people are divided into two test groups. One group is the "experimental" group: they are given the new diet to eat over several years. The second group is the "control" group: they continue to eat their normal diet. At the beginning of the study, both groups are tested for various health indicators, such as blood pressure, cholesterol levels, weight, and so on. They are then retested at intervals as time goes by. Often these studies go on for five or ten years, during which there will also be some deaths.

Thousands of clinical trials have tested various hypotheses about food and how it affects health and life span. The results of such studies give us very clear indications as to what is right for human beings to eat and what is not. Quite understandably, we have not the space here to go into the detail of all these studies. We will therefore cite one powerful example and then give a summary of the overall picture that the collection of studies paints for us.

Under chief researcher Serge Renaud, the Lyon Diet Heart Study involved a group of 606 heart attack patients living in Lyon, France. It was equally divided into a control group and an experimental group.[24] The control group followed the conventional advice of the hospital dietitians based on the American Heart Association (AHA) diet. The experimental group was told to adopt a Cretan-type diet: more green vegetables and root vegetables, more fish, less meat, and replace beef, pork, and lamb with poultry, no day without fruit, and replace butter and cream with a special margarine made from canola (rapeseed) oil. Olive oil and/or canola oil replaced all other fats. Moderate wine consumption was allowed.

After 27 months, the experiment was stopped early: members of the control group on the AHA diet were dying at a much faster rate than those on the Cretan diet. There were 16 deaths on the AHA diet compared to just three on the Cretan diet. The AHA group was also suffering a much higher rate of second heart attacks: they had 17 non-fatal heart attacks compared to just five on the Cretan diet.

The French Paradox

In most countries where the population has a high intake of saturated fat, there is a corresponding high death rate from heart disease. However, the situation in France does not conform to this pattern. The French have a high intake of saturated fat, particularly in cheese where they consume three times as much as Americans, but they have a low death rate from heart disease. It is the so-called French paradox.

Professor Serge Renaud dug deeper and found that there were strong regional differences. In Toulouse, in the southwest of France, a Mediterranean-type diet was practised. While not consuming much olive oil, the Toulousains did use duck and goose fat rather than butter. He found that they drank red wine copiously—up to one bottle per person per day (it is the Bordeaux region after all). In contrast, in the northern city of Strasbourg, on the border with Germany, the diet is more "Anglo-Saxon": the population drank much more milk, used butter for everything, and drank beer rather than wine.

In comparison with the United States, Dr. Renaud found that the pattern of French alcohol consumption was quite different. For the French, wine is 58% of alcohol consumption (in the U.S., 11%), beer 23% (U.S., 57%), spirits 19% (U.S., 37%). Plus, the French mostly consume their wine as an agreeable accompaniment to a meal, whereas in many other countries binge drinking is common and alcohol is consumed in order to get drunk.

Paradoxes like this are useful tools to identify such mysterious factors. They are the clues we need in order to understand what really makes our bodies work properly. Paradoxes also remind us that nothing is as simple as it seems: that, in matters like health and nutrition, there is rarely a straight line from cause to effect. We will see later how the French paradox might be explained and how it gives us more clues about our ancestral, naturally adapted diet.

It is not as though the AHA diet was bad—it was certainly better than how the patients were eating before the start of the study—but the Cretan diet proved to be exceptionally superior even to the conventional dietary treatment recommended by the American Heart Association. The committee charged with looking after the welfare of the groups swiftly decided to stop the trial early so that the AHA group of patients could benefit from the study's insights and adopt the Cretan diet if they so desired.

Summary—Population Study Clues

Researchers have carried out thousands of similar clinical studies on a huge range of different dietary factors. It is an exciting story in itself, but it is not the purpose of this book to relate them in detail. However, the results of such studies do fill in some important gaps in the "Owner's Manual." To save the reader so much detail then, we distill these results into generalized summaries. They highlight the foods linked to disease and the foods linked to health. This is a broad-brush approach, but the circumstantial evidence is pointing strongly to lifestyle patterns close to our ancestral, naturally adapted ones. In order to live in the modern world, we need to understand what to make of this evidence, which is the purpose of the latter part of the book.

HELPFUL FOODS		
FOODS	**DISEASES ENCOURAGED**	**DISEASES INHIBITED**
Fruit		Arthritis
Non-starchy vegetables		Bowel diseases
Salads		Cancers
Tubers (non-starchy)		Constipation
Berries	None	Diabetes
Nuts (in moderation)		Heart disease
Seafood and oily fish (in moderation)		High blood pressure
Wild animal protein (in moderation)		Indigestion
Low-fat poultry (in moderation))		Infectious diseases
		Obesity
		Osteoporosis

HARMFUL FOODS		
FOODS	**DISEASES INHIBITED**	**DISEASES ENCOURAGED**
Bulk vegetable oils		Allergies
Dairy products		Autoimmune diseases
Farmed "red" meat		Cancers
Grains		Constipation
Saturated fats	None	Heart disease
Hydrogenated fats		High blood pressure
Trans-fats		Indigestion
Sugars		Infectious diseases
Starchy vegetables		Obesity
Meat (high-meat diet)		Osteoporosis
		Stroke

BIOCHEMICAL CLUES

We turn now to the study of the tens of thousands of chemicals that swirl around our bodies. It is also the study of how they are orchestrated into this incredibly complex system that, day after day, makes our bodies function. It is the science known as biochemistry. A knowledge of how human biochemistry operates will provide us with valuable clues as to what dietary factors fuel the system as nature designed it.

With advancing research, we are realizing just how incredibly complex are the workings of the body. It is a classic case of the more we know, the more we realize how little we know. Biochemists call our body's biochemistry a "chaotic" system in the mathematical sense. That is, it obeys all physical laws, yet the outcome of any particular action is mathematically impossible to predict. The weather is another chaotic system—even if we knew everything about barometric pressure, temperature, and so forth, there is no way of accurately predicting the weather. We now understand that, when we try to intervene in our body's operations, we can never predict the outcome with certainty either.

There is a myriad of chemical processes going on in the body all the time. It is mind-bogglingly complex, like a three-dimensional chess game. We have to just understand that it is an unmanageable network. A very important lesson is this: an action today will sometimes have the opposite outcome to the same action yesterday; it all depends on what other processes are happening in the body at the same time.

To take one example: a teaspoon of evening primrose oil taken yesterday might calm inflamed joints; today, it might make them worse. What causes this disquietingly unpredictable result? It all depends on what else you have eaten in the last few hours. A glycemic food (one that causes blood sugar to spike abnormally) increases the body's production of an enzyme called delta-5-desaturase. This in turn flips a switch: evening primrose oil now makes chemicals that inflame joints rather than calm them. This is just one of a huge variety of inputs for which we cannot second-guess the outcome.

Indeed, this is one of our central messages: we cannot micromanage our body's operations. However, this is what people are trying to do all the time, and we end up driving a truck through the delicate minuet being danced by our body's biochemistry. We meddle in things we only partly understand with consequences that can be the opposite of those intended. I call it the Sorcerer's Apprentice syndrome. In the 1940 Disney film *Fantasia*, Mickey Mouse knows the magic spell to animate the broom to fetch water from the well to fill up the kitchen sink. However, he doesn't know the magic spell to make the broom stop fetching water. Result? The broom goes out of control filling up first the sink and then the house with a nightmarish, unstoppable flood of water. The lesson to learn is this: our own body is the best manager of itself—we just have to get out of the way and give it the tools to do the job.

We have known for a long time that some saturated fats are harmful to the smooth functioning of our bodies. Already, the message has gotten through that old friends like cream, butter, and fatty meat are not to be trusted. Health professionals have been proclaiming for decades that we should avoid them. Recent discoveries are dispelling other myths: cholesterol consumption of itself is not threatening to health; cholesterol only becomes a problem when it attaches itself to the artery walls. Why does it do that? One immediate reason is that immune system cells on one side of the wall are trying to pull the cholesterol molecule through from the other side, and it gets stuck. The question is: what provokes immune cells into doing something harmful like that?

In other words, our biochemistry needs to work to a very specific pattern. It has firmly defined characteristics that provide strong clues to our naturally adapted diet. We will now examine four of them to see how they illuminate our understanding of the "Owner's Manual": blood sugar control, essential fatty acid hormones, the salt/potassium ratio, and the acid/alkali balance.

Blood Sugar Control and Carbohydrates

People generally understand that carbohydrates are starchy foods like bread, pasta, potatoes, cookies, and cereals. Technically, however, the term *carbohydrate* is much broader: it also includes a whole spectrum of vegetation (such as lettuce, broccoli, and apples) to starches and sugars (such as sugar itself, honey, confectionary, and maple syrup). In fact, carbohydrate molecules are nothing more than glucose molecules strung together in a multitude of different ways. Most creatures, even carnivores like dogs, are equipped to digest sugars and starches. Our bodies can unzip the starch molecule back into glucose molecules very quickly by using special helpers known as enzymes. Enzymes have the power of speeding up chemical reactions by thousands of times. Other carbohydrates, such as the material that makes plant walls, can take much longer to digest—these are known as "very complex carbohydrates."

What are Carbohydrates?

Carbohydrates used to be classed as either simple or complex. Simple carbohydrates were sugars and were considered "bad" for blood sugar control. Complex carbohydrates included everything else from starches to broccoli and were all considered "good" since they were thought to be easier on blood sugar control. We now realize that this was too simplistic, because starches aren't all that complex either and are "bad" as well. In common parlance, starches are still called complex carbohydrates; however, a new category of "very complex carbohydrates" has been created for foods such as broccoli, lettuce, and so on, and these now inherit the mantle of "good" carbohydrates.

The body converts all carbohydrates, sometimes quickly and sometimes slowly (according to their type), into sugar (glucose) in the bloodstream. The body needs to maintain blood glucose levels within very narrow limits, which it does by a seesaw mechanism using hormones released by the pancreas. The pancreas is an organ that has many functions: it secretes a wide variety of hormones and digestive enzymes under instruction from other parts of the body.

If blood sugar is low, the brain instructs the pancreas to release the hormone glucagon into the blood. Glucagon is an "unlocking hormone" that instructs the fat cells to release fat, convert it into glucose, and push it into the bloodstream. In contrast, if the glucose level is too high, the brain instructs the pancreas to release the hormone insulin into the blood. Insulin is a 'locking up' hormone that instructs the fat cells to take the excess blood glucose and store it as fat. In other words, excess glucose equals excess body fat.

In a normal glucose reaction, the body carefully masters the rising level of glucose in the blood and brings it under control. There is no abnormal peak of glucose and the level never drops below the normal fasting level. In a bad reaction, we eat a food that gives us a "sugar rush." The arrival of glucose is too rapid, and the pancreas cannot maintain this orderly processing. Instead, glucose levels spike sharply to overdose levels about 20 to 30 minutes after eating the food. This condition is known as hyperglycemia, and when this happens, nerve endings are killed off and blood vessels are damaged.

The state of hyperglycemia lasts about 30 minutes, during which we do not feel anything special, and then the pancreas catches up. But it overshoots the mark—the pancreas overcompensates and clears too much glucose from the bloodstream. By 2 to 3 hours after eating the food, there is now a deficiency of glucose in the blood. This deficiency, known as hypoglycemia, provokes feelings of drowsiness, dizziness, irritability, exhaustion, cold sweats, depression, headaches, and a desperate craving for something sugary. Many readers will be familiar with this phenomenon: the mid-morning or mid-afternoon "slump," which happens a couple of hours after a copious bad-carbohydrate meal.

In this way, abnormally high blood sugar levels mean abnormally high insulin levels. Most Americans are putting their bodies under this kind of stress on a daily basis. This is a biochemical disaster: insulin is a powerful hormone and having it floating around in abnormal quantities (hyperinsulinemia) upsets all other kinds of hormonal reactions.

For example, insulin instructs the liver to make cholesterol. The more abnormal the insulin level, the more abnormal the cholesterol production. The reason most people have high cholesterol levels is not because they are eating it, but because their body is making abnormal quantities of it. In a similar way, abnormal insulin levels provoke abnormal levels of other hormones, which cause abnormal blood clotting (leading to strokes and thrombosis), abnormal clogging and inflammation of arteries, abnormal suppression of the immune system (allowing cancers to grow), and even increased sensitivity to arthritis, allergies, and asthma. The problem with hyperinsulinemia is that you do not even feel it. It goes about its work silently and you notice nothing until it is too late—you have the stroke, the heart attack, the cancer, and the sludged arteries.

The end result of this abuse of the blood sugar mechanism is often diabetes. Diabetes is a condition in which one of two things happens: either the pancreas cannot keep up with the demand for insulin and so the insulin production machinery goes into failure or the fat cells stop listening to insulin's instructions and fail to absorb sugar out of the bloodstream. Either way, there is then an excess concentration of sugar in the blood. Diabetes sufferers, even if medicated, are vulnerable to heart disease, kidney failure, blindness, and gangrene in the feet and hands.

Sugar for Fat Equals Fat

Americans now worry about fat in the diet and seek out fat-free and low-fat foods. The food manufacturers have been only too happy to oblige. But almost always in such foods, they have increased the sugar content to compensate. Unfortunately, fat-free but sugary foods can be just as fattening. But the hormone insulin is then released to take the excess blood sugar and store it as fat. This insulin mechanism is the major reason why Americans are still getting fatter, even if they are trying to reduce their fat intake. Of course, when they eat fat, insulin sweeps that into the fat cells too.

This illustrates another curiosity of human biochemistry—fat by itself does not increase insulin levels. Therefore, fat eaten in the absence of either carbohydrates or protein is not easily absorbed into the fat cells. This explains how the Cretans could consume a jigger of olive oil on an empty stomach and not get fat.

Think of abnormal insulin levels like the iceberg that sank the Titanic. You see very little on the surface, but underneath lurks danger. You just see apparently disconnected peaks—heart disease, thrombosis, artery disease, cancer, allergies, depression, arthritis, obesity—but a looming mass of ice (representing abnormal insulin levels) interconnects them under the surface.

Glycemic Index and Glycemic Load

Until the 1980s, medical knowledge about how diet affects and controls diabetes was surprisingly imperfect. Then, Canadian researcher David Jenkins developed a breakthrough concept—the glycemic index.[25] He fed various foods to volunteers and measured their blood sugar over a period of time, usually two hours. He then did the same with glucose. Blood sugar is, in fact, glucose and so glucose is thought to be the most "glycemic," that is, it creates the most powerful sugar rush. Jenkins compared the spikes in blood glucose caused by the test foods against the spike for glucose, and the ratio of the two, on a scale of 0 to 100, gives the glycemic index.

The results surprised him and surprised those doctors who took notice. This new way of looking at what carbohydrates do to blood sugar control turned conventional medical ideas upside down. A whole range of foods that doctors thought safe, particularly for diabetics, Jenkins found to be decidedly dubious. Over the years, researchers have tested many more foods and they found that most processed foods have consistently the same index. However, fresh fruits and vegetables, which are naturally variable, can have quite a wide range of index. Even so, when all is considered, the glycemic index measure brings completely new insights into what type of foods are right for humans: we now understand that nature did not design the human body to handle foods that give a blood sugar rush.

In this book, foods that have an index in the range of 61 and above, we call "bad" carbohydrates: they consistently produce an unhealthy sugar spike. Foods with an index between 31 and 60, we call "borderline" carbohydrates: they produce sugar surges which, in a healthy person, the body controls, but only at the price of unnecessary stress to the body. Foods with an index from 0 to 30, we call "favorable" carbohydrates: they produce blood sugar levels that are within the body's normal range for comfortable, unstressed handling.

TYPICAL GLYCEMIC INDEX		
FOOD	GLYCEMIC INDEX (GLUCOSE = 100)	CATEGORY
Maltose	110	Bad
Cornflakes	85	Bad
Potato, baked	85	Bad
Bread, whole-wheat	70	Bad
Sugar	65	Bad
Pineapple	65	Bad
Rice, brown	55	Borderline
Spaghetti	45	Borderline
Banana (unripe)	40	Borderline
Raspberries	25	Favorable
Fructose	20	Favorable
Walnuts	15	Favorable
Tomato	15	Favorable
Lettuce	15	Favorable

Glycemic index scores present a few surprises. Starchy foods like bread (even whole-wheat) and breakfast cereal (corn flakes) are "bad" carbohydrates. Fruits are all over the place: pineapple is "bad," banana is "borderline," and raspberries are "favorable." Unsurprisingly, non-starchy, non-sugary foods like most nuts, salads, and vegetables fit into the "favorable" category.

Another surprise is the special type of sugar called fructose—it has a favorable glycemic index and does not raise blood sugar levels unhealthily. Fructose is common in fruit, so it is not a surprise that human bodies are very well adapted to it. Fructose is not converted to glucose straight away by the digestive system; it has to pass through the liver for conversion. This slows down the rate at which it hits the bloodstream. Finally, it's a surprise to find another sugar, maltose, that is more glycemic than glucose itself. Maltose is made of two glucose molecules joined together and, as its name suggests, is the chief sugar in malt.

There is another factor that makes a difference: the concentration of sugars and starches in the particular food. Will just one cornflake or one pineapple chunk set off a bad glycemic reaction? One supposes not, but to find out, some researchers have developed the concept of the "glycemic load." This is an attempt to define how much of a food needs to be consumed before it triggers a glycemic reaction. They take the glycemic index (GI) of a food and combine it with the amount of carbohydrate in a standard U.S. Department of Agriculture (USDA) serving size to get the glycemic load (GL) score. A GL of 20 or more is "high," a GL of 11 to 19 is "medium," and a GL of 10 or less is "low."

Of course, everything depends on the serving size that is actually consumed by a person. That is why even the concept of glycemic load has its limitations—this factor is only valid if one consumes a standard serving size. The USDA sometimes has absurdly low "normal" serving sizes. For example, a serving of spaghetti is 2 ounces (57 g) of dry weight. Most home cooks use double that quantity when serving spaghetti.

Insulin Index

Measuring the glycemic power of foods is a useful guide and it has a direct bearing on the damage that glucose can do to our health. Nevertheless, it is one stage removed from a worse villain: abnormally high insulin levels. Because of insulin's potential for creating havoc with our biochemistry, researchers such as human nutrition expert Susanna H. Holt have established insulin indexes for many foods.[26] She did it in a way similar to the process for glycemic indexes: volunteers ate different foods and had their insulin levels measured over several hours.

Insulin indexes usually, but not always, rise and fall in the same rhythm with the glycemic index. Once again, there are some real surprises—some foods that might pass muster on a glycemic basis fail on an insulinemic basis. There is one further factor: proteins might not raise blood sugar levels, but they *do* raise insulin levels, some very sharply—notably, yogurt. Worse, if proteins and carbohydrates are eaten together, then the insulin raising power of the combination is much greater than of the two ingredients separately.

The table gives some typical values for an insulin index.[27] It can be seen that potato and yogurt are exceptionally "insulinemic"—that is, they have a powerful insulin-raising ability. Beef, fish, and eggs have a normal insulin-raising ability. Information like this helps build a picture of the foods that we should consider eliminating from the Savanna Model candidates.

INSULIN INDEX		
FOOD	INDEX	CATEGORY
Potatoes	124	Abnormal
Yogurt	115	Abnormal
Bread	100	Abnormal
Rice	79	Abnormal
Fish	59	Normal
Beef	51	Normal
Eggs	31	Normal

We're Not Designed to Consume Sugars

We saw in Chapter 1 how the San were measured as having a low "insulin response": this means that their fat cells do not react quickly to the instructions given by insulin. Another way of saying it is that their bodies display "insulin resistance." Insulin resistance occurs when the body needs to produce "abnormal" levels of insulin to deal with high-glycemic foods. Australian professor Jennie Brand-Miller is the icon of glycemic index research. She and Stephen Colagiuri of the University of Sydney, Australia, argue that insulin resistance is actually the naturally adapted state for human beings.[28] All peoples used to living on a primitive diet, such as the Australian Aboriginal, the Native American, and the African Pygmy, all display insulin resistance. This is normal, since the forager's food supply does not contain glycemic foods.

In fact, this insulin resistance is helpful for reproduction. During pregnancy, glucose needs to be diverted to the fetus. Insulin-resistant females automatically maintain glucose in circulation so that the fetus can benefit from it, rather than locking it up in her own fat stores. Furthermore, during breastfeeding, the breasts develop insulin sensitivity, which encourages the uptake, by breast tissue, of glucose for conversion into the milk sugar lactose.

Most primal peoples are terribly vulnerable to the Western diet and rapidly develop diabetes, obesity, and heart disease. In a classic study, Australian researcher Kerin O'Dea returned diabetic Aboriginals to their traditional lifestyle.[29] Just a few weeks of living like this brought their diabetes, obesity, and poor cardiovascular vital signs back to normal.

The research on blood sugar control and insulin resistance provides powerful insights into the naturally adapted diet for humans. Clearly, nature did not design us to consume sugars and starches. This is a startling revelation for we are so used to the idea that starchy foods, such as grains and potatoes, should be part of the diet. We also see that not all fruits are entirely innocent: some of today's fruits clearly conform to our ancestral diet and some do not. It's clear that we have to look past the stereotypes, and at the details about what we eat, in order to understand how to navigate through our food options.

Fats and Oils

Fats and oils ("oils" are fats that are liquid at room temperature) were divided into three types: saturated, monounsaturated, and polyunsaturated. All three types are made up of fatty acids, the building blocks of all fats. Primal humans subsist on a very low-fat diet. Even so, human nutrition requires a fat intake of some kind, because the body sickens and dies if certain fatty acids are not in the diet. These are known as essential fatty acids (EFAs), and all are polyunsaturated fats. This family can be divided into two classes called omega-3s and omega-6s.

Omega-3 EFAs are found in plants and animal matter. In plants, the most common form is alpha-linolenic acid (ALA), found particularly in walnuts, flaxseed, hempseed, and rapeseed (canola oil). In animals, omega-3 oils are particularly found in "oily" fish, such as sardines, salmon, trout, and tuna. The most common omega-3 EFAs in fish are docosahexaenoic acid (DHA) and eicosapentaenoic acid (EPA). Omega-6 EFAs are chiefly found in oilseed plants: for example, corn oil, sunflower oil, safflower oil, peanut oil, and soybean oil. There is only one, main omega-6 which is called linoleic acid (LA).

The body only needs these two classes of fat in small quantities of a gram or two (about $1/2$ tsp) from all food sources combined per day. They are important because they act rather like vitamins. Indeed, at one time, we called them vitamin F1 and F2—it is a pity that we dropped this designation, because it gives us an idea of their powerful effect on the body. The body converts these EFAs into potent types of hormones called prostaglandins. Prostaglandins are powerful agents that cause the body to do things like thicken or thin blood, increase or decrease bone building, depress or boost the immune system, and a host of other effects.

The first important feature is that what one omega type of EFA does, the other omega type does the opposite. Plus, they both use the same biochemical machinery to do their work. If one is using it, the other cannot; that is, one of them can monopolize the process to the complete exclusion of the other. This leads to a third important feature: they need to be present in the diet in a proportion of about 1 to 1—they need to be balanced. If not, one of them dominates and produces prostaglandins that, in abnormal quantities, cause sickness and disease. In the American diet, this is indeed the case. It is estimated that the ratio of omega-6s to omega-3s is about 32 to 1 instead of the ideal 1 to 1. These abnormal quantities of omega-6 fatty acids produce volumes of "bad prostaglandins" that are in part responsible for many of the diseases we see today.

Diseases Provoked by Bad Prostaglandins

Bad prostaglandins increase:

- Blood clotting (thrombosis)
- Bone destruction (osteoporosis)
- Inflammation (arthritis)
- Histamines (allergies)
- Pain sensitivity
- Vasoconstriction (high blood pressure)
- Autoimmune reactions (arthritis, lupus, multiple sclerosis)
- Hypertension (high blood pressure)
- Bronchial restriction (asthma)

Bad prostaglandins depress:

- Immune system (cancer)
- Bone building (osteoporosis)

Fatty Acids and the Ancestral Diet

Earlier in this chapter, we touched on this subject with the Eskimo. The Eskimo diet is overbalanced in favor of the omega-3 oils, the opposite to that of the western diet. This causes overproduction of compounds that abnormally *reduce* blood platelet stickiness and blood clotting, which explains the Eskimo's unstoppable nosebleeds and immunity to heart disease.

However, most people in the West have the opposite problem: they have sticky blood liable to clot when it is not supposed to. This phenomenon can lull Western surgeons into a false sense of security—they find that bleeding is easily controlled. Steven Gundry, medical director of the International Heart Institute, in Palm Springs, relates how American surgeons could not understand the difficulty that Japanese surgeons had in controlling bleeding under the surgeon's knife.[30] Belatedly, they realized that this is the normal condition for healthy people: the Japanese, with their diet rich in oily fish, have the omega-3/omega-6 balance about right.

How does this fit in with what we know about essential fatty acids in our ancestral diet? The vegetation was indeed rich in these fatty acids. In turn, the creatures such as antelope that ate the vegetation, and the animals (such as lions) that ate the antelope, were all rich in these fatty acids. Even more remarkable, the omega-3 and omega-6 fatty acids were present in a ratio of around 1 to 1. In fact, we should not be surprised that these fatty acids are *essential*—our bodies never had to learn how to make them, just like our bodies have lost the ability to make vitamin C because it was always present in our diets of fruits and plants. Carnivores, such as lions, cheetahs, and cats do not eat fruits and plants and so their bodies make their own vitamin C. In contrast, carnivores are dependent on a wider range of fatty acids in their diet.[31]

Companion animal researcher Michael G. Hayek points out that cats, for example, cannot transform alpha-linolenic acid (usually from plants) into another essential compound, arachidonic acid (AA).[32] Cats get a wide range of necessary fatty acids from their prey, such as arachidonic acid (AA), gamma-linoleic acid (GLA), and eicosapentaenoic acid (EPA). Plants do not have them. This is another sign that hunted meat could not have formed a significant part of the human diet, otherwise, as with cats, our bodies would have lost the ability to make these fatty acids.

A large number of favorable factors must come together for humans to have evolved as they did. Humans are peculiar because of their large brains, so one of those factors must have been an abundant supply of brain-building material. Two polyunsaturated fats, arachidonic acid and DHA (docosahexaenoic acid), make up the bulk of brain and central nervous system tissue. C. Leigh Broadhurst, a nutrition scientist, and others have wondered where early humans got these fats in the diet, since they are not abundant in the ordinary savanna landscape.[33] However, these fats *are* abundant in fish and shellfish. Humans evolved in an area, the African Rift Valley, that was endowed with lakes and streams. Humans of that time freely consumed shellfish, fish, wading birds, and ducks and their eggs. Leigh Broadhurst calculates that the quantities consumed did not have to be large—just 6% to 12% of calories.[34]

Fatty Acids in the Body

There are dozens of fatty acids, most of which are either neutral or harmful to health. Saturated myristic acid and palmitic acid are aggressive to arteries. They are particularly found in butter, cream, cheese, beef, pork, and lamb. Palmitic acid is also the chief component of palm oil, which is used in processed foods. However, the body converts another saturated fat, stearic acid (particularly found in cocoa butter), into oleic acid (as found in olive oil). Oleic acid, which dominates the family of monounsaturated fats, is neutral on the body. Olive oil is "good" because it does no harm.

When it comes to consuming fats and oils, we have to realize that in nature they come as a cocktail of many varieties. For example, the chief components of pork fat are the saturated fats palmitic acid (24%), stearic acid (13%), and myristic acid (2%); the monounsaturated fats oleic acid (41%) and hexadecenoic acid (2%); and the polyunsaturated omega-6 fat linoleic acid (4%). In other words, it is mainly composed of fats that are innocuous—just the palmitic and the myristic acids, totaling 26%, are harmful. However, that is enough for damage to be done.

Fatty acids are present in our bloodstream bound up into a compound called a triglyceride. A triglyceride is composed of a molecule of glycerol to which three fatty acids are attached. When we eat a triglyceride molecule, digestive enzymes split it apart into its component fatty acids (plus the glycerol). These components pass through the gut wall into the bloodstream, where the body reconstructs the fatty acids into a *different* triglyceride.

Depending on the fatty acid's position (1, 2, or 3) on the original molecule, it is more or less "bioavailable."[35] In human biochemistry, fats in position 2 are very easily absorbed, while the others in positions 1 and 3 are not. Pork fat finds 66% of its worst fatty acids in position 2, which is why pork fat is so much more harmful than a simple analysis of its saturated fat content would suggest. The same is true for butter and cream. On the other hand, cocoa butter, which contains 60% saturated fat, finds 95% of it parked harmlessly in positions 1 and 3.[36] Harmless monounsaturated fats occupy 85% of position 2, from where fatty acids are easily absorbed. That is why cocoa is far less cholesterolemic than a simple examination of its saturated fat content would suggest.

Calcium in the gut also combines readily with fatty acids to form insoluble compounds that cannot be absorbed into the body. This is the fate of much of the calcium in milk—it is locked up with the milk fats and both are passed out in the stools. In cheeses, researcher Serge Renaud has shown that this appears to be the mechanism where unhealthy saturated fats are shown the back door.[37] This seems to be one part of the explanation for the French Paradox: most of the "bad" cheese fats are not absorbed into the body

Humans in our ancient homeland did not find much fat in their diet, so they never developed a mechanism for knowing when they had eaten enough. Because some fats are essential, we have a well-developed mechanism to keep eating them for as long as supplies last. However, our bodies do not know how to discriminate between what is essential (and beneficial) and what is nonessential (and often harmful), and we pay the price. Fatty foods taste good and trigger the approval mechanism in the brain, which gives us that feeling of comfort.

We've seen that humans are adapted to a low-fat diet, but what fat there is should be of two particular kinds, omega-3 and omega-6. Moreover, these two types of fat should be consumed in the ratio of about 1 to 1. In recent years, our pattern of fat consumption has changed dramatically, with the arrival of omega-6 vegetable oils on the market. Their dominance over omega-3 is responsible, at least in part, for the rapid increase in a range of diseases.

Salt/Potassium Ratio

The Savanna Model diet is low in sodium and rich in potassium. Sodium, of course, is the active component of salt. Potassium is an element mainly found in plant foods, chiefly fruit. To expand on what we said under "Salt" in Chapter 3: The evolutionary nutritionist Boyd Eaton estimates that the typical consumption in Pleistocene times was about 1 grams of sodium to 5 grams of potassium.[38] Consequently, this ratio is important for the proper functioning of our biochemistry, particularly at the cellular level. Today, the average American has reversed this ratio and consumes 6 grams of sodium to 2.5 grams of potassium—and it matters!

Medical researcher Louis Tobian shows that salt damages arteries even if blood pressure is not raised.[39] High salt levels irritate and scar the arteries, making it one more factor in the development of atherosclerosis.

High sodium levels also affect the way calcium is mobilized by the body. Canadian researchers have shown that over-consumption of salt drains calcium out of the bones.[40] Other studies confirm that potassium and sodium imbalances destroy bone building.[41] This is just one more example of how today's dietary practices are greasing the slippery slope toward osteoporosis.

As with fats, salt is a compound that our brains tell us to eat while the going is good. That is because in our evolutionary past salt was never abundant and it was impossible to overconsume it. It is only in recent times that salt has passed from being a rare luxury to an all-pervading flavor enhancer. In the quantities that we consume today, salt is one of the many factors undermining our health. Salt is yet another food where we have defeated nature's discipline of natural scarcity, so we should be exercising self-discipline to reinstate scarcity in our diets.

Acid/Alkali Balance

Acids are compounds that taste sour and eat away at metals. Examples are the citric acid in lemons, acetic acid in vinegar, and sulfuric acid in car batteries. Alkalis (also known as "bases") are the opposite; in a way, they are the antidote to acids. For example, the stomach contains hydrochloric acid, which sometimes causes indigestion; the antidote is an alkali (or "antacid"), such as sodium bicarbonate and magnesium hydroxide. When acid and alkali cancel each other out, the result is neutrality—the blood is neither acid nor alkaline.

All foods, once digested and absorbed into the bloodstream, will cause the blood to be either more acidic or more alkaline. Clinical researcher Anthony

Sebastian confirms that nature designed human biochemistry to work on a broadly neutral diet.[42] This is not like a cat, for example, which functions best on an acid diet, nor like a horse, which prefers an alkaline diet. In humans, the body is constantly juggling to restore a neutral balance.

What are alkali-forming foods? They are ones that have a predominance of the metallic elements potassium, sodium, iron, and calcium—chiefly fruit, salads, and non-starchy vegetables. This demands an explanation, because many of these foods, notably fruit, *taste* acid but are, nevertheless, alkalizing in effect. For example, grapefruit, although acid to the taste, is strongly alkalizing. The answer to this paradox lies in what happens after the digestive system has broken down the acid into its parts.

The acid taste of many fruits is due to the presence of organic acids, such as citric acid and malic acid. This acid stays intact through the mouth, the stomach, and into the intestine. Up to this point, the effect on the digestive process and lining is acidic. But in the intestine, the organic acid passes through the intestinal wall into the bloodstream. Here, it is broken down into two parts: carbonic acid, which is blown out of the body through the lungs in the form of carbon dioxide, and the alkaline portion, which is left behind to alkalize the body.

What are acid-forming foods? Not foods that taste acidic, but rather the ones that after digestion and metabolism have the effect of acidifying the body. They are foods that contain sulfur, phosphorus, and chlorine—found chiefly in proteins like meat, fish, eggs, and cheese. For example, bland roast chicken is one of the most acidifying foods around. Starches like bread, flour, pasta, and cereals are also acid forming.

The body compensates for an acid diet by drawing down reserves of calcium, sodium, and potassium to neutralize the acid and excreting the waste through the kidneys. The average person eating a Western diet has chronically acidified his body, disrupting many biochemical mechanisms. For example, an acid diet irritates the kidneys into abnormally leaking calcium into the urine. This phenomenon, known as protein-induced calciuria, is a major mechanism for bone demineralization. Considering the epidemic proportion of osteoporosis in this country, it is a vital fact that too few people know. This knowledge also explains how, on a high-meat, highly acidic diet, the Eskimo suffers from osteoporosis even though he has a high calcium intake.

The Eskimo's high-meat diet provides protein in excess of the body's requirements. The body cannot tolerate excess protein in the bloodstream, so it immediately mobilizes the kidneys to get rid of it. In turn, the kidneys have to extract more water from the bloodstream to provide the necessary fluid for flushing the waste proteins out in the urine. This has two consequences. This extra urination leads to dehydration and abnormal feelings of thirst—the reason why Eskimos were driven to downing vast quantities of water on their high-meat diets. Second, nature did not design the kidneys to work like this on a continuous basis. Waste protein cells and calcium-bearing cells crystallize into hard nodules. These are the kidney stones that block kidney ducts and cause immense pain.

Many other organs, including the pancreas, lymphatic system, thyroid, intestines, and liver are either dependant on or responsible for a neutral environment. They are put under abnormal stress and can fail if they continually have to compensate for an unrelenting acid diet.

Nutrition researchers Robert McCance and Elsie Widdowson formed a remarkable partnership for over 60 years. They established the specifications for British wartime rations during World War II and the British nation has never been healthier since that time, when the portions of food were metered with tight discipline and only foods essential to the human body were made available. McCance and Widdowson worked out indexes of acidity and alkalinity for many foods.[43]

SELECT ACID/ALKALINE INDEXES		
LEVEL	FOOD	INDEX
Very Alkaline		
	Almonds	18.3
	Avocados	10.7
	Grapefruit	6.4
	Tomatoes	5.6
	Cucumber	3.2
	Apples	3.0
Neutral		0
	Bread, toasted	−2.6
	Cheese, cheddar	−5.4
	Spaghetti	−7.5
	Peanuts	−11.6
	Bacon	−17.0
	Chicken, roasted	−25.4
Very Acid		

So, what pattern of eating does this imply? Notice that the acid-forming foods (mainly proteins) are *dense* compared to the alkali-forming ones (mainly non-starchy plant food). That is to say, the plant food is more watery than the proteins. We also see how in today's diet, starches, which are acidic, displace other kinds of plant foods that are alkalizing.

On average, it takes three times as much plant food as protein to maintain a neutral balance; in other words, about 75% by weight of plant food to 25% of protein in the diet. This same ratio also provides the right amount of protein in the diet, neither an excess or a deficit. Have we seen this ratio before? It is not a coincidence that both the San and the Australian Aboriginal consumed a very similar ratio of plant food to animal food. This is another piece of evidence confirming the natural adapted eating pattern for human beings—one in which non-starchy plant food occupies about three-quarters of what we eat and foods of animal origin about one-quarter.

Summary—Biochemical Clues

We have delved into how the food we eat is a major influence on the human body's biochemical processes. It is a complex subject and our knowledge is far from complete. We cannot predict with certainty that what we do today will have the same results tomorrow. This reinforces our idea that, perhaps, we should not even be trying to micromanage these processes. Instead, we should simply consume the foods that our body expects and it will sort these matters out for itself.

5. The Science II— Digestive System and Dietary Clues

In the last chapter, we looked at scientific studies on human populations around the globe and investigated how their different diets affected their health and life span. We also looked at the way our biochemistry is supposed to work and the consequences for our food choices. Here, we examine the way nature has designed our digestive system to work and what this tells us about the foods we should be eating. Then, we will look at what our modern diet is doing to us.

DIGESTIVE SYSTEM CLUES

What process can be more intimate than this: absorbing foreign agents into the most secret parts of our bodies? It is remarkable how little we think about this process, for that is what eating is—infiltrating stuff from our mouths into the very fiber of our being. The mechanics are performed by the digestive system, which can be thought of in two major parts: the physical digestive tract (mouth, stomach, and intestines) and the complex array of enzymes, juices, and hormones (secreted by the pancreas, liver, and the digestive tract itself) that make it all work.

We've talked previously about the "chaotic" complexity of our body's systems, and the digestive system is no exception. Signals reverberate between the digestive tract, the pancreas, liver, and brain. Hormones and nerves are constantly relaying messages to our brain and back again to the digestive system, and organs communicate with each other using hormones and nerve signals. It all works automatically, entirely without our knowledge. When it works well, our bodies hum along like finely tuned machines. However, when it goes wrong, then we can learn from the dietary errors that caused the malfunction. By looking at the digestive tract and how nature intended it to work, we can draw lessons about how we should be eating.

The digestive tract of all mammals, including humans, is built to the same basic plan—it begins at the lips and ends at the anus. Digestion begins in the mouth with its teeth, for grinding the food, and its tongue, which kneads the food and mixes it with saliva. It then sends the pellet of food down to the stomach. On its way there, it passes through the long tube called the esophagus or gullet. At the entry to the stomach, the food passed through a non-return valve. This is to stop the stomach contents from accidentally passing back up into the mouth, although in emergencies this mechanism is suspended to reject any substances that the stomach detects as harmful.

The stomach is basically a holding reservoir where the food is churned with hydrochloric acid to kill any harmful bacteria. A secondary role is to secrete a mixture of enzymes to begin digestion of proteins and fats. From there, the mixture (chyme) passes through another non-return valve (the pylorus) into the small intestine. Once past this gate, it is impossible for the chyme to come back into the stomach. The small intestine is just over one inch in diameter and about 23 feet long. Here, most of the food is mixed with various digestive juices and enzymes and absorbed into the bloodstream. The remaining, unabsorbed food residues pass through another non-return valve into the large intestine or colon, which is about 5 feet long. Here, excess water and various nutrients are absorbed into the bloodstream.

The Underrated Colon

The colon until recent years has been a much underrated organ, even thought to be dispensable. We now know that the colon performs many essential functions when in a proper state of health. Today, diseased colons cause a wide range of illnesses. So, we now examine what makes the colon function properly and, in this way, better understand what kinds of food residues we should be putting there.

We are all walking around with 3 to 5 pounds of living matter ("biomass") in our colons: bacteria, yeast, and fungi. Collectively, they are known as gut "flora" (from the Latin word for the Roman goddess of flowers). There are over a trillion bacteria alone, of many and varied species. Most of them are "anaerobic"—they do not need oxygen in order to survive. They live on the food residues that arrive in the colon. For example, many kinds of carbohydrates survive digestion, particularly plant fiber and the very complex carbohydrates.

Through fermentation of these food residues, this biomass produces all kinds of useful compounds. Fatty acids called butyric acid and propionic acid are absorbed through the colon wall into the bloodstream, where they carry out important functions in the body, such as boosting immune function and controling cholesterol. Gases like hydrogen, carbon dioxide, and methane are also produced and, in part, pass into the bloodstream. (The other part is passed as wind.) From the blood, the gases pass to the lungs where they are breathed out. However, even bacteria have difficulty breaking down some indigestible compounds, such as lignin (a woody fiber) and cellulose. These are passed out, unaltered, in bowel movements.

We should consider this biomass as an important organ. French gut specialist and researcher M.C. Moreau says that the mucous membrane lining the gut is the largest immunological organ of the body.[1] Remarkably, these gut organisms communicate with elements of the immune system, a phenomenon known as "cross-talk." For example, lymphocytes are white blood cells of the immune system that do not mature and work properly unless the colon flora stimulates them.

For the colon's cargo of flora to thrive, it needs to be fed with plant fiber: viscous (soluble) fibers such as pectin, guar gum, and beta-glucan, which are the building materials of plant cell walls. We are not talking about insoluble fiber as found in cereal brans (a partial exception is oat bran). Researchers have discovered the many benefits of a high consumption of viscous fiber from plants:[2] it has a lowering effect on "bad" LDL cholesterol levels and it reduces mutant cells in the bowel and free radical damage.

Free Radicals and Antioxidants

Free radicals are highly aggressive molecules that the body creates continuously as a by-product of various chemical reactions. Outside agents such as ultraviolet rays, tobacco smoke, and alcohol also trigger them. Free radicals can cause a lot of damage to cells and DNA.

A free radical is a molecule that contains at least one electron that is looking for a partner. Because of this, free radicals vigorously react with whatever they encounter. At worst, they tear open intact molecules, cannibalizing parts of them to complete their own electron partnership. This creates new partnerless electrons and so the attacked molecule becomes a new source of many free radicals. In this way, an exploding chain reaction is set in motion that can cause damage out of proportion to the initial provocation.

The body quenches free radicals by the use of antioxidants: micronutrients that neutralize free radicals and the damage they cause. There are many antioxidants in plant foods but they are rarely found in animal products. Antioxidants have the ability to put a stop to the free radical chain reaction. Food antioxidants include vitamin C, vitamin E, zinc, and selenium. Other antioxidants are "background" micronutrients, such as quercetin, resveratrol, and anthocyanine.

The benefit is a reduced risk of colon cancer. Bowel movements are more massive and they pass more quickly through the system: constipation is eliminated and diverticulosis (abnormal balloonings in the gut wall) is avoided. The viscous fiber also locks up harmful compounds and evacuates them. For example, estrogen isoflavonoids are chemicals in plants that can affect the same tissues as human estrogen, but can produce very different effects.[3] They are found in some plants such as soy. These phytoestrogens are not always such a good thing, for they are implicated in lung and breast cancers. However, in a high-fiber diet, these phytoestrogens are safely ushered out of the body.

Other foods, like hot peppers, cause the lining of the intestine to become more porous, a condition known as leaky gut syndrome. It does not take much: the gut wall is as thin as tissue paper and that is all that separates the sludge in your gut from your blood circulation. Even under good conditions, there are always some bacteria that pass through into the blood. For example, primitive herders knew to starve a beast for 24 hours before slaughter, because there would be fewer bacteria generalized throughout the carcass and the meat kept longer.

Herbs and Spices

Herbs and spices are usually rich in aromatic micronutrients, which accounts for their pungent flavor. This is all to the good, yet normally the quantities we eat are an insignificant part of the diet. For this reason (we suppose), the U.S. Department of Agriculture diet guide for 2005 has nothing to say about them. We do not give them a high profile either.

Nevertheless, there is one class that has powerful effects on our digestive system: the hot pungent ones, such as chili pepper, cayenne pepper, and paprika. Austrian researchers found that chili has a provocative effect on irritable bowel disease.[4] Dr. Rodriguez-Stanley found that heartburn ("acid reflux") was acutely increased too.[5] Dr. Erika Jensen-Jarolim found that chilies, and to a lesser extent paprika and cayenne pepper, make the colon "leaky."[6] She found that large molecules could then pass through the colon wall into the bloodstream, giving rise to allergies, a depressed immune system, and increasing chances of colon cancer. However, black pepper was harmless.

Chilies are native to Mexico and were brought to the rest of the world by the Portuguese 400 years ago, to places like India and Thailand. There, curries and hot dishes were enthusiastically developed. The reality is that the human body is not adapted to hot spices and they have a number of serious drawbacks. Chilies and other hot red peppers are not human foods.

The body deals with infections and injury with a reaction called inflammation. This is a not only normal but necessary for healing to take place. Inflammation is characterized by heat, redness, swelling, and pain. In part, this reaction is set in motion by special immune system cells called mast cells. Many mast cells line the intestine, where they stand guard watching out for harmful foreign bodies trying to enter the bloodstream. Mast cells deal with infections by releasing chemicals that have the effect of increasing the permeability of blood vessels (leading to swelling), contraction of smooth muscles, and increasing mucus production.

Antigens in the diet wreak havoc on our bodies by causing a savage malfunction of mast cells. Antigens can trick the mast cells into thinking they need

Villi

Villi (singular, villus) are tiny hair-like projections in the intestine wall. There are 6,000 to 25,000 per square inch, giving the wall a velvety texture. Each villus is supplied with a microscopically thin artery, vein, and lymphatic capillaries and 600 tiny projections called microvilli. These incredibly delicate and precisely adjusted structures are responsible for absorbing nutrients and fluid from the digestive system into the bloodstream and lymphatic system. They are remarkably fine-tuned to take in just what is right for the body and to act as a barrier to harmful substances. Any disruption to their proper functioning undermines the health of the whole body.

to start an inflammatory reaction. So, consumption of food antigens can lead to increased swelling and constricted muscles (for example, those involved in asthma), and cause mucus membranes to discharge (such as in the nose). In other words, by malfunctioning, mast cells cause an allergic reaction.

Also under the action of antigens, the tiny, delicate villi lining the intestinal wall are withered or destroyed. The colon is lined with millions of tiny pockets called crypts, which are in turn lined with stem cells. Antigens provoke abnormal growth of the stem cells, increasing the risk of cancer. An important function of the colon wall is to secrete mucus, potassium, and bicarbonate and to absorb sodium and chloride. Antigens disrupt the transport of these substances across the intestinal wall and the colon becomes more porous. What foods contain these antigens? The biggest culprits are grains, particularly wheat, and dairy products.

Food Choices and the Health of the Colon

Do you ever wonder why the contents of your bowels sometimes smell like sewage sludge? Researchers found that this was due to the abnormal presence of alien, harmful bacteria known as sulfur-reducing bacteria.[7] They flourish on sulfur-containing foods, mainly animal proteins. These alien bacteria create the gas hydrogen sulfide, the compound that gives rotten eggs their overpowering smell. To humans, hydrogen sulfide is as toxic as cyanide; in water, it rapidly becomes corrosive sulfuric acid. Ulcerative colitis, a serious inflammatory bowel disease, is directly linked to the dominating presence of sulfur-reducing bacteria in the colon.[8] Worse, the toxic sulfides released by these bacteria promote cancerous changes in gut cells by damaging their DNA. All this helps to explain why heavy meat eaters are more vulnerable to colon cancer. Proteins from plants usually do not contain sulfur.

The other major source of sulfur in the Western diet is the food preservative collectively known as "sulfur dioxide." Sulfur, in many forms, is found everywhere in processed food—in packaged salads, jams, hamburgers, sausages, instant soup, beer, and wine. People who eat a lot of processed foods not only promote sulfur bacteria in their gut, they also raise their sensitivity to allergic reactions.

The human gut clearly needs a plentiful supply of plant foods to operate healthily. The San consumed a very high-fiber diet and their plant matter was naturally very fibrous. In Chapter 1, we saw how the examination of 11,000-year-old fossilized feces showed that our ancestors were consuming 130 grams per day of plant fiber. The average American only consumes a tenth of that amount, 13 grams per day, and way below even the modest target set by various authorities of around 30 grams per day. Most of today's salads, vegetables, and fruits are less fibrous and contain around 2 grams of fiber per 100 grams, and nuts contain around 8 grams per 100 grams. Thus, one way to get to 30 grams per day is to consume, for example, 1 pound (450 g) of salad, 1 pound (450 g) of vegetables, 1 pound (450 g) of fruit, and $1/4$ pound (4 ounces, 100 g) of nuts.

In this book, we will argue that we need to be aiming higher. When the intake of plant fiber is up to at least 60 grams per day, then passage of food through the digestive tract is prompt, and the friendly bacteria get a rich, nutritive diet. Friendly bacteria are methanogens, producing methane in the gut. Under the right conditions, they thrive, multiply fast, and greatly increase the bulk of the feces. They also gobble up the "bad" sulfur-releasing bacteria.

Let us now look at what happens when we eat starches and sugars. Under normal, healthy circumstances, starches and sugars are mostly digested and absorbed into the body before they reach the colon. However, with the way we eat today, starches and sugars reach the colon in significant quantities. Because "bad" gut flora, particularly fungi like *Candida*, thrive on them, they quickly overgrow and flood into the bloodstream through the "leaky gut." Plus, the high insulin reaction from all the sugar provokes a condition called "digestive neuromuscular disease," in which the gut muscles go haywire, leading to cramps, diarrhea, and bloating.[9]

Today, our dietary errors vastly increase both the porosity of the gut and the microorganism load flooding into the body. In this way, abnormal quantities of digestive toxins, bacterial and fungal toxins, and the bacteria and fungi themselves, pass into the bloodstream. They can be the origin of various allergies, autoimmune responses, poisoning of various bodily functions, headaches, arthritis, tiredness, irritability, and depression.

The colon is a hive of activity—in hundreds of ways, it affects the health of the whole body. Our guts are also the scene of intense warfare between "friendly" organisms and unfriendly ones, but it does not have to be like this. We can be reasonably sure that the San's colons functioned as nature intended. All is not well with the way we eat today. We are sending down residues that our intestines do not recognize and that promote malevolent gut flora. Passage through the intestines is slow and consists of foods that destroy the delicate gut wall and undermine the immune system.

The Immature or Baby Digestive System

Mammals, such as cows, sheep, goats, chimpanzees, and humans, give birth to their young, in a sense, prematurely. The newborn bodies are underdeveloped and not yet fully functional, they do not have the full range of digestive arrangements, and the nutrients required to develop their bodies are impossible to find in the external environment. For example, a human baby's brain has to double in size in just a few months—to do this it needs a massive intake of specific kinds of fats, some of them saturated. Similar needs have to be satisfied for bone building, energy, muscle building, nerve building, and the growth of various organs.

For this reason, the baby of the species has special needs for substances like calcium, lactose (a sugar), fatty acids, and protein. They get these things from their mother's milk. Moreover, the mother's milk has a composition that is right for that particular species. For example, cow's milk is formulated to build big horns and small brains. It might seem obvious to say so, but nature designed milk for mammal mothers to feed their *own* young.

However, the differences go much deeper than the ingredients. A human baby has immature organs, notably kidneys and liver. It has a different biochemistry and digestive arrangements compared to a person over 4 years old. Curiously, a baby's throat is so arranged that it can breathe and suckle at the same time. After about 12 months, the breathing tube descends to the position it will keep for the rest of its life.

Only a baby's stomach can secrete the special enzyme, rennin, which is responsible for separating the mother's milk into curds and whey. The curds are composed chiefly of fats and the milk protein called casein, and digestion of the curds takes place slowly in the baby's stomach. Only babies secrete the special stomach enzymes to digest the fats and protein in the curd. The whey, freed by the rennin from the curds, passes quickly into the intestines for absorption into the body. Whey is a watery mixture containing dissolved compounds essential for a baby's growth. It is rich in micronutrients, immune system antibodies, a soluble protein similar to egg-white called lactalbumin, and the milk sugar called lactose. The baby's intestine secretes a special enzyme, lactase, to digest the lactose. After the age of about 4, all these processes stop. In other words, we should think of an infant up to the age of 4 as requiring a different feeding pattern to older children and adults.

Human bodies over the age of 4 are not designed to absorb human milk. What, then, about the milk of cows, goats, sheep, and other creatures? The effects of dairy consumption on the human body will provide important clues when we assemble the evidence for the "Owner's Manual," the guide to the true eating pattern for human beings.

Proper Food Combining

Our forager forebears only ate from two food groups, non-starchy plants and animal matter. Even their fruits, being fibrous, oil-rich, and with a low sugar content, were included with the non-starch plant foods. The digestive system has to break down a variety of foodstuffs, each requiring a different process, into their useful component parts. Remarkably, it can perform this feat, but not simultaneously, because the processes are conflicting.

This leads to the concept of eating food in batches that require the same chemical and mechanical treatment in the digestive tract. It is known as the principle of proper food combining. The question never arose in our formative past because the two food groups that humans ate—non-starchy plant material and animal matter—combine just fine. Today, we have complicated and confounded the process by introducing new types of food into the diet, notably starches, dairy products, and fruits with a distorted sugar profile.

Most of us picture our stomachs as a kind of cauldron into which we can haphazardly toss a variety of ingredients at random. The mixture bubbles away and the body gradually absorbs it all. We now know that this is quite wrong. We would all be a lot healthier if we did not put our digestive system through these gymnastics and returned to sending down just the two foods groups for which it is designed. With regard to modern fruits, we can make small adjustments so that we extract their health benefits without compromising digestion. We begin by describing in some detail the gruesome truth of what goes on in your guts when you send down bad food combinations.

Starch/Protein Combinations

The digestion of starches begins in the mouth with the enzyme ptyalin secreted in saliva. Starch digestion is stopped by the acid in the stomach and is then continued in the small intestine, under the action of enzymes like amylase secreted by the pancreas down the pancreatic duct.

Proteins, and particularly animal proteins, undergo a prolonged churning and exposure to the acids and enzymes present in the stomach. It can be several hours before the stomach releases the resulting chyme into the small intestine. The digestion then continues in the small intestine under the action of enzymes like protease, again secreted by the pancreas.

Unlike the chicken, which has three pancreatic ducts, the single human pancreatic duct is a bottleneck. The pancreas has to choose which enzyme to secrete first.[10] If the starch/protein combination contained predominantly starch (90%) or predominantly protein (90%), then the choice is easy, and digestion proceeds as nature intended. If the meal is an equal mix of starch and protein, then enzyme secretion by the pancreas is perturbed.

The imperfectly digested remains travel with difficulty through the digestive tract. The highly sophisticated machinery of enzyme activity, hormonal feedback, and nutrient absorption is impaired. The balance of the intestinal flora is disturbed—bad bacteria multiply and helpful bacteria are discouraged. The intestinal wall can become porous and bacteria, fungi (such as *Candida*), and undigested food particles travel through the bloodstream, creating mischief wherever they go. Dyspepsia, ulcerative colitis, liver disorders, demineralization, depression of the immune system, candidiasis, allergies, and general bad health can be the result.

Proteins, like starch, also provoke the secretion of insulin. When starches are ingested at the same time, insulin secretion is multiplied. All the bad effects of abnormal insulin levels are multiplied, increasing the risk of heart disease, atherosclerosis, obesity, and cancer. Worse, in the Western diet, fat is usually present in large proportions with protein. This fat gets stored immediately and preferentially into the fat cells. So, starch/protein combinations multiply the fattening effect of fat!

Remembering that starch is not a great thing to be putting in the body, let us keep things in perspective. There are occasions when there are small amounts of starch in a protein dish, like a few bits of sweet corn in a tuna salad. This is unimportant provided that the protein dominates. The trouble arises when the proteins and starches are equally balanced and they fight each other for priority. This is the case with so much of what we eat today—for example, steak and french fries, hot dogs, hamburgers, and tuna sandwiches. Starch/protein combinations cause trouble when they are present in nearly equal proportions and they fight each other for dominance.

Fruit/Protein and Fruit/Starch Combinations

Eaten on their own, fruits pass quickly through the stomach and are rapidly digested in the small intestine. On the other hand, if fruit is eaten at the end of a meal, it is kept waiting in the stomach. If this happens, most modern fruits will start to ferment and produce gases and harmful compounds, such as fusel oil. Digestive processes are also disrupted and the fruit's nutritive value is compromised. This is a main cause of digestive upsets, gas, headaches, and gastroesophageal reflux disease (GERD).

Fruits have a predominantly acid nature. Acid inhibits ptyalin production in the mouth, thus conflicting with starch digestion, and inhibits gastric acid production in the stomach, interfering with protein digestion. Fruit and starch combinations lead to disoriented digestion and the arrival in the colon of poorly digested, *Candida*-feeding starch particles. Fruit is best eaten on an empty stomach.

Milk

Milk forms a bad combination on its own. After the age of about 4 years, a human does not have the enzymes to properly digest dairy products. Notably, we do not secrete the enzyme rennin to separate milk into curds and whey. As a result, the half-curdled mixture proceeds through the digestive system, improperly digested and causing mischief on the way. In most adult humans, the milk sugar lactose arrives in the colon undigested, where it feeds bad bacteria, producing gas. The body perceives lactose as an antigen, so it also creates mischief with allergic reactions, such as damage to the colon lining, headaches, and diarrhea. More subtly, lactose is strongly suspected of playing a role in autism, chronic fatigue syndrome, and attention deficit disorder (ADD).

Milk fat is also largely undigested, because the adult digestive system fails to separate the fat (in the curds) from the calcium (in the whey). The two combine to form insoluble solids that pass, unchanged, the full length of the digestive tube and out the other end. In this way, the calcium in milk is largely lost to the body.

Summary—Digestive System Clues

From this quick appraisal of the digestive system, focusing on just a few key areas, we throw into high relief the factors that are beneficial to it and those that are harmful. From our study of colon health, we find that a high non-starch plant food diet is healthy. On the other hand, starches, sugars, grains, dairy, and a high-meat, high-sulfur diet are unhealthy.

We have seen that babies are well adapted to consuming the milk of their species, but the adults are not. This notion is reinforced by a look at food combining. Nature did not design our digestive systems to cope with starches, dairy, and sugary fruits. This strongly reinforces earlier clues from other fields of enquiry. Now, we'll look at these food items individually to find out what creates these problems.

DIETARY CLUES

Grains (Cereals)

All grains are mostly composed of starch. White wheat flour is about 75% starch, whole wheat flour is 67%, rye flour 75%, white rice 85%, oatmeal 65%, and corn flour (maize) 92%.[11] The products made from them are also mostly starch: spaghetti is 71% starch, corn flakes 77%, white bread 46%, and whole-grain bread 40%. Starches from all grains are rapidly converted to glucose, provoking an unhealthy glycemic and insulin reaction. So, when you look at a slice of bread, think 4 teaspoons of sugar; a cup of cornflakes is equal to 5 teaspoons of sugar; and $1/2$ cup of rice is 6 teaspoons of sugar.

Primatologist Katharine Milton has studied the foods eaten by apes and monkeys in the tropics and draws comparisons with how human food must have been in our evolutionary past.[12] She finds that grains are a poor source of micronutrients. Grains have massively displaced more nutritious plant foods from our modern diets. This is why makers of breakfast cereals are obliged by law to "fortify" their products with a long list of classic micronutrients. Of course, this is no substitute for the rich variety of background micronutrients found naturally in many plant foods, all working with each other in harmony to nourish our body in the way it recognizes.

Cereals, like many other plants, have developed defenses against being eaten. These defenses take the form of antinutrients, toxins that are designed to upset the biochemistry of the creature that eats them. Seed-eaters (from fungi to bacteria to insects and birds) have developed resistance to these antinutrients, but primates (man included) have never been grain eaters and have low resistance to cereal toxins. It may come as a shock to learn that cereal toxins have been undermining human health for millennia. In this book, we call these "background" toxins: they do not kill you right away and often they do not produce any obvious symptoms, but silently, in the background, they are undermining our health. Researchers Loren Cordain[13] and the Dane H. Frøkier[14] have studied and reported on their effects. Let's look at four types of antinutrients.

Lectins. Lectins can batten on to carbohydrate-containing molecules anywhere in the body. They pass easily from the gut into the bloodstream and disrupt the work of any body cell to which they attach themselves. They are powerful provokers of all kinds of autoimmune diseases, including allergies, asthma, lupus, and arthritis, and are even suspected of causing autism in susceptible children. Lectins cause the gut to be more porous, allowing bacteria, fungi, and food particles to flood into the bloodstream and create mischief. Most Americans, with their depressed immune systems and vague headaches and allergies, are unknowingly suffering from this effect. In extreme cases, a porous intestine develops into leaky gut syndrome.

Alpha-amylase inhibitors. Alpha-amylase inhibitors interrupt the activity of the starch-digesting enzyme amylase and damage the pancreas. In addition, they are strong allergens, which explains the "baker's asthma" referred to in Chapter 3.

Protease inhibitors. Protease inhibitors interrupt signals from the intestine telling the pancreas to reduce secretion. As a result, the pancreas continues churning out the hormone cholecystokinin like a runaway flywheel. This disrupts normal digestive processes and the stress on the pancreas can lead to abnormal enlargement and cancer.

Alkyl resorcinols. Alkyl resorcinols disrupt a wide range of body functions: they disintegrate red blood cells, disrupt DNA maintenance, abnormally increase blood clotting, and depress production of human growth hormone (HGH). HGH is needed, even in full-grown adults, for cell renewal and to maintain health as we age. Depressed HGH might also be part of the explanation why humans lost stature when they took up farming (see Chapter 3).

We introduced the most powerful allergen in grains, the gluten complex, in Chapter 3. Recent research finds that one in 133 Americans has a full-blown gluten allergy called celiac disease.[15] Japanese researcher Hideaki Tsuji finds that it is the portion called gliadin that is responsible for celiac disease.[16] In addition, it causes killer lymphocytes to malfunction and damage the delicate mucous membrane lining the intestine. It withers away the villi and provokes crypt cells to proliferate in a pre-cancerous way.

Apart from gluten, there are dozens of allergenic substances in many types of grains, including rice, barley, and corn. Some people suffer allergic reactions, even anaphylactic shock, to the barley present in beer. Tsuji says that rice is the foremost allergen in Japan. He describes eight major allergens in wheat, four in barley, three in rice, and two in maize.

Heirloom Grains: Quinoa and Amaranth

The grain quinoa has a particularly high content of the poisons cyanide and saponin. Saponin is a heart-stopper related to digitalis; Amerindians used the concentrated extract on their poison arrows. Amaranth accumulates poisonous levels of nitrates and oxalates, toxins that cause inflammation and may lead to swelling of the throat to the point of suffocation.

Vegetables, Starchy

In the modern diet, there is only one big player in the category of starchy vegetables—the potato. But in passing we mention that parsnips, sweet potatoes, yams, and plantains are also starchy and give "bad" blood sugar spikes; that is, they are high glycemic. Carrots and beets are not starchy but, depending on their age, variety, and other factors can have a high sugar content. They, too, can be unhealthily glycemic.

The potato is a newcomer to the human diet and it is starchy. In all its forms (baked, boiled, mashed, fries, and so on) it is strongly glycemic, so it is classed as a bad carbohydrate. Its ability to raise insulin levels is even greater than the glycemic index would suggest. These properties alone make the potato a poor food for humans.

Potato is a poor source of micronutrients as well. This might not be important if Americans consumed potatoes frugally and rarely, but they consume it in vast quantities every day. In this way, it shoulders aside the consumption of much more nutritious non-starchy plant foods. The U.S. Department of Agriculture (USDA) classes potatoes as a vegetable, as though it has equal nutritive value as, say, a tomato. Americans are thus led to believe that they have filled their vegetable quota by filling up on french fries. They are mistaken: filled with potato, the population is nevertheless starving for all those ingredients needed in trace amounts from authentic non-starchy vegetables.

As with cereals, we have to wonder about the presence of plant toxins in potato to which humans have no resistance. Agricultural researchers Leslie

Plhak and Peter Sporns have studied and reviewed this interesting question.[17] Potatoes fall under suspicion because they are part of the same plant family (Solanacea) as the poisonous and narcotic plants henbane, deadly nightshade, belladonna, and mandrake. It turns out that potatoes are charged with many background toxins, of which the most potent are glycoalkaloids. Potatoes have been responsible for a number of human poisonings—up to 30 deaths and over 2,000 cases of non-fatal poisonings have been documented. The *British Medical Journal* observes that there is certainly a vast reservoir of unreported cases.[18]

Symptoms of potato poisoning include vomiting, diarrhea, drowsiness, confusion, weakness, and coma. In those cases where people have died, it has been from strangulated bowel, respiratory failure, and cardiac arrest. From these unfortunates, it has been possible to calculate the fatal dose. Researchers estimate that the safety factor is just four-fold against toxic poisoning for a one-pound serving.[19] It should not be surprising that episodes of glycoalkaloid poisoning, some fatal, have occurred.

Glycoalkaloids do their damage on several fronts. First, they can form a soapy lather that destabilizes membranes, particularly those lining the intestinal tract. They inhibit production of the nerve enzyme cholinesterase, which is a likely cause of their neurological effects. Finally, they encourage mutations in the cells of the liver, nerve tubes, and immune system.

Vegetables, Non-Starchy

We do not generally think of plants as a meaningful source of protein, yet indeed they are. Young leaves routinely eaten by primates in the tropics contain 10% to 20% of protein dry-weight[20] and gorillas build and maintain their muscles entirely on plant protein. In contrast, modern species of intensively cultivated plants tend to have lower protein content, but there are exceptions: Brussels sprouts contain 24% protein per 100 grams dry-weight.

Monocot and Dicot Plant Foods

Humans and other primates find their plant food mainly from the class of plants called angiosperms, which are flowering species. Angiosperms are, in turn, divided into two main classes, monocot and dicot. Monocot species includes grains, cereals, and other grasses like alfalfa. Dicot species include what we think of as salads and colored vegetables.

Can humans get enough protein from plant foods alone? We need less protein than we think—about 75 grams per day for an average 165-pound adult. That equates to about 2 pounds (1 kg) of Brussels sprouts per day. Not impossible! This book is not about making us all vegetarians, but it is useful to see how plant food is adding to our protein intake, which implies that we do not need as much high-protein food as we think.

Wild leaves typically have a high percentage of indigestible cell wall material, up to 35%. It is almost entirely the types of soluble fiber called "unlignified hemicelluloses and cellulose." Such fiber is common in dicot vegetables. The human gut is good at degrading this type of fiber, which is found in carrots and cabbage, for example. The human gut is much less efficient at degrading the fiber from monocot plants, such as wheat bran. According to Dr. Milton, most primates focus almost entirely on the dicot plants with their soluble fiber.[21] This is just the type of fiber that our bodies need and the low intake of fiber today has serious consequences for human health. Non-starchy plants are, of course, naturally rich in micronutrients, notably the myriad "background" micronutrients that are so important to our biochemistry.[22]

Finally, in regard to essential fatty acids, wild plants show a roughly equal balance between linoleic acid (23%) and alpha-linolenic acid (16%). Most cultivated plants that Americans eat are notoriously poor in alpha-linolenic acid. However, there is one plant that grows as a weed all over the southern United States; one that the '49ers of the California gold rush consumed so much that it was dubbed "miner's lettuce"—that plant is purslane. It contains 8% fats, of which 50% is omega-3 oil.[23] Here, we finally uncover the last secret to the Cretan diet: they were one of the few peoples eating a proper balance of omega-6 to omega-3 fatty acids, thanks to the high volumes of purslane they were consuming. It is no coincidence that the San also ate the same plants in our African homeland.

Fruits

Modern fruits have, by and large, quite different characteristics to those of our African homeland. Dr. Milton finds that wild fruits as eaten by primates and our ancient ancestors do not have a Technicolor, super-sized, and plump appearance. They have a much higher seed-to-pulp ratio and are less sweet, they have a high roughage content composed of woody seeds and fibrous strands, and they have higher protein levels, micronutrient levels, and pectin (a soluble fiber) levels. As eaten by primates in the jungle, they frequently contain tiny insects and larvae, which are eaten inadvertently.[24]

Wild fruits (and plants) are much richer in micronutrients than cultivated ones—particularly in minerals (notably iron, copper, and calcium) and the vitamins C, E, and K, beta-carotene, and folic acid. Dr. Milton estimates the vitamin C intake of a human-size ape to be 2–6 grams.[25] Contrast that with the recommended dietary intake of 60 mg for an adult human, or 100 times less! Research indicates that wild plants are also much richer in the millions of other "background" micronutrients essential to good human health, such as bioflavonoids, terpenes, phenols, carotenes, and many more.

Cultivated vs. Wild Fruits

Compared to cultivated fruits, wild fruits are:

- Low glycemic
- Less watery
- Low in sucrose
- Less sweet
- Richer in fiber
- Richer in micronutrients

Dairy Products

We've seen how dairy products are implicated in a wide range of diseases. For example, the milk sugar lactose is an antigen undermining our bodies in many subtle ways. There is now a huge body of knowledge linking milk and dairy consumption to an incredible range of diseases. In addition to lactose, the proteins in milk (casein and lactalbumin) are among the most powerful allergens known. Casein also raises cholesterol levels.[26] In a controlled study on autistic youngsters, Dr. Ted Kniker found that when dairy is eliminated from the diet, there was dramatic improvement.[27]

The Nurses' Health Study, begun in 1976, is a national survey of more than 121,000 female registered nurses, 34 to 59 years old, which analyzes diet and health data every two years. In a stunning counterblast to conventional wisdom, lead researcher Diane Feskenich found that those nurses who drank two or more glasses of milk per day were 40% *more* likely to suffer hip fractures than those who drank less than one glass.[28] Here we have the explanation for why Norwegian women suffer more from hip fractures than Spanish women: traditionally, Norwegians are high consumers of dairy products, Spaniards hardly at all.

Dairy consumption is also linked to cancers of various kinds. As part of the Physicians' Health Study, epidemiologist June M. Chan investigated the connection between dairy products and prostate cancer in a large group of male U.S. physicians. Compared with the men who consumed less than half a serving of dairy products daily, men who consumed more than 2.5 servings had a 34% higher risk of developing prostate cancer.[29] Cancer researcher Eduardo De Stefani found that Uruguayans consuming dairy products increased lung cancer risk by 2.5 times.[30] Researcher Helena Liljeberg Elmstahl found that dairy is linked to abnormal insulin levels.[31]

Dr. Guy Abraham, a professor of gynecologic endocrinology at the University of California, sees a connection between dairy consumption and premenstrual tension.[32] Dr. Honglei Chen, of the Harvard School of Public Health, finds that men have an 80% increased risk of Parkinson's disease with dairy consumption of all kinds.[33] Gastroenterologist A.M. Riordan of Cambridge University found that remission rates for Crohn's disease were doubled when both dairy and cereal were excluded.[34]

Milk fat (butter and cream), while good for baby cows, is not good for humans. It raises blood pressure and cholesterol, hardens the arteries, and increases heart disease and the risk of stroke. Even the fat-free varieties are not safe: milk lactose and milk calcium alone are enough to calcify arteries, the most dangerous form of arteriosclerosis.[35]

Many people think that yogurt is healthy and that organic milk is best. They believe that milk from other species such as goat, buffalo, sheep, camel, or even humans is superior. In fact, the drawbacks to dairy from cows apply equally to dairy products from all these other creatures, and that includes yogurt, buttermilk, cheeses, and milk, whether full fat or non-fat.

Summary of Diseases Linked to Dairy Consumption

- Abnormally high insulin levels (hyperinsulinemia)
- Allergies
- Autism
- Breast cancer
- Crohn's disease
- Hardening of the arteries (arteriosclerosis)
- Lung cancer
- Osteoporosis and hip fracture
- Parkinson's disease
- Premenstrual tension
- Prostate cancer

Meat, Poultry, Eggs, and Fish

The problem with so-called red meats—beef, lamb, and pork—lies with the amount and types of fat they contain. In part, this is just an accident of breeding, because down the millennia the breed has changed. Some breeders are now trying to breed these animals back to a much lower fat percentage and to a better fatty acid profile. Mostly, however, the problem is with the food the beasts are given to eat. Cattle are naturally "browsers": they eat from a huge variety of bushes, flowers, and other vegetation. Today, ranchers feed them on grass or, even worse, corn and soybeans.

As long ago as 1968, Michael A. Crawford, zoologist at the London Zoological Society, was raising the alarm. He studied the difference in beasts living free-ranging lifestyles in African woodlands compared to the same species living in captivity on grassland.[36] He found that the meat of free-living cattle had fatty acid profiles in line with the Savanna Model, whereas cattle fed on grassland had the "bad" fatty acid profile that we associate with beef today. That is, high in the saturated fats palmitic acid and myristic acid.

Pigs (and the wild boar from which they are descended) are creatures that browse freely in woodlands, even digging up earthworms and truffles. Today, pigs are fed on anything from restaurant scraps to time-expired processed foods. Sheep actually prefer eating the type of plant called "forb," which is any kind of herbaceous plant *except* grass. Today, perversely, sheep are fed only on grass (if they are lucky) or otherwise on artificial concentrated feed made from rejected grains, vegetable oils, and soybean waste. Japanese researchers have demonstrated that sheep, cattle, and pigs have a "good" fatty acid profile if they feed in their natural habitat, whereas they have a harmful fatty acid profile when fed conventionally.[37]

Dr. Artemis Simopoulos of the Center for Genetics, Nutrition, and Health, in Washington, D.C., is one of the foremost advocates of the need to incorporate omega-3 oils in the human diet. He observes that "on the Ampelistra farm in Greece, purslane is plentiful and grows wild; the chickens make a feast of it, along with insects and lots of fresh green grass, supplemented with fresh and dried figs, barley flour, and small amounts of corn. . . . As we expected, the eggs contained substantial amounts of omega-3 fatty acids."[38] The Greek egg had an omega-6 to omega-3 ratio of 1.3 to 1, whereas a supermarket egg has a ratio of almost 20 to 1. The point is that many animal products have become unhealthy because the feed given to the animal bears no resemblance to the natural feeding pattern of the creature. As a result, the flesh and eggs are devoid of omega-3 oils.[39]

The food industry should correct this imbalance. One of the secrets to the Greek free-range egg is the omega-3-rich purslane that the chickens were eating. Now some egg farmers are producing omega-3 rich eggs by feeding the chicken on flaxseed, which is itself rich in omega-3s.

So much for the eggs, but what about the flesh of the chicken? According to Dr. Crawford, chickens are much fatter than 35 years ago: they contain 24 g of fat per 100 g compared to just 8 g in 1970. "Chickens used to roam free and eat herbs and seeds. Now they are fed with high-energy foods and even most organic chickens don't have to walk any distance to eat." It is likely that the Greek free-range birds had very little fat, of which a high percentage was omega-3s. This is the direction our food supply needs to go.

The situation is slightly different with other types of poultry. The fat from goose and duck is semi-liquid at room temperature, which tells us that there is not much saturated fat in it. The fat of these birds has a high percentage of monounsaturated fat. This seems to be one more element helping to explain the French Paradox—the people of Toulouse use these fats in preference to butter, thus increasing their intake of monounsaturated fats.

Some species of oily fish contain high levels of omega-3 oils as well, particularly wild salmon, sardines, herring, mackerel, tuna, and wild trout. Here, we have another secret to the long-lived and healthy Cretans and Japanese—their diets were rich in fish, many of them oily species. The Okinawans were eating 144 g (5 ounces) per day, six times the average American consumption. The high omega-3 intake increased the hormones that reduce abnormal blood clotting. Creatures like seal, walruses, and whales that eat these fish also have high omega-3 content, and this is the main source in the Eskimo diet.

However, all is not well with farmed fish, such as salmon and trout: their omega-3 content depends on what they are fed. Even though they are carnivores, farmed salmon are fed with pellets made of grains, fish meal, and vegetable oil, and so their flesh is often deficient in the omega-3 oils.

Animal matter can provide the same micronutrients as plants, such as calcium and vitamin A, but there is one essential micronutrient that has to be obtained from animal matter—vitamin B_{12}. It is only needed in tiny amounts and it is easily obtained from eggs, fish, poultry, and meat. However, without it, we sicken and die, unlike the vegan gorilla who can manage without it. This is yet one more clue that animal matter must have been a constant part of the human ancestral diet.

Legumes

Legumes are notorious for being "gassy." They contain a high percentage of indigestible carbohydrates called oligosaccharides, notably one called raffinose. When they arrive in the colon, still undigested, the bacteria feed on them, producing hydrogen, carbon dioxide, and methane—up to 5 gallons of flatulence per day in extreme cases. Humans simply do not have the digestive enzymes necessary to comfortably digest legumes.

Legumes are also not exempt from the same kinds of antinutrients, particularly lectins, found in cereals. Lectins in winged, kidney, mung, lima, and castor beans are toxic in their raw state. The lectins bind with the wall of the intestine, causing lesions and abnormal development of the microvilli. Nutrient absorption is impaired and the intestine wall becomes porous to bacteria, bacterial toxins, and lectins themselves. They pass into the lymphatic system and bloodstream to cause havoc directly.

Baking or vigorous boiling will deactivate some of these poisons. Our prehistoric ancestors had no way to boil water and could only bake with difficulty. We can be sure that our Pleistocene ancestors had less troublesome foods to eat. Had it been otherwise, our bodies would be immune to these toxins. Neither the Aboriginals nor the San ate beans of this nature.

In Victorian times, castor bean oil was administered as a purgative and it became a byword for vile taste. Today, we know that the castor bean harbors one of the most toxic poisons known, one that has been developed into a chemical warfare agent—ricin. This poison causes severe vomiting and diarrhea, dehydration, shock, kidney failure, liver failure, and fatal stomach hemorrhaging. Ricin is also toxic to the heart and bursts red blood cells.[40] When ricin is inhaled, lung disease follows.[41] Lentils, soybeans, and peas contain a related lectin that interferes with the membrane of immune system lymphocytes.[42]

Soy is loaded with antinutrients, such as genistein, daidzein, trypsin inhibitors, allergens, and phytoestrogens. The wonders of marketing have turned these drawbacks into advantages: women are sold soy as a remedy for female conditions such as hot flashes and PMS. It is even sold as having anti-cancer properties when in fact it increases the risk of uterine cancer[43] and breast cancer.[44] Soy gives you allergies: over 16 allergens have been identified, of which at least three are considered "severe."[45] Soy's antinutrients genistein and daidzein attack thyroid function,[46] which can lead to goiter and, in extreme cases, thyroid cancer.

Soy gives you brain atrophy: the more people eat soy bean curds (tofu), for example, the more likely they are to have senile dementia in later life. Dr. Lon White, a researcher on aging, studied Japanese Americans in Hawaii and found that consumption of only two portions of tofu a week raises the chances of getting dementia by 50% compared to those who consume no tofu at all.[47] Here is a probable explanation why, more than anyone else, the tofu-eating Okinawans lose their mental faculties in old age.

Soy also disrupts gastric function. Trypsin inhibitors disrupt the pancreas, causing it to secrete out-of-control quantities of cholecystokinin (a gastric hormone).[48] The result is withering of the pancreas and even cancer.

Soy is not good for babies. New Zealand researcher Cliff Irvine finds that babies fed on soy-based formula receive the adult equivalent of five birth control pills per day.[49] Children of both sexes suffer disproportionately from extreme emotional behavior, asthma, immune system problems, pituitary insufficiency, thyroid disorders, and irritable bowel syndrome.[50] Soy-fed baby boys sometimes fail to develop proper male traits later in life; girls can enter puberty earlier than normal.[51] In a study of over 13,000 schoolchildren in Britain, researchers found that children who were fed soy-based formula as babies were 2.5 times more likely to suffer peanut allergy than other children.[52] The New Zealand Government already issued a warning in 1998 about the use of soy in infant formula. Britain's Food Standards Agency (FSA) raised the alarm in 2003 about feeding soy to babies.[53] It calls upon the Department of Health to revise its guidelines to say that soy-based infant formulas be fed to infants only when the doctor says it is safe to do so. They cite one study where such babies were five times more likely to have genital abnormalities.

The peanut is now one of the most prevalent allergenic foods, having shown a notable increase in recent years.[54] It is probably not a coincidence that mothers have been increasingly using soy formula over recent years. It is now estimated that 6% to 8% of children, and 2% of adults, suffer from these allergies. About 30,000 cases of anaphylaxis (extreme sensitive reaction) occur annually, resulting in 2,000 hospitalizations and 200 deaths.[55]

Because of their antinutrients, legumes—and soy, in particular—are not miracle foods. They are beans to which humans have never become naturally adapted, and it matters. Their anti-nutrients are diverse kinds of poisons or toxins that disrupt many bodily processes, undermining our health in ways never before suspected. Since they work slowly and in the background, it is only recently that these harmful properties are being uncovered.

Sugar

In just the last three centuries, humans have dramatically increased consumption of this totally new food—sugar. Sugar consumption contributes to dysfunctional blood sugar control and all the degenerative diseases that follow: obesity, diabetes, cardiovascular disease, stroke, arthritis, osteoporosis, and many more. Dr. William Grant estimates that sugar is killing 150,000 Americans a year.[56] In addition, sugar is empty calories—it provides nothing in the way of micronutrients and it displaces traditional nutritious foods.

Sugar (sucrose) is, of course, a naturally occurring substance. Nevertheless, many health-conscious people think that there is something unnatural about it and choose to sweeten with "natural" honey or maple syrup. But consumption of these sources of sweetness is tiny compared to that of sugar. However, even here there is no escape: maple syrup is at least 90% sucrose[57] and has a "bad" glycemic index.[58] The composition of honey is different and varies more widely. It is composed mainly of the sugars fructose (48% to 67%), glucose (38% to 48%) and maltose (3% to 15%). Commercial, blended honey has a "bad" glycemic index of 62 to 72.

However, Professor Jennie Brand-Miller has studied Australian eucalyptus honey, where the bees collected the nectar only from specific flowers. She finds an extreme case of a low–glycemic index honey obtained from the yellow box flower: it has a GI of only 35 and an insulin index of only 40.[59] This honey is particularly rich in the low-glycemic sugar, fructose. As such, it hovers on the borderline of "favorable" carbohydrate and has a "normal" insulin index. This is the way of the future, where foods like honey from particular flowers will be labeled with their glycemic index, enabling the consumer to make informed choices.

Beverages

Beer is brewed using the sugars from malted barley, so there is a percentage of the highly glycemic sugar, maltose. There is usually about 4 grams per 100 ml, which translates to about 3 teaspoons of sugar per 12 ounce can. Beer is in itself a "bad" carbohydrate with a high glycemic index. That is why big beer drinkers tend to suffer from the various sugar diseases—and put on a beer belly—when wine drinkers do not.

Dry wine, such as Bordeaux, is not glycemic. In particular, red wine contains a number of antioxidants like tannins and resveratrol. Dr. Serge Renaud, after numerous studies and analyses, came to the conclusion that it was these antioxidants in red wine that preserved the Toulousains from heart disease. So, this is perhaps the final element in explaining the French Paradox.

Regular carbonated drinks contain high levels of sugar: a can of cola contains 5 teaspoons of sugar. Carbonated drinks of this nature are "bad" carbohydrates. There is a further drawback with colas—they are rich in phosphoric acid, and high phosphoric acid consumption upsets the normal functioning of the parathyroid gland. Because parathyroid hormone regulates bone building, cola consumption has the net effect of demineralizing the bones.

Tea, whether black or green, contains a wide range of "background" micronutrients. Many studies have shown that tea helps combat cancer,[60] heart disease,[61] heart attacks,[62] hardening of the arteries,[63] and many other conditions. Coffee, particularly the weak American coffee, has no particular virtues or vices. Fruit juices are almost always glycemic, which is their big drawback.

PUTTING THE SCIENTIFIC CLUES TOGETHER

We have looked at various extremes of lifestyle around the world, from the Eskimo to the Okinawan. We learn from the Eskimo that a low–plant food diet is harmful but one high in essential fatty acids (particularly with the omega-6 to omega-3 ratio in balance) is healthful. The Eskimo does not suffer from cardiovascular diseases, but he does suffer from osteoporosis and premature aging due to his highly acidic, low-micronutrient diet. The Japanese, Cretans, and Okinawans are getting a lot right. The pointers are all toward a low calorie intake, a low fat intake (but sufficient intake of essential fatty acids), a low starch intake, a good intake of plant food, but low or zero intake of dairy products and red farmed meat.

In the biochemistry section, we saw how foods that spike blood sugar are bad for our bodies. They lead to high cholesterol, poor bone-building, cardiovascular disease, and cancers. We saw how the essential fatty acids omega-3 and omega-6 produce powerful hormones that affect the proper working of our bodies. Salt and its relationship to potassium intake is a fundamental factor affecting the efficiency of our very cells. In the segment on acid/alkali balance, we saw how acid-forming foods now dominate our Western diets. This too provides problems for our bodies, leading to kidney stones, bone demineralization, and stressed-out organs, such as the lymphatic system, liver, and pancreas.

We have learned the lesson, too, that it is impossible to second guess the way our bodies work. It would be wise to avoid the temptation to micromanage its internal processes—just give it the right fuel and let it manage matters for itself.

We looked at our digestive system and featured a much neglected area: colon health. By understanding what foods nourish friendly gut flora, we obtain strong clues to the kinds of residues we should be sending down there. Nature intended the incredibly delicate lining of the gut to resist a great deal of wear and tear, but the gut is defenseless against some of the residues we send down.

They are highly aggressive to the gut lining and destroy its ability to keep bad agents out of the bloodstream.

We also looked at two other interesting aspects: the immature or baby digestive system and the phenomenon of food combining. Babies have digestive arrangements which nature designed to work on mother's milk; adult digestive systems are not designed to handle milk. We found that the digestive system works fine on the two food groups present in our ancestral food supply. The introduction of new foods groups, notably starchy foods, dairy, and many modern fruits poses digestive problems both when they are eaten in combination with each other and also with the ancestral groups.

We also looked at our modern food supply. Until very recently, we ignored many straws in the wind because they did not fit into our Western cultural preconceptions. For instance, we think most peoples around the world are abnormal because milk makes them feel bad. The milk sugar, lactose, gives them allergic reactions, such as diarrhea, rashes, and headaches, and doctors say that they are "lactose intolerant." This is a looking-glass view of the world. Most peoples of the world are lactose intolerant because it is *normal;* even the San bushmen are lactose intolerant. In spite of the blandishments to consume milk "to build strong bones," milk consumption actually destroys bones.

Celiac disease is an allergic reaction to gluten, a compound found in cereals. We think that it is a "disease" because we cannot imagine that humans are not supposed to be eating grains. However, we now know that it is *normal* to react badly to cereal gluten.

Many plants contain poisons that the human body does not know how to handle. This fact gives us strong clues as to the kinds of foods that are right for humans. This leads to another surprise: legumes such as lentils, soy, and other beans contain antinutrients that undermine our health in many subtle ways; the same applies to potatoes and grains. Nature did not design humans to consume legumes, potatoes, or grains.

On the other hand, the body does need a good supply of micronutrients: not just the few dozen "classic" micronutrients, but tens of thousands of "background" micronutrients. Non-starchy plant foods and fruits supply these in abundance, in the variety needed and in ways where they pull together as a team.

This overview of the science gives us the main signposts, but when it comes to food choices, we need to have a knowledge of the details as well. Our ancient ancestors had the skills to survive in the jungle. They knew which mushrooms were poisonous and when a tree would be fruiting. We will need to learn the same level of skill when navigating our way through the supermarket jungle today. However, we can finally declare that we have enough evidence to describe the basic specification for the diet that is right for the human species. That is, we can now write the "Owner's Manual."

6. The Owner's Manual

At the beginning of this book, we painted a picture of our naturally adapted lifestyle. We saw how our ancient environment conditioned our bodies—and our very natures—for life on the savannas of east Africa. We called this lifestyle the "Savanna Model" and outlined how our ancient ancestors fed themselves for thousands of generations. This outline gives us the key to how we should be feeding ourselves today.

It's as if our bodies are an incredibly complex machine for which we have lost the operating instructions or "Owner's Manual." We can visualize the Owner's Manual as an ancient parchment that generations of scribes have overwritten many times. By carefully clearing away the more recent layers, we can rediscover the original scripture. The purpose of subsequent chapters was to explore these newer layers and find out how they came to be there. By this means, we reveal the underlying message.

In Chapter 2, we saw how the naturally adapted feeding pattern changed dramatically with the farming revolution 11,000 years ago. Governments intervene to regulate our food supply with the laudable intention of keeping it "fit" for "human consumption," but they've only had partial success. Governments also took it upon themselves to advise us how and what to eat, but much of this advice is flawed. In Chapter 3, using our own, redefined food groups as a framework, we looked at the history of our current food supply. This examination highlighted just how far we have distanced ourselves from our ancestral origins and the consequences of this departure. In Chapters 4 and 5, we looked at how other populations (Eskimos, Japanese, Cretans) around the world fare with their different diets. We put the microscope on how our bodies and biochemistry operate. By seeing what works well—and what works badly—we get strong pointers to the ideal feeding patterns for the human organism.

We have now done enough to clear away all the overwritten layers of our Owner's Manual. In this chapter, we show how the original scripture is revealed.

THE IDEAL HUMAN FEEDING PATTERN

There is no way that we can go back to eating the identical foods of our ancient ancestors or even those of today's San bushmen. We are totally dependent on the modern supply chain that brings us foods from near and far, most of it farmed. The species of plant food and animal matter are quite different too: we are not going to find caterpillars, mongongo nuts, or grewia berries in the supermarket any time soon! The way forward is to define the essential, fundamental characteristics of the Savanna Model eating pattern and then apply them in the modern world. When we put together all that we know—from foragers and foraging theory; from what goes wrong when we don't fuel our bodies correctly; from what we know about our biochemistry; from information gleaned from population studies and clinical studies—we can identify basic characteristics of the ideal human feeding pattern, for eating the way nature intended.

Blood Sugar Control

We saw that the San have a diet that is rich in plant food, yet there are no starches and very little sugar. Their digging sticks produced plenty of tubers but very few of them are starchy. Consequently, the San insulin response is slow. Our closest cousins in the animal kingdom, the chimpanzee and the gorilla, have similar diets. Starches and sugars badly disturb our blood sugar control. This in turn disrupts our biochemistry, leading to numerous diseases and eventually death. We come to the inescapable conclusion that nature designed the human frame for what we call a low-glycemic diet: that is, one that does not produce abnormal blood sugar spikes. The Western diet is the opposite—it produces high blood sugar surges. Abnormally high (and harmful) levels of insulin are the major consequence of high blood sugar levels. However, other factors too can aggravate high insulin levels, notably foods that are "high insulinemic" (see Chapter 4).

Owner's Manual: Focus on low glycemic, low insulinemic foods.

Acid-Alkali Balance

The San ate a diet that was roughly 75% plant food, which is alkali-forming, and 25% animal matter, which is acid-forming. They ate no grains or dairy products, which are both acid-forming. The net result is a diet that creates a neutral state in the blood between acidity and alkalinity. This is the ideal state for human biochemistry to function properly. Unfortunately, the average Western diet is strongly acidic.

Owner's Manual: Keep protein consumption modest (25% by weight) and keep non-starchy plant food and fruit consumption high (75% by weight).

High Volumes of High-Fiber, Low-Density Foods

Our evolutionary past designed our digestive systems to have high volumes of plant food passing through them. These non-starchy plant foods were, by nature, low density: that is, they had few calories for their volume. A lettuce leaf, for example, is 95% water (the remaining 5% is a wonderful cornucopia of vital nutrients). In addition, plant food is rich in soluble plant fiber, the sort that our colons are designed to work with. The typical Western diet is the opposite: energy dense and low in fiber.

Owner's Manual: Consume high volumes of non-starchy plant foods and fruits.

Low Sodium to High Potassium Ratio

We saw that salt, until very recent times, was a scarce commodity. In our ancestral homeland, it was unknown. Humans and other creatures only absorbed sodium from what was innate to the food they were eating. For example, uncooked broccoli contains, quite naturally, 27 milligrams of sodium per 100 grams. Similarly, it contains 325 milligrams of potassium per 100 grams. This ratio (about 1 to 12) of sodium to potassium is of fundamental importance for our body cells to function properly. Today, we have reversed this ratio to about 6 sodium to 1 potassium.

Owner's Manual: Avoid added salt in cooking, in processed foods, and at the table.

Healthy Fatty Acid Profile

All the evidence we have seen indicates that the human organism should not be eating much fat on a regular basis. A rough guideline suggests that maximum intake should not exceed 10% of calories from all sources. However, the little fat that we do eat should be of specific kinds. We looked into the vital role that the various fatty acids play in manipulating our biochemistry. There are 25 different fatty acids and most play no significant part in human nutrition. However, a handful that should not be there create havoc with the body's workings, and some that we desperately need are absent. We can summarize the position quite simply: the only fatty acids that we need to be consuming are omega-3 oils and omega-6 oils. Furthermore, ideally, they should be in the ratio of 1 to 1.

Nevertheless, we need to note one further phenomenon. Depending on what creature or plant they come from, some particular fatty acids are readily absorbed by the body, and they are said to be "bioavailable." There are other foods that contain unsafe fatty acids, but these are not bioavailable. We will make use of this knowledge when deciding what foods are safe and which are harmful. This can produce surprising results, sometimes contrary to what a simplistic analysis of their fatty acid composition might indicate.

Owner's Manual: Eat no more than 10% of calories as fat/oil. Focus on consumption of bioavailable omega-3 fatty acids, reduce consumption of bioavailable omega-6 fatty acids, and avoid foods with bioavailable "bad" fatty acids.

High Micronutrient Content

When we talk about micronutrients, we include not only all the familiar vitamins and minerals but also the thousands of "background" micronutrients. These are found predominantly in non-starchy plant food. We realize that many diseases, vague ills, and premature aging are symptoms of micronutrient deficiency. Today, micronutrient-poor starchy plant foods such as grains, rice, and potatoes have crowded out micronutrient-rich non-starchy plant foods. We saw how, in the Savanna Model, our ancient food supply contained both high concentrations and high volumes of micronutrients. This is the situation we need to return to today.

Owner's Manual: Consume non-starchy plant food and conforming fruits.

Low Plant Poison (Antinutrient) Levels

Earlier, we revealed that many of our commonly consumed foods contain sublethal doses of plant poisons or antinutrients. Our ancestral diet did not contain such foods and our bodies do not know how to deal with them. We will all find better vitality and health when we eliminate such foods from our diets.

Owner's Manual: Avoid grains, legumes, and potatoes, which contain antinutrients.

Low Antigen Content

Many of our commonly consumed foods contain harmful doses of immune system saboteurs or antigens. Our ancestral diet did not contain such foods—and our bodies do not know how to deal with them. We need to eliminate these foods from our diet.

Owner's Manual: Avoid dairy and grains, which contain antigens.

Feel Hungry Regularly

The San, Japanese, Okinawans, and Cretans were all skinny people. They ate sparingly and they often felt hungry, yet these peoples were all remarkable for their good health and longevity. The slimmer you are (without being emaciated), the longer you are likely to live and the less disease you will suffer. All the evidence points to this factor as being an essential characteristic of a healthy, naturally adapted lifestyle.

However, even if we cannot be skinny, there is a halfway house we should try to achieve to make sure that the blood sugar control machinery functions smoothly. Insulin is the sugar "locking up" hormone and its counterpart, glucagon, is the sugar "unlocking" hormone. Glucagon instructs fat cells to convert fat into sugar and release it into the bloodstream. Lack of use often atrophies this vital function of our biochemistry. Blood sugar levels have to be low and maintained low for the glucagon mechanism to swing into action. That means feeling hungry for about 30 minutes on a regular basis. Older people will remember that this happened several times a day before a main meal. Today, if people feel slightly hungry, there is always a sugar-boosting snack within easy reach.

Owner's Manual: Feel hungry for 30 minutes two or three times a day.

OWNER'S MANUAL TABLE OF CONTENTS

Here, we pull together all the arguments, evidence, and reasonings to draw up the broad outlines of the feeding pattern that is ideal for the human species. These, then, are the contents of the Owner's Manual.

Basic Specifications

Nature designed the human feeding pattern to:

1. Be low glycemic.
2. Be low insulinemic.
3. Have acid/alkali ratio in balance.
4. Have a high volume of high-fiber, low-density foods.
5. Sustain a low sodium (salt) to high potassium ratio.
6. Sustain a healthy fatty acid profile.
7. Provide high micronutrient content.
8. Provide a low plant poison (antinutrient) level.
9. Have a low antigen content.
10. Produce hunger some of the time.

Overview of Implementation

When we put together these criteria with what we know about certain groups of foods, these are the broad outlines for implementation of the Savanna Model.

• Consume a weight of conforming colored plant food that is about three times the weight of conforming protein-rich food. This means consume an abundance of non-starchy, colored plant foods and low-glycemic fruits, while consuming protein-rich foods modestly.

• Eliminate salt added at the table and in processing or cooking.

• Consume fats and oils generally sparingly. In addition, eliminate saturated fats in non-conforming foods, drastically curtail omega-6 oils, and boost consumption of omega-3 oils.

• Eliminate grains in all their forms.

• Eliminate potato in all its forms.

• Eliminate dairy products in all their forms.

• Eliminate processed foods.

• Feel hungry for at least 30 minutes two or three times a day.

Next, we will discover which are the "conforming" plant foods and "conforming" protein-rich foods that are readily available to us today. We will answer the challenge of how to adapt the Savanna Model to the food supply in the modern world. The choices are not always as obvious as we might think.

THE SAVANNA MODEL TODAY

For this information to be useful, we need to relate it to our everyday lives. Our Pleistocene ancestors had incredible jungle survival skills and we have to develop the same level of skill for survival in the supermarket jungle. There is not a single food that we eat today that our forager forebears would have recognized in the African savanna. So, for example, even when we talk in broad terms about eating fruits, our ancestors' fruits were different species, with somewhat different nutrient profiles, from our apples, oranges, and pears today. That is why we have to be well-informed about everything we eat and why we go into some detail to explain how to make wise food choices.

We will categorize foods according to how closely they conform to the Savanna Model. The classification is based on a traffic light system: Green means "Go," Amber (yellow) means "Caution," and Red means "Stop." We introduce finer gradations, such as "Green-Amber," which means "Go, but proceed with caution." Green-Green means "Go-Go!"—these are superfoods which are particularly healthful.

- **Green-Green:** Perfect—in perfect conformity with the Savanna Model.

- **Green:** Conforming—in close conformity with the Savanna Model.

- **Green-Amber:** Comfort Zone—within the margin of tolerance for everyday consumption by a healthy person.

- **Amber:** Slight Lapse—acceptable for a healthy person to consume on a regular basis, provided the rest of the diet is conforming.

- **Amber-Red:** Modest Lapse—acceptable for a healthy person to consume on an occasional basis, provided the rest of the eating pattern is conforming.

- **Red:** Bad Lapse—not acceptable; avoid.

Grains

This is the great shock to conventional nutritional ideas: grains are not the best thing since sliced bread! Grains are not a natural human food and they do nasty things to our bodies. They cause the human organism a number of problems, from unhealthy blood-sugar spikes to plant toxins (antinutrients) and immune system depressors (antigens). They are poor in nutrients and crowd out more nutritious foods.

Grains include wheat, rice, rye, barley, and oats, as well as the "ethnic" grains such as amaranth and quinoa, and "authentic" grains such as einkorn and emmer wheat. We also include the products made from grains: bread, spaghetti, pizza, croissants, cookies, and so on.

In making this blanket condemnation, we hear protests in the background. What about whole grains? What about oats, which the manufacturers sell as lowering cholesterol? The reality is that marketing forces have distorted the true perspective. Whole grains may contain useful nutrients, such as wheat germ, but they are just as glycemic, the bran contains even more antinutrients and antigens, and their content of harsh insoluble fiber is not what the intestines need.

Oats, of all the grains, contain rather more soluble fiber than average, a quality that manufacturers promote as cholesterol-reducing and therefore heart healthy. This, nevertheless, is not a valid argument: they are still glycemic, contain antinutrients and antigens, and are deficient in micronutrients. Oats are no alternative to proper plant food like lettuce and avocado.

The human diet is far better off without any cereals and their products. However, not all grains have all the same drawbacks and the way they are prepared modifies, for better or for worse, these drawbacks. The criteria used to categorize the Grains Group are: their effect on blood sugar surges, their antinutrient content, their gluten content, and their allergen content. They are all classified as "Red" in some degree. The purist will not have them in the house.

FOOD GROUP 1 GRAINS		
AMBER		
GRAIN SEEDS barley, pearl pumpkin seed sesame seed	**GRAIN PRODUCTS** **Seeds** Tahini (sesame seed butter)	
AMBER-RED		
GRAIN PRODUCTS **Bakery** pumpernickel vollkornbrot black bread	Breakfast Cereals All Bran oatmeal porridge	Pasta spaghetti (whole wheat)
RED		
GRAIN SEEDS barley, cracked bulgur wheat corn (maize) corn on the cob	oat bran oats rice, brown rice, instant	rice, white rye sweet corn (mature) wheat

FOOD GROUP 1 GRAINS *(continued)*		
RED *(continued)*		

Speciality Grains amaranth buckwheat einkorn emmer wheat quinoa spelt wild rice *(Zizania aquatica)* **GRAIN PRODUCTS** **Bakery** all (except "Amber-Red") including: bagel baguette bread, rye bread, wheat bread, white bread, whole wheat bread, buckwheat bun, hamburger bun, hot dog buns, generally cakes	cookies crackers, water crackers, wheat crispbread croissant Danish pastry gateaux muffin pastry, generally pizza, all kinds pretzels tarts wafers **Breakfast Cereals** all (except "Amber-Red") including: bran cereals bran flakes bran, oat Cheerios corn flakes hominy muesli	Rice Krispies Shredded Wheat Weetabix **Sundry** corn starch couscous pancakes pie crust popcorn rice cakes rice pudding semolina waffles **Pasta** all (except "Amber-Red") including: gnocchi lasagna linguine macaroni noodles spaghetti (white)

Starchy Plant Foods

Starchy plant foods are high glycemic (they cause unhealthy blood sugar surges), and for this reason alone you should avoid them. In addition, the most important of these foods in the Western diet, potatoes, are exceptionally bad for you: they are not only highly glycemic, they are highly insulinemic and also contain "background" poisons. Other starchy plants are parsnip and rutabaga, and these are best left out of the diet too.

There are some vegetables that are sugary, notably carrots and beets (beetroot). For this reason, they were included with the starchy vegetables. The glycemic index of carrots can vary considerably, but if they are raw and mature, they have only a modest impact on blood sugar levels. This is where we deploy the concept of glycemic load. Carrots have a low calorie density, so you have to eat quite a lot before triggering a glycemic reaction. Therefore, because we want to take in their good micronutrients and fibers, we allow the carrot a small place in our diet. Be wary, though, of carrot juice: it is more glycemic and, because it is possible to quaff down a tumblerful in one go, it is easy to overdose with carrot sugar. Beets are quite glycemic, but since they are rich in certain antioxidants, they just creep into the "Amber" category.

FOOD GROUP 2	VEGETABLES, STARCHY	
AMBER	**AMBER-RED**	**RED**
beets, red (beetroot)	parsnip	potato, baked
carrot, cooked	sweet potato *(Ipomoea batatas)*	potato, boiled
yam *(Dioscorea)*	tapioca	potato, chips
	pumpkin	potato, French fries
	rutabaga (swede)	potato, instant
		potato, mashed

Non-Starchy Plant Foods

With this group, we finally come in contact with foods that are in conformity with the Savanna Model. Ideally, we would eat these raw. However, if you choose to cook, always employ the gentlest cooking methods.

Since we are recommending that you consume an abundance of conforming non-starchy, colored plant foods, what plant foods are "conforming"? They are foods that are low glycemic, rich in micronutrients and fiber, and harmless with regard to antinutrients and antigens. Broadly, they include most salad foods, such as lettuce, onions, cucumber, radish, and mushrooms, and they also include colored vegetables, such as broccoli, green beans, bell peppers (sweet peppers), and Brussels sprouts. These are considered "Green-Green," "Green," and "Green-Amber." Under "Green-Green," we have separated out the vegetables that have the high concentrations of background micronutrients that our ancient ancestors delighted in. You can have unlimited consumption of these foods, and the ideal is up to 2 pounds (900 g) per day.

Note that we include "baby" sweet corn as a good salad vegetable. Unlike its mature form, the grains in baby corn have not yet formed and it is neither starchy nor glycemic. Tomatoes, because of their mild background antinutrients, only receive qualified approval in the "Green-Amber" category. Chili pepper and curry powder (particularly the "hot" variety) are to be used sparingly if ever at all; they damage the colon and make it leaky. Sauerkraut and other pickles receive a poor rating because of their high salt content. Ketchup has several possible ratings. The best is our own Savanna Model recipe (see our companion cookbook). If not, speciality ketchups are commercially available which use "safer" ingredients: tomatoes, canola oil, and fructose.

We also include a meat substitute made from fungus known as "mycoprotein." The manufacturer, Quorn, makes it available either in the raw state as a kind of ground meat look-alike or made up into veggie burgers, frankfurters, and so on. Mycoprotein is by far the best meat substitute when compared to soy protein or gluten protein. It is a high-protein vegetable product, so it should be consumed in restricted quantities, just like other high-protein products.

FOOD GROUP 3   VEGETABLES, NON-STARCHY

GREEN-GREEN

beet greens	cauliflower	**Herbs**
broccoli	kale	parsley
Brussels sprouts	Swiss chard	garlic
cabbage, red	turnip greens	ginger
cabbage, white		

GREEN

alfalfa sprouts	fennel	summer squash
artichoke	garlic	sweet corn, baby
asparagus	green beans	turnip
avocado	Jerusalem artichoke	water chestnut
bean sprouts	kohl rabi	watercress
bell pepper	leeks	zucchini courgette
bok choy	lettuce	
celeriac	mushroom	**Condiments**
celery	okra	All other herbs
chicory	onion	vinegar, all kinds
coleslaw	green onion	lemon juice
cress	palm heart	**Sauces and Dips**
cucumber	radish	guacamole
egg plant	spinach	**Meat Substitute**
endive	sugar snap peas	mycoprotein (Quorn)

GREEN-AMBER

tomatoes	**Pickles**	**Sauces**
Condiments	onions, pickled	ketchup, made with
mustard		fructose and canola

AMBER

Condiments	**Pickles**	**Sauces**
curry, mild	gherkins, low-salt	salsa, mild
	olives, rinsed	ketchup, regular

FOOD GROUP 3	VEGETABLES, NON-STARCHY *(continued)*	
AMBER-RED		
Condiments curry, medium	Pickles sauerkraut gherkins, salty olives, salty	Sauces salsa, hot
RED		
Condiments chili pepper curry, hot	Sauces Tabasco	

Fruits

Fruits today have quite different nutritional characteristics to those of our ancestors of the African Pleistocene era. The most troubling difference lies in the sugar content: it is often high and it is often glycemic. Even if they are not glycemic, the fructose content can be at worrisome levels. Some sugars, like fructose, do not raise blood sugar levels, but in large quantities upset other aspects of our biochemistry (see inset below). In other respects, fruits are generally a rich source of valuable micronutrients, so we need to prioritize which fruits to focus on.

• **Low-Glycemic Fruits.** Fruits that are both low glycemic and low sugar are "good" to eat without restriction. Fruits in this category are gooseberry and raspberry. Tomato, which is technically a fruit, is also included. There are other low-glycemic fruits, such as cherries and grapefruit, which nevertheless have a significant content of various sugars. You should go easy on these fruits if your doctor is asking you to restrict your intake of fructose or glucose.

Fructose

Fructose, although kind to blood sugar levels, is not without dangers. Professor George Bray estimates that as long ago as 1997, the average American was consuming 60 grams of fructose per day and rising.[192] Researchers find that a diet high in fructose has drawbacks. By "high in fructose," they mean a massive intake of 100 grams (20 teaspoons) per day. Many teenagers can get to this level by the consumption of just four 12-ounce cans of cola. At this level of consumption, fructose undermines blood sugar control, provokes diarrhea and bloating, and drives up glucose intolerance, blood pressure, cholesterol, triglycerides, and insulin resistance.[193] And let us not forget that fructose is empty calories—the more you consume, the more likely you are to get fat.

- **Borderline Glycemic Fruits.** These fruits tend not only to be relatively glycemic, but they also often have a correspondingly high sugar content. It is good to incorporate them into the daily diet, but keep their consumption modest. Examples are apple, pear, orange, and strawberry.

- **High-Glycemic Fruits.** Many fruits, often of tropical origin, are high glycemic. They are not pariahs, but we should not go out of our way to obtain them. If you find a morsel or two in your fruit salad, swallow it down, it won't poison you. But do not consume these regularly or copiously. Examples are watermelon, pineapple, and ripe banana.

The fruits classified as "Green" are mostly low-sugar berries; they are often exceptionally good sources of antioxidants too. Cranberries, in the raw state, are extremely nutritious and low in sugar. Unfortunately, they are so astringent as to make the lips pucker up. For this reason, cranberries are nearly always heavily dosed with sugar, either as a jelly or stewed in sugar. This process converts a great fruit into a bad one. Bananas become more sugary as they ripen; the greener you can stand them, the better.

FOOD GROUP 4 FRUITS		
GREEN		
bilberry	cranberry, fresh	raspberry
blackberry	elderberry	redcurrants
blackcurrants	gooseberry	strawberry, wild
blueberry	grapefruit	whitecurrant
cherry	nectarine	
GREEN-AMBER		
apple	guava	pear
banana, green-tipped	orange	plum
dates, fresh	peach	strawberry, cultivated
AMBER		
apricot, dried	kiwi	pineapple
apricot, fresh	mango	watermelon
banana, ripe	melon, cantaloupe	persimmon (sharon, kaki)
custard apple	melon, horned	pomegranate
grapes, red or white	papaya	prickly pear
AMBER-RED		
cranberries, sweetened	figs, dried	raisins
dates, dried	prunes	sultanas

Dairy Products

Dairy products are a biochemical disaster for the human organism—we do not have the digestive enzymes to assimilate them properly and they contain a range of compounds that bring bad health. Chief among them is lactose (which is highly allergenic), but we can also cite dairy fats (saturated and artery clogging) and dairy proteins (allergenic and cholesterol disrupting). Whether "raw" or processed, from cows or goats, whether turned into yogurt or cheese, dairy products are all classified in various degrees of "Red."

Cheese lovers have a slight consolation, as cheese is the least harmful: they have less lactose and, seemingly, their bad fats are not readily absorbed by the body. Cheese can be consumed modestly on the rare occasion. When you commit this offense against the Savanna Model, make sure that it is worth it—that the cheese is a really good one—and savor every nibble slowly, spreading it carefully around the palate. However, no platform of bread or cracker!

FOOD GROUP 5 DAIRY		
AMBER-RED	**RED**	
cheeses, all kinds	buttermilk	milk, cow's, skimmed
	ice cream	milk, goat's
	ice cream, low-fat	milk, sheep's
	milk, buffalo	whey
	milk, cow's, condensed	yogurt, full fat
	milk, cow's, evaporated	yogurt, reduced fat
	milk, cow's, full fat	yogurt, all varieties

Meat, Poultry, Eggs, and Fish

Animal matter has formed a moderate part of the human diet for an evolutionarily significant part of human history. As we have seen, the type of animal matter was rather different. Here we make judgments about the animal matter available to us today. The chief criterion is the fatty acid profile—the quantity of fat and the types of fatty acids. In addition, some variety meats (offal) can contain unhealthy amounts of some substances; for example, iron and vitamin A in liver.

• **Farm Meat.** Common farm meats, such as beef, pork, and lamb, have become problem foods. The difficulty is their high fat content and the harmful nature of the fat. Stockbreeders are beginning to work on improving the nutritional nature of their herds, but for now we are better off avoiding these meats and everything that is made from them. In contrast, an uncommon farm animal, the goat, is acceptable.

• **Wild Game.** In most instances, meat from various wild creatures has a conforming fatty acid profile. Truly wild game that feeds off what it finds in its natural habitat is an approved animal matter and is fine to consume in moderation. It will be low-fat and should have a good fatty acid profile. This includes wild boar, moose, caribou, and bison.

• **Variety Meats (Offal).** Our Pleistocene ancestors ate all parts of a slain animal, but this did not happen all that often. Many of the internal organs have wildly varying nutrient composition, depending on a number of factors: what the animal ate recently, how it was raised, and even its state of health. It is difficult, therefore, to generalize about variety meats. They are usually rich in micronutrients not found in such high concentrations in other sources. Variety meats are normally all right to consume in moderate quantities on an occasional basis.

Kidney, tripe, and liver are low-fat meats, but liver in particular is heavily loaded with vitamin A and arachidonic acid, both of which are harmful in high doses; you should consume it with caution. Tongue, heart, and brains are high-fat meats, with much of the fat saturated, and brains are particularly rich in cholesterol; eat these only occasionally.

Not many Americans eat variety meats as such, but they are still consuming them without even realizing it. That is because meatpackers disguise them as salami, hot dogs, luncheon meats, and sausage. These products should definitely be avoided because they are high fat (most of it unhealthy), salty, and often doctored with sulfur compounds to preserve them.

• **Exotic Animal Matter.** This category includes such creatures as alligator, ostrich, emu, kangaroo, frogs' legs, and escargots (snails). The last two have a long, honorable tradition in France and they all correspond very well to the kind of animal matter that our Pleistocene ancestors ate all the time. Other exotic foods are making their appearance, particularly bush tucker from Australia, which corresponds to the food traditionally eaten by the Australian Aboriginal. My wife and I have sat down with aborigines in Central Australia to eat one of their delicacies, witchety grub. Lightly roasted in the embers of a fire, the 3-inch-long caterpillar tastes rather like sweet corn.

• **Poultry (Farm and Wild).** The low-fat parts of farm fowl, such as skinless chicken and turkey breast, are good in modest quantities. You should reduce consumption of other parts as much as possible. All parts of duck and goose are fine. Wild birds such as pheasant, grouse, and pigeon are fully conforming.

• **Eggs.** Our Pleistocene forebears consumed all kinds of eggs: ostrich, bustard, duck, and anything else they could find. Hen's eggs come close, with a proviso—seek out eggs that are rich in omega-3 oils and it is preferable if they are also free range and organic. Duck, turkey, quail, and goose eggs are good too. Industrially produced eggs are a poor substitute and should not be consumed on a regular basis.

• **Seafood.** All seafood is an acceptable component of the Savanna Model feeding pattern. The "oily fish," rich in omega-3 oils, are best, such as wild salmon, sardines, and mackerel. Other fish and shellfish have an excellent essential fatty acid profile and are also good.

FOOD GROUP 6 MEAT, EGGS, AND FISH		
GREEN-GREEN		
Eggs eggs, omega-3 **Fish, finfish** herring mackerel	salmon sardine trout tuna	**Fish, shellfish** clam oysters shrimp squid
GREEN		
Meat, farmed goat rabbit **Meat, offal** tripe kidney **Meat, game** bison boar, wild buffalo caribou deer (venison) elk horse moose **Meat, exotic** crocodile escargots (snails) frog's legs turtle **Poultry, farmed** chicken, breast, skinless turkey, breast, skinless duck	goose emu ostrich **Poultry, wild** partridge pheasant quail duck, wild goose, wild pigeon **Fish, finfish** all other fish including: carp caviar cod eel haddock halibut monkfish pike pollock roe roughy, orange sea bass	sea bream shark skate swordfish turbot **Fish, shellfish** all shellfish, including: calamari crab crayfish cuttlefish lobster mussels octopus prawns scallop whelks **Eggs** all other eggs including: eggs, chicken eggs, duck eggs, goose eggs, quail eggs, turkey
AMBER		
Meat, offal brains	heart liver	thymus tongue

FOOD GROUP 6 MEAT, EGGS, AND FISH *(continued)*		
AMBER-RED		
Meat, farmed veal	**Poultry, farmed** chicken, buffalo wings chicken, drumstick	chicken, wings turkey, drumstick turkey, wings
RED		
Meat, farmed beef, all kinds beef, spare ribs beef, steaks lamb, all kinds lamb, chops lamb, leg pork, all kinds pork, bacon	pork, chops pork, ham pork, leg **Meat, processed** beef burger bologna bratwurst cold meats	frankfurter hamburger luncheon meat meat paste pate de foie gras salami sausage Spam

Legumes

Legumes are newcomers to the human diet and there are major drawbacks to consuming them: the body is not equipped to handle their plant poisons (antinutrients) and antigens. Only from time to time may you include a moderate portion of legumes in your diet; the purist will avoid them altogether. Examples of legumes are lentils, beans, peas, and peanuts. Peas are a slightly different case: they contain fewer antinutrients, but on the other hand they are starchy and glycemic. In addition, we single out the soybean for special mention because of its false reputation as a miracle food—avoid soy and all its products (tofu, soy protein burgers, tofu-substitute yogurts, and so on).

FOOD GROUP 7 LEGUMES—DRY BEANS, PEAS		
AMBER-RED		
hummus (chickpea dip)	noodles, Chinese bean	peas
RED		
beans, all, including: beans, adzuki beans, baked, canned beans, fava	beans, baked, low sugar/salt beans, broad beans, garbanzo beans, haricot	beans, kidney beans, mung beans, navy beans, pinto beans, refried

FOOD GROUP 7 LEGUMES—DRY BEANS, PEAS *(continued)*		
RED *(continued)*		
beans, white	peas, mushy	soy, milk substitute
chickpeas (garbanzo)	pease pudding	soy, protein
lentils, green	soy, all, including:	soy, tofu
lentils, red	soy, bean	soy, yogurt substitute
peanut butter	soy, cheese substitute	vetch
peanuts	soy, meat substitute	

Nuts

Nuts are a natural food for humans to be consuming. All tree nuts are generally fine. Examples are walnuts, almonds, Brazil nuts, and filberts. However, chestnuts and coconut do not fit into this tree nut category. Chestnuts are mainly starch and so are included in the starchy vegetable group; coconuts are mainly oil and are included in the fats and oils group. Peanuts are a legume and are included in the previous group.

Nuts should be raw and fresh. Regrettably, food manufacturers usually roast and salt nuts to improve shelf life and taste. However, this destroys useful nutrients and the salt is an unwelcome burden to the diet. Around half the weight of a nut is oil, much of it omega-6 fatty acids. Nuts are therefore calorie-dense and tend to upset the omega-3 to omega-6 balance. For these reasons, nuts should be consumed in moderation. Those classified "Green-Green" have a high omega-3 content. We make special mention of walnuts, which have the exceptional property of being rich in omega-3 oil. However, it is essential that the walnuts be fresh, because their omega-3 oil turns rancid very easily and becomes an oxidized fat particularly harmful to cardiovascular health.

FOOD GROUP 8 NUTS		
GREEN-GREEN		
flaxseed	hempseed	walnut
GREEN		
all other nuts including:	cashew	pecan
almond	filbert (hazelnut, cobnut)	pine
brazil	macadamia	pistachio
Note: All nuts must be fresh, raw and unsalted.		

Fats and Oils

In nature, fats and oils do not occur on their own: they are always part of something else. The Bushman could not eat the mongongo oil without eating the nut; he could not eat the animal fat without eating the animal. Fats and oils in their separated state are in a very concentrated form and therefore more potent. That is why they should always be treated with caution.

As a rule of thumb, oils that are solid at room temperature are suspect, as they are almost certainly unhealthy, saturated fats. Examples are butter, lard (including bacon fat), and tallow (beef and sheep fat). Artificial saturated fats are equally unhealthy, such as trans fats and hydrogenated fats. They are present in many processed foods and in margarines and spreads. In other words, all fats should be avoided.

The general injunction is to consume oils sparingly. We should focus on omega-3 oils. A prime example is canola (rapeseed) oil, which is readily available in supermarkets. However, we recommend going for cold-pressed, organic canola oil, if possible. Flaxseed oil has the highest concentrations of omega-3s and is preferred if you can afford it. The oil is fragile and needs to be kept in the refrigerator and consumed within a few weeks. Other options are hempseed oil and walnut oil (make sure it is not made from roasted walnuts).

All these omega-3 oils should only be used cold, for example, in a salad dressing. Omega-3 oils do not resist heat very well and the oil oxidizes and becomes toxic. If you need to heat the oil for cooking, then a monounsaturated (and thus inert) oil is best, such as olive oil.

The human organism also needs a second class of oil, the omega-6s, in a balanced ratio with the omega-3s. The trouble in the modern diet is that omega-6 vegetable oils are in everything and thus overwhelm our omega-3 consumption. We must therefore avoid any unnecessary intake. For this reason, you should strictly avoid knowingly consuming omega-6 oils, such as sunflower oil, safflower oil, peanut oil, and corn oil.

The criteria we have used in our classification are: omega-3 content; omega-6 to omega-3 ratio; and presence of harmful fatty acids, such as palmitic acid and myristic acid. In addition, we have taken into account the bioavailability of the "good" fatty acids and the "bad" fatty acids. That is to say, the position of these fatty acids (1, 2, or 3) on the glycerol molecule is an important factor as we saw in "Fatty Acids in the Body," Chapter 4. In this way, for example, cocoa butter has a more favorable category than a simple examination of its saturated fat content would have predicted. In all cases, fats and oils should be consumed with restraint. We have included mayonnaise and spreads, but it makes a big difference which oils they are made from. Check the labels and reject products that are "Amber-Red." Watch out for hydrogenated fats in spreads and all kinds of processed foods.

FOOD GROUP 9 FATS AND OILS		
GREEN-GREEN		
Plant Oils Canola (rapeseed) oil flaxseed oil hemp oil walnut oil	**Fish Oils** all fish oil, including: cod liver oil herring oil menhaden oil salmon oil	sardine oil **Marine oils** all marine oils, including: seal oil whale oil
GREEN		
Plant Oils almond cream mayonnaise, canola	mayonnaise, olive oil olive oil	spread, canola spread, olive oil
GREEN-AMBER		
Plant Oils cocoa butter coconut cream	coconut oil soybean oil	**Animal Fats** duck fat goose fat
AMBER-RED		
Plant Oils corn oil mayonnaise, lite	mayonnaise, not "Green" peanut oil safflower oil	spread, not "Green" sunflower oil
RED		
Plant Oils hydrogenated oil, *all* margarine palm oil	transfats, *all* **Animal Fats** butter cream	lard shortening tallow drippings

Sugars and Sweeteners

Sweet-tasting foods were a rarity in our ancestral diet. Consumption of any of these items should be restrained. The various sweetnesses available to us today fall into three main categories: high-glycemic sugars, low-glycemic sugars, and artificial sweeteners. We have seen how most sugars, the high glycemic ones such as table sugar and most confectionary, are harmful for us. They must be ruthlessly removed from the diet. More surprising for many of you is that the "natural" sugars, honey and maple syrup, are to be equally avoided. Some dried fruits have high sugar content and are highly glycemic; for example, dried figs, dried dates, and sultanas. They should also be avoided.

A second class of sugars is based on fructose, a naturally occurring, low-glycemic sugar. They are not glycemic and are admissible in moderation. Fructose itself is available in powder and liquid form in many supermarkets and in health food stores. It is present to a greater or lesser degree in honey. That is why, depending on which flower the honey comes from, the honey changes classes. The sugar from the agave plant is almost entirely fructose and has a very low glycemic index. In contrast, high-fructose corn syrup is a misnomer: it is as glycemic as table sugar itself. It is easy to overdose even on fructose, so its consumption should be kept moderate.

What about artificial sweeteners? Researcher William Grant estimates that 150,000 American deaths a year can be attributed to sugar consumption. This is a massive figure and it would be even more if the true causes of all heart attacks, cancers, and other illnesses could be identified. Just imagine the outcry if just one death could be attributed to the use of an artificial sweetener. In a world where we sometimes have to choose the lesser of two evils, substituting an artificial sweetener for sugar, as a first step, is a move in the right direction. From a theoretical point of view, Aspartame, saccharine, and other artificial sweeteners never formed part of the Pleistocene diet. Nevertheless, government authorities around the world have exhaustively tested them. If sugar had been obliged to pass the same regulations as artificial sweeteners, the authorities would have banned sugar as a dangerous substance. The purist will wish, understandably, to eliminate all artificial sweeteners from the diet. However, it is our view that they can form a very useful support when weaning from sugar itself.

Chocolate which is made with a high percentage of cocoa solids (and therefore little sugar) is low glycemic and contains many useful micronutrients; it can be consumed in restrained quantities. Most other confectionary items are high glycemic and devoid of useful nutrients; they usually contain bad fats and dairy as well—the dreaded "Red" column for them. Watch out for manufactured foods that claim to have "no sugar added." Often you are being duped: they are sweetened with apple or grape juice concentrate, which are just as bad.

FOOD GROUP 10	SUGARS AND SWEETENERS	
GREEN		
Confectionary chocolate, 85% cocoa solids		
GREEN-AMBER		
agave "nectar" fructose	Confectionary chocolate, 75% cocoa solids	Sugar Replacements isomalt lactitol

FOOD GROUP 10 SUGARS AND SWEETENERS *(continued)*		

GREEN-AMBER *(continued)*

Sugar Replacements	Artificial Sweeteners	saccharin
maltitol	acesulfame K	stevia
mannitol	aspartame	sucralose
sorbitol		
xylitol		

AMBER

honey, locust flower	honey, yellow box	

RED

apple juice concentrate	sugar, brown	**Confectionary**
barley malt	sugar, Demerara	candies
blackstrap molasses	sugar, icing, frosting	chocolate (all except "Green"
cane sugar	sugar, table	and "Green-Amber")
date sugar	sugar, white	energy bars
fruit sugars	treacle	fudge
golden syrup		granola bar
grape juice concentrate	**Sugar Aliases & Variants**	jelly beans
high fructose corn syrup	dextrose	life savers
honey, all, except Amber	galactose	M&Ms
honey, commercial blend	glucose	Mars bar
invert sugar	lactose	muesli bars
malt	levulose	Nutri-Grain bar
maple syrup	maltodextrin	sweets, boiled
molasses	maltose	toffee
raw sugar	saccharose	
	sucrose	

Salt and Sodium

Salt needs to be ruthlessly eliminated from the diet. By far the biggest source is in processed foods; seemingly innocent foods like cornflakes contain more salt than seawater, for example. The examples are legion in manufactured food, so the best rule of thumb, as ever, is to avoid them altogether.

Our preoccupation is with the salt-to-potassium ratio. As we have previously described, salt has moved from being absent in the human diet to massively contaminating all aspects of our food supply. We are therefore obliged to adopt a strategy of avoiding all salt, whether incorporated in processed foods or added at the table or in cooking. These measures, together with the high consumption of plant foods (which are rich in potassium), will ensure that an optimum sodium-to-potassium ratio is maintained.

Here, we focus on external sources of salt. Not everyone realizes that garlic salt is plain salt with garlic flavoring; regular stock cubes are over 50% salt; soy sauce is just liquid salt fermented with soybeans. The "Amber" column contains some low-salt seasonings and also salt substitute. Salt substitutes are based on potassium chloride rather than sodium chloride. There are dangers in over-consuming potassium chloride too, so although there is little or no sodium in salt substitutes (check the ingredients label), they should only be consumed sparingly.

FOOD GROUP 11 SALT AND SODIUM		
AMBER	**AMBER-RED**	**RED**
salt substitute	celery salt	bicarbonate of soda
yeast extract, Marmite	garlic salt	coarse salt
yeast extract, Vegemite	seasoning, Maggi	MSG (monosodium
stock cubes, low salt	soy sauce	glutamate)
	stock cubes, classic, incl.:	rock salt
	stock cubes, Knorr	salt, table
	stock cubes, Maggi	sea salt
	stock cubes, Oxo	

Beverages

Earlier, we cast doubt on the current preoccupation with guzzling water at every opportunity. The slogan "drink 8 glasses a day" is a highly misleading piece of marketing by the mineral water companies. Other water manufacturers jumped on the bandwagon with so-called special property waters—mineralized, ionized, magnetized, polarized—a whole range of sales gimmicks to gull the public. We now live, quite falsely, in terror of not drinking enough water. Just know that if you follow the Savanna Model to the full, you will be getting 4 pints (64 ounces) of water just from what you eat. The bottom line is that we need only drink when thirsty. By all means, drink bottled water, but water out of the tap is probably just as good.

Do not forget that tea, herbal teas, and American coffee are valid thirst quenchers.[3] Cocoa is fine too, but make it with 100% cocoa powder (not chocolate mix) combined with water or almond milk. If you like, use a "Green-Amber" sweetener.

The "Amber-Red" and "Red" columns are dominated by high-glycemic drinks, such as beer and colas, and by milk in its various forms. Milk is simply not human food and is harmful to our biochemistry. The milk of almonds (and other nuts) is a great alternative to regular milk, particularly in cookery. Fruit juices, even when freshly made, are glycemic—for this reason they get the "Amber" classification; it is much better to eat the fruit itself. Watch out for tomato juice: choose brands that are made from pure tomatoes and no salt. Sugar-sweetened carbonated drinks and colas are high glycemic and disrupt bone building.

Some alcohol drinks can be tolerated, but do not go out of your way to start consuming them if they are not already part of your diet. Beer is highly glycemic and potentially allergenic. Dry wine is acceptable and particularly red wine is mildly healthful when consumed in moderation. One might be surprised at the moderate classification of spirits like gin and whiskey. Most spirits are all right, especially if diluted in a suitable, low-sugar mixer (for example, whisky and soda, gin and diet tonic). Bear in mind that alcohol is empty calories and it disrupts your body's ability to burn fat, so you will struggle to lose weight if you consume alcohol.

FOOD GROUP 12 BEVERAGES		
GREEN		
almond milk	tea, herbal	water, mains potable
cocoa, unsweetened	water, distilled	water, purified
tea, black	water, mineral	wine, dry, red
tea, green		
GREEN-AMBER		
cocoa, artificial sweetener	sodas, non-cola, diet	wine, dry, white
coffee, Americano	tomato juice, unsalted	wine, dry, champagne
grapefruit juice	water, mineral, high sodium	sherry, dry
AMBER		
apple juice, fresh	fruit juices generally	soy milk substitute
cider, dry	orange juice, fresh	spirits: gin, whiskey etc
coffee, espresso	pineapple juice, fresh	tomato juice, salted
coffee, strong	port	wine, dessert
colas, diet	sherry, sweet	wine, sweet
AMBER-RED		
beer, ale	beer, porter	fruit drinks
beer, lager	beer, stout	liqueurs
beer, lite	cider	perry
RED		
chocolate "drinks"	milk, full fat	colas, classic
cappuccino	milk, skimmed	fruit juices, sweetened
coffee, milk	yogurt drink	sodas, classic
milk shake		

THE GOLDEN RULES FOR TODAY'S SAVANNA MODEL

A simple rule of thumb is to choose foods from the "Green" classes: "Green-Green," "Green," and "Green-Amber." Of these, Food Group 3 (Vegetables, Non-Starchy) has no restriction on consumption. "Green" classes in the other food groups should be consumed in controlled amounts.

1. The food to which as a species we are primarily adapted is plant food. Think big when planning volumes of salads and vegetables. Eat a minimum of one large mixed salad per day. Consume up to 24 ounces (900 grams) of salads and colored vegetables per day. Put vegetables at the center of the plate ("Green" classes, Food Group 3).

2. Prefer raw vegetables to cooked. When cooking, use steaming, blanching, or stir-fry methods.

3. Eat fruit every day. Consume at least 12 ounces (400 grams) of fruit per day, but spread it out over several eating sessions ("Green" classes, Food Group 4).

4. The food to which as a species we are secondarily adapted is animal matter. Think modest when planning servings of meat, poultry, eggs, and fish (Food Group 6).

5. Avoid red or fatty meat and their products ("Red" classes, Food Group 6).

6. Don't overeat protein: limit consumption to about 10 ounces per day of protein-rich foods. Concentrate on sources of "good" proteins ("Green" classes, Food Groups 6 and 8).

7. Avoid dairy products (All classes, Food Group 5).

8. Be frugal with fats and oils, even the "Green" classes. If cooking at high temperatures, only use olive oil. Replace "Red" classes of fats and oils with "Green" classes such as canola (rapeseed) oil, walnut, hemp, and flax oils (Food Group 9).

9. Avoid the use of salt in cooking and at the table (Food Group 11).

10. Avoid all manufactured (processed) food. Be wary of anything that comes in a packet, can, jar, bottle, or box. Be wary of anything that has an ingredient label—read the fine print on the label and act on it!

11. There is no need to count calories with the Savanna Model. You can eat to satiety provided these rules are followed. Your body, now receiving the correct fuel supply, will do the rest.

12. Feel hungry for at least 30 minutes two or three times a day.

7. Eating the "Savanna Model" Way

Our Pleistocene ancestors were not following any feeding strategies—they just followed their instincts. Their eating patterns would have changed from day to day according to the hazards of foraging. From season to season, they would have changed according to the availability of flora and fauna in the environment. Even so, the possible variations would have fallen within fairly strict limits.

Today, "what is there" is mostly artificial. The artful food manufacturers are masters at giving us taste without food value at all, and our instincts are readily duped by the divorce of taste from nutritional quality. The fluctuations of "what is there" fall within much wider limits. There is virtually no external discipline of what, and how much, we eat. So, we are obliged to adopt eating strategies.

Here, we look at ways for realizing the Savanna Model pattern. The objective is to give an example of the thought processes, the questioning, and the discipline that it is necessary to adopt it. Do not get fixated on the patterns described here. Within the boundaries of the Owner's Manual, there is a wide variety of ways you can organize your eating day. Use the examples given here to limber up the brain and begin working in a new paradigm. This is one aspect of the "Bond Effect," the art of putting the Savanna Model into practice.

We favor eating at home whenever possible, because you have the most control over your food supply. Nevertheless, there will be times when you are obliged to eat away from home—in restaurants or at the homes of friends and family. Try to rid yourself of notions about which foods are to be eaten at which meals: for example, eggs are often thought of as being purely a breakfast food. In fact, you can eat them at any meal. The same goes for just about every dish: they can be eaten at any time of day. The following strategies are to help you make these changes to your way of eating. Refer back to the Owner's Manual in Chapter 6 for specific information on food groups.

EATING AT HOME

Morning

Our Pleistocene ancestors would rouse themselves with the sunrise and gradually get organized for the day. By mid-morning, the first groups, having set off on foraging expeditions, would start to feed on what they found. We should be doing the same: not rush into eating a heavy, early breakfast. Don't worry about hunger cravings—there won't be any unless your blood sugar is out of control (in which case you need to be particularly careful to follow these recommendations). Suppress any prejudices you may have about the desirability of eating a "hearty" breakfast. Commercial interests, perhaps more than for any other meal, have manipulated our ideas of breakfast. Just in the last 50 years, public relations consultants have manipulated the American public into accepting corn flakes and bacon as breakfast foods.

A common reaction when people hear about the Bond Effect for the first time is: "What on Earth can we now have for breakfast?" In fact, there are many options, many of them being simply a return to what our grandparents ate as children.

Breakfast Ideas

Strategy A—Eat Conforming Fruit (Food Group 4, "Green"). A good time to eat fruit is a short time after waking up in the morning. Your stomach is empty (or should be). You can then eat small portions of conforming fruit all through the morning until lunch time. You will feel a little empty as the morning progresses, so you can then eat another portion of fruit. Eat until the feeling of emptiness is gone. You may have eaten a little or a lot, but it doesn't matter because nobody is counting. Remember that an important part of feeling satisfied has to do with putting our eating apparatus to work. That is, feeling the fruit on the lips and teeth; tearing a bite out, chomping it, grinding it in our mouths, and feeling the sensation against our tongues, gums, and mouth linings.

Strategy B—Eat Conforming Vegetables (Food Group 3, "Green"). An alternative that is practiced in many parts of the world is to start the day with a vegetable stir-fry. This is what many societies in Asia do. Just take a bag of frozen, mixed vegetables and cook it in a saucepan using the "oil and water" method. Don't forget, you are using large quantities—at least 12 ounces per person. If you like, you can add a few shrimp, for example.

"Oil and Water" Cooking Method

Try this quick (5 minute) method of cooking vegetables. Many vegetables soak up oil and this method greatly reduces the quantity of oil absorbed. Put $1/4$ inch of water into a saucepan with a clove of sliced garlic and a bay leaf (or a pinch of oregano). Add a tablespoon of canola oil. The boiling water forms an emulsion with the oil. Add vegetables (fresh or frozen). Heat moderately with the cover on, but stir frequently too. The vegetables cook fast, partly by boiling and partly by steaming. At the end, when the vegetables are close to done, heat vigorously and stir continuously until all the water has gone. They will be a beautiful golden brown when the water has evaporated. Always use plenty of herbs.

Strategy C—Eggs Any Style. Omega-3-rich, free-range eggs any style are fine to start the day. Make a hearty vegetable-filled omelet or grill some tomatoes and mushrooms with eggs any style. Don't forget that plant food should form the major part of the meal, and no backsliding—definitely no bread.

Strategy D—Salad. The idea of eating salad for breakfast does indeed run counter to our Western cultural programming, but it is something that many societies do, notably in Africa. A copious mixed salad with some avocado, tuna flakes, or shrimp makes a great start to the day. Again, make it a large portion—at least 1 pound per person. It is not really so much: one large tomato, one cucumber, some onion, and some lettuce leaves make 9 ounces of plant food. Round it off with 3 ounces of canned tuna and you have a hearty breakfast.

Strategy E—Old-Fashioned Haddock Breakfast. This used to be a good stand-by in many parts of the English-speaking world. Many people are old enough to remember, perhaps, when their grandparents used to eat like this. They would lightly poach a piece of haddock (or kipper or any other appropriate fish) in simmering water for about 5 minutes. They would accompany it with lashings of sauteed onion, grilled tomatoes, and mushrooms.

Strategy F—The Savanna Model Continental Breakfast. In the companion food preparation book (see Resources), we present a number of recipes to make conforming dishes. They are all free of flour, dairy, butter, and sugar and are fully safe, even for diabetics. Some of these, such as chocolate brownies, orange cake, and Nicole's apricot tart make excellent and tasty substitutes for croissants or Danish pastry.

Mid-Morning

Depending on how you started the day, you can snack on an avocado, a handful of raw unsalted nuts, or a big bowl of homemade vegetable soup. Select vegetables from Food Group 3 (Vegetables, Non-Starchy). Get used to making extra large quantities of everything and make sure that the fridge/freezer has a ready supply of easily accessed foods.

Lunch Time and Afternoon Tea

A suitable choice for lunch is a mixed salad, and an appropriate quantity might be 12 ounces. Weigh foods until you are used to estimating the quantities by eye—it's larger than you are used to. Get in the habit of thinking that a salad is often in two parts: the salad vegetables, comprised uniquely of foods from Food Group 3 (Vegetables, Non-Starchy), and some additions of protein-rich foods from Food Group 6 (Meat, Poultry, Eggs, and Fish). You can add tuna or chicken breast, for example, to the salad or eat as a side dish. Use a homemade vinaigrette.

Preferably, eat the salad before the side dish, because your appetite will be more readily satisfied by the bulkiest part of the meal. Eating the low-density plant food takes time. This gives time for the complex signaling from stomach to brain to catch up and tell you to feel satisfied.

Through the afternoon, you may begin to feel hungry. Keep ready prepared in your fridge some raw broccoli, cauliflower, and baby carrots, and also have some containers of preservative-free dips such as guacamole. That's all you'll need—a raw vegetable dip. Get used to taking your fuel with you when you are away from home for several hours. Above all, overcome any inhibitions you may have about pulling it out and eating it when the occasion calls.

Homemade Tuscany Vinaigrette

This is a very simple dressing that you can mix in 5 minutes. It has a robust taste and you can use it directly on all salads. The quantities here are to make up about a pint. Store it in the refrigerator and use as needed.

1 cup (225 ml) Canola oil, cold pressed, organic if possible
1/4 cup (55 ml) Walnut oil, cold pressed, organic if possible
1/4 cup (55 ml) Balsamic vinegar
1/4 cup (55 ml) Lemon juice
4 tsp. Garlic paste
2 tsp. Mustard paste
1 tsp. Ground black pepper

Vigorously mix all the ingredients together and store in a suitable glass, stoppered bottle.

Dinner Time

Dinner involves the same decision-making process as at lunchtime. This time you decide to do some cooking. Maybe 12 ounces per person of stir-fried vegetables accompanied by two eggs, any style. Or a grilled trout with a head of steamed broccoli. It's as easy as that. The stir-fry can be ready frozen; season with garlic, lemon juice, and herbs. Note that we are escaping the tyranny of the starter, main course, and dessert regimen. Instead, it's just the one course. As ever, try to eat the vegetables before anything else. A glass of dry, red wine is okay too.

Bedtime (Supper)

For a snack before bedtime, if there has been a sufficient gap after the last meal, eat a low-glycemic fruit (as much as you like). If not, try 2 ounces of nuts. Avoid bad carbohydrates this late in the day—they provoke a hormonal reaction that disturbs sleep and interferes with the body's nighttime repair processes. If you fancy it, have a mug of cocoa or 1 ounce of dark chocolate (at least 75% cocoa solids).

Trout Marrakech

Trout is classed as an "oily" fish, rich in omega-3 oils. We recommend its consumption on a regular basis. The following recipe combines the simplicity of baked fish with the mysterious flavors and spices of the East. This is a good, conforming fish dish in the Moroccan style.

FISH:
1 trout (approx. 1 lb.), cleaned
5 oz. (145 g) red onion, thinly sliced
4 Tbsp. (60 ml) white wine
2 pinches saffron

STUFFING:
2 Tbsp. (30 ml) olive oil
1 Tbsp. (15 ml) water
1 Tbsp. fructose
1 tsp. cinnamon
2 oz (55 g) almond flakes
2 tsp. (10 ml) orange blossom water (optional)
Lemon juice, pepper

Season the trout on the inside with salt and pepper (moderately). Set aside. Lay out the onion in a baking dish lubricated with olive oil. Mix the white wine with the saffron and pour equally over the onion. For the stuffing, in a bowl, mix all the ingredients together. Put half of the stuffing inside the trout and place the trout on top of the onion in the baking dish. Spread the remaining stuffing over the top of the fish. Cover with aluminium foil and bake in a hot oven at 380°F (190°C) for 10 minutes. Uncover and continue baking for a further 20 minutes, approximately. Serves two.

EATING AWAY FROM HOME

It is one thing to be organized at home for eating in accordance with the Savanna Model, but it is quite another matter when away from home. However, by planning ahead, being assertive, and being prepared, it is quite possible to stay close to the ideal regimen.

Restaurants

In reasonable quality restaurants, it is relatively simple to find items on the menu that can form the basis of a meal. "Form the basis" because there will still be clarifications and negotiations to be conducted with the waiter. You have to ask questions and request changes: "What exactly does the salad have in it? I

don't want any croutons, pasta, rice, or fruit." So it goes, until you have selected the starter, main course, and dessert.

Pay close attention to the vegetables that accompany the main course and
refuse potatoes, french fries, and rice, which the restaurant often offers as "vegetables." If green beans, broccoli, spinach, or any other green vegetable is available, ask for double portions. You will firmly wave away the bread basket and
leave on the plate any sweet corn that may have intruded in spite of the negotiations. Most of the desserts will be off limits. When you have finished such a
meal, you can congratulate yourself—you have eaten healthily and within the
margins of tolerance.

Eating in fast-food restaurants is just the same, only harder. Resign yourself
to ordering the burger and throwing away the bun. Find a salad, if you can, but
discard the packet of salad dressing (consider carrying a bottle of your own
vinaigrette). Or eat the all-day breakfast: eggs with tomatoes and mushrooms
are acceptable, but avoid the sausage, steak, hash-browns, toast, waffles, syrup,
and muffins.

Many fast-food restaurants have salad bars. This is good news and, with
care, one can eat reasonably correctly. They do tend to drench the salads in
sweetened dressings. Often they mix in fruit or combine starches and proteins.
Be selective: pick out and put aside the offending ingredients. Be suspicious of
all salad dressings—the manufacturers invariably make them with low-quality
ingredients, fillers, and sugars. Do the best you can.

Dinner Parties

In some ways, this is the hardest situation to manage. You don't want to put
your hosts under pressure and you want to be invited another day. If you
know your hosts well, it is all right to call in advance and mention that you
have special dietary requirements. Say that you prefer fish over red meat or
that you don't like to eat fruit after a meal. Mention that you like green salads
and lots of green vegetables. Then, dig into your meal and enjoy it for what it
is. You will certainly have to compromise, but then your basic eating habits are
natural and healthy and the occasional lapse is not going to be the end of the
world.

If you don't know your hosts well, or the dinner party has a set menu, then
it is best to act defensively. You don't want to go hungry and you don't want to
be churlish. So, before setting off, eat a light meal of conforming plant food
(salad, vegetables, nuts, and so on). Then, when you get to your dinner, eat
lightly—enough to preserve appearances and to flatter the cook. The "allergy
excuse" is always accepted when you want to leave a significant portion on
your plate. People also understand if you are watching your waistline and
don't want to eat much of the dessert. You can escape from this challenge in
pretty good order.

COOKING AND FOOD PREPARATION

In our African Pleistocene past, our ancestors did indeed have fire, but they had no way to boil water. They generally ate plant food raw, although they sometimes roasted nuts and other materials. Animal matter, according to convenience, type, and body part, was eaten raw or roasted. Eggs were also eaten raw. These are generalities, but we can combine this with what we know about how cooking affects nutrition.

In the Savanna Model, the emphasis is on keeping meals simple and cooking as little as possible. Vegetables should be used as fresh as possible. Store them in a cool, airy place like the vegetable rack of the refrigerator. Most vegetables can (and should) be eaten raw. Frozen vegetables are acceptable. Canned vegetables are acceptable in controlled situations where the convenience outweighs the nutritional drawbacks. Canned tomatoes, for example, are still quite wholesome and are useful in "quick-fix" dishes. Think big for your utensils. The food quantities are at least double what you are used to. Get a really large salad bowl, frying pan, and saucepan.

With regard to plant food, it is always best to eat it as soon as possible after harvesting and to eat it raw. That is why we put the emphasis on the consumption of salads and for them to be as fresh as possible. Be imaginative—many vegetables can form part of a mixed salad, including chopped broccoli, cauliflower, cabbage, zucchini, and leeks. With that big salad in place in your diet, it is acceptable to consume cooked vegetables too. However, the process should be quick to avoid leaching of nutrients. Always use the minimum cooking possible so that the vegetable is still "al dente," that is, cooked to keep its crunchy texture.

The best method is steaming or blanching. For example, you can cook broccoli florets in boiling water for 3 minutes and that will minimize nutrient loss. Microwave steaming is acceptable, although it is more aggressive on nutrient loss. Light stir-frying is also an acceptable cooking method. Stir-frying in the traditional Chinese method uses no oil, just a couple of teaspoons of water. Steaming, steam microwaving, and blanching are all good ways to cook vegetables. Avoid lengthy boiling, deep frying, and roasting.

Frozen, chopped vegetables are a good standby. They can be stir-fried, just as they come, in their own juices. No need to use a wok—just heat rapidly and stir constantly for 5–6 minutes in a large saucepan. Always use plenty of herbs. The basic stir-fry herb mixture contains oregano, crushed bay leaves, basil, and thyme. You can make up your own mix using equal parts of these herbs, or find a product that conforms closely to this recipe. Use the "oil and water" cooking method.

Foods of animal origin can be cooked. In general terms, there are few nutrients that might be destroyed by heating. Even oily fish retain their good omega-3 oils intact after baking, grilling, or barbecuing. One of the reasons we recommend avoiding red meats is not only their high content of fat (particularly bad fats) but that the fat oxidizes under high heat. Oxidized fat is a biochemical disaster for health. Meat, poultry, eggs, and fish (Food Group 6) can be cooked using the most appropriate method: microwaving, steaming, grilling, baking, or sautéing. Avoid deep frying. If using oil, just use a light coating of olive oil.

You do not need to make fancy dishes every day. In fact, we encourage you to eat simply. Nevertheless, there are many occasions when such dishes are appreciated, particularly for dinner parties and even as useful snacks at home, school, or work.

Preserved Foods

"Fresh is best" is a familiar slogan and it is good for us too. However, that is not always possible, so how do we prioritize? Broadly speaking, the "least bad" alternative to fresh plant food is frozen. Frozen plant foods, such as cauliflower, spinach, and chopped onion, have been quickly prepared in the field, and then blanched and frozen nearby. Blanching is designed to destroy certain enzymes that cause discoloration, softening, and bruising. It is likely that these are background micronutrients that are useful to the human body and which we lose in the process. So, here we make a compromise: in the absence of an alternative, freezing is the least of all evils.

The other methods of preserving plant food are to be avoided: freeze-dried (packet soups), canned (peas, green beans), pickled in salt (gherkins), syruped (fruit jams and jellies), and fermented (sauerkraut). That is not to say you can never eat these things, just do not think that they are proper food. Foods pickled in vinegar (such as onions) have lost many nutrients, but at least the pickling does not add undesirable chemicals.

With regard to animal matter, many methods of conservation are acceptable. Canned oily fish (such as sardines) are, in nutritional terms, just as good as fresh. Just choose the versions that are preserved in olive oil, canola oil, or unsalted water. Smoked salmon or kipper are good, although watch out for high salt content. Frozen poultry, fish, seafood, and exotic meats are fine too. Pickled fish (like herring) are acceptable, but be watchful of the salt and sugar content. Cured meats (such as bacon, ham, sausage, and bologna) are to be avoided simply because they contain high levels of fat, bad fats, and sulfites.

Processed and Manufactured Foods

Eat food that is the least processed as possible. Processing destroys fibers and leaches out valuable micronutrients. Processing increases the glycemic index and almost always means the addition of unwanted, useless, and sometimes harmful compounds—artificial coloring, artificial flavoring, preservatives, emulsifiers, stabilizers, and fungicides (like sodium propionate). Harmful ingredients like sugars, salt, trans-fats, and hydrogenated fat are frequently added.

The manufacturers adulterate and thin down their products with a variety of junk fillers like whey, modified starch, and unbleached wheat flour.

Government authorities allow meat packers to inject saltwater into products like ham, bacon, and chicken breasts. You do not need the salt and you might object to paying up to 25% of the price just for water. Take your fine reading glasses with you to the supermarket (even health food stores are not necessarily safe) and read the ingredient labels. Avoid the bad carbohydrates, shy away from products that have lengthy ingredient lists, and avoid oils and fat additives, particularly animal fats and hydrogenated fats. As a rough guide, if a product is sold with an ingredients label, then it is processed and you should thoroughly vet it.

Genetically Modified Organisms (GMOs)

Biotechnology companies have genetically modified plants for many reasons but rarely to increase nutrition. Governments and the industry hasten to reassure the public that genetically modified organisms (GMOs) are safe, but that is not the point. Volcanic ash might be safe to eat, but is it food? Already our current food supply is too far removed from the Savanna Model. After all, we are organic creatures that have grown up in harmony with a particular pattern of naturally occurring vegetation and fauna.

Most Americans do not realize how much of their food supply is infiltrated by GMOs—some 60% of it—in particular, anything containing tomato, soy, and corn (maize). In America, no authority requires the presence of these GMOs to be labeled. In contrast, the European Union (EU) requires all foodstuffs containing GMOs to be so labeled. However, all is not lost for Americans. After an outcry from consumers, the U.S. Department of Agriculture (USDA) backtracked and agreed that the "organic" label could not be applied to genetically modified foods.

As things stand, genetically modified food is probably "safe" and nutritionally similar to plants produced by regular intensive farming, but no one knows for sure. Nevertheless, avoid GMOs where you can and consume them when you must. There is also a stronger reason to avoid GMOs: the ethical one of combating the agro-industry mentality that recklessly dumps fake food onto our plates.

Organic Foods

Organic plant food is usually much richer in micronutrients than food from intensively farmed plants.[1] It is less likely to contain pesticides and other chemicals. Moreover, its production methods are kinder to the landscape and its animal husbandry practices are usually more caring. Organic foods of the Savanna Model will always be best. But is "organic" the first priority? Not necessarily. One of the greatest dietary errors in the West is the low consumption of plant food. The adverse health consequences are grave and measurable; the consequences of eating agro-industrial versions rather than organic are smaller. Therefore, the highest priority is to eat more Savanna Model food from whatever source. Eating organic is better, but it is a second order of priority.

A second point is that the designation "organic" does not turn a bad food into a good one. Organic sugar, organic milk, organic butter, and organic pork are all just as bad as the regular sort. Does a cigarette smoker worry if his tobacco is organic? Of course not—the main problem is the tobacco itself.

So, choose organic when you can, otherwise select conventionally produced foods when you must. For this to happen, your attitudes will have to change. In particular, be prepared to pay a little more. Also, be prepared for produce that is more misshapen, bruised, and discolored—buy organic and shun the Technicolor perfection of supermarket produce. You will be rewarded by glorious, rich flavors and the comfort of knowing that you are nourishing your body with genuine nutrients.

DIETARY TIPS

Fruit

As a general rule, fruit should not be eaten at the end of a meal. However, strawberries and raspberries seem to be an exception and most people do not have any digestive difficulty with them. You can make them, therefore, into attractive desserts. Cooked fruit, while less nutritious, is not problematic. Many people have digestive difficulties if they drink on top of fruit. Definitely avoid drinking tea, as it contains certain compounds that reduce the effectiveness of the range of micronutrients in fruits.

We do not recommend that you liquidize fruits. Juicing, pasteurizing, concentrating, and reconstituting are processes that destroy the nature and utility of the natural fibers, strip out the nutrients, and increase the glycemic index. It is much better to eat the fruit itself: when we eat an apple, for example, it requires chewing and it takes time. As a result, our brains register the process at its true value, gastric juices are mobilized, and we feel satiated more easily.

You should treat dried fruit (raisins, currants, dates, figs, apricots, peaches, etc.) as sugars. They are, therefore, bad carbohydrates. In addition, the drying process destroys some of the micronutrients, so in no way can dried fruit be a substitute for the fresh variety.

Candy

Almost all confectionary is high in sugar and you should avoid it. However, all is not lost: cocoa powder is low glycemic. Moreover it is a "Green" plant food, rich in a wide range of antioxidants and other micronutrients. If cocoa is combined with "safe" ingredients, it can make an excellent chocolate. The dark, bitter chocolate made with a minimum of 75% cocoa solids is low glycemic. Read the fine print—if "cocoa solids" come before sugar on the list, then this is probably acceptable. Really good varieties will have the exact percentage of cocoa indicated. You can eat this kind of chocolate safely at the end of a meal, but discipline yourself to eat just a couple of squares (about 1 ounce). Some enterprising makers of diabetic chocolate (sweetened with "Green-Amber" sugar alcohols) have rebranded their chocolate as a "low-carb" or "diet" chocolate; these are fine in moderation.

Caffeine

Caffeine is sometimes demonized in health circles. Nevertheless, almost all vegetation contains some caffeine and the body is quite capable of processing it without distress. It is only in certain plants that the concentrations reach mind-altering proportions. In modest quantities, caffeine can give increased mental performance and improve mood. Increasing the dosage doesn't bring increased benefit and some unpleasant symptoms start to appear: irritability, anxiety, jitteriness, headaches, and insomnia. In addition, at higher doses, caffeine drives up insulin levels, increases insulin resistance, and makes it harder to lose weight.[2] However, the harmful effects of caffeine are reduced when it is present in tea or coffee. Scientists speculate that other beneficial nutrients in these beverages compensate. Researchers have also found that a high consumption of micronutrient-rich plant food mitigates the harmful effects of caffeine on its own.

So, how quickly do we reach this safe limit? The average cup of American coffee contains 100 milligrams (mg) of caffeine, whereas coffeehouse strength can be 180 mg. The caffeine content of tea varies, but it averages about 40–50 mg. There are also about 40 mg of caffeine in a 12-ounce can of cola. In a cocoa drink (2 teaspoons of pure cocoa powder), there are only 10 mg. Our view is that caffeine in modest amounts is well within the normal range for human consumption. For a 165-pound adult, that works out to 4 cups of American coffee per day or 8 cups of tea. Be sensible about it, watch how your caffeine intake affects your mood, and avoid overdosing. If you are diabetic, caffeine in the form of moderate tea or coffee drinking might even be helpful.[4]

What is "Modest" Caffeine Consumption?

A modest consumption of caffeine means about 2.75 milligrams (mg) per pound of body weight per day for the average adult. This works out to 450 mg for a 165-pound person. Children should be restricted to 1 mg per pound per day (70 mg per day for a 70-pound child) and reproductive-age women to 2.1 mg per pound per day (260 mg per day for a 125-pound woman). At these dosages, the drawbacks to caffeine use are minimal.[3]

What about Supplements?

Many people think that it is a good idea to take supplements, particularly if they have a medical condition, but this is a very narrow way of looking at nutrition. There are thousands of compounds that are important to the harmonious functioning of the body, and they all need to be working together. It is unrealistic to think that we can compensate for dietary errors by cherry-picking this or that supplement.

Worse, dosing up on one compound can have unforeseen and detrimental ramifications. This is the Sorcerer's Apprentice syndrome mentioned in Chapter 4. Nevertheless, we are obliged to eat foods that are produced chiefly by agro-industrial methods. Farmers grow lettuce hydroponically (the technique of growing plants with their roots not in soil but in nutrient-dosed water), only using nutrients that are essential to lettuce. Ordinary soils too might have reduced levels of micronutrients, either from intensive farming or just because they are made that way. Does it matter? When we say "reduced levels," that still means that there are enough nutrients. The main problem with the average Westerner is that he or she is only consuming about 12% of the ideal amount of plant food. Just by doubling consumption, this will double the intake of micronutrients and they will be a lot better for it.

If you are eating according to the Savanna Model, what is the likelihood that you are suffering any deficiencies? The answer is, highly unlikely. You will be consuming eight times the weight of non-starchy plant food compared to the average American. So, even on plant foods with "reduced levels" of micronutrients, your intake will be well into the healthy intake comfort zone. (The one nutrient that it is hard to get this way is omega-3 essential fatty acids.)

The central tenet of the Bond Effect is that we will find all the nutrients we need by eating the right kinds of foods in the right patterns. The whole thrust of our message is to discourage people from the prevailing idea that they can avoid hard choices, keep their bad eating habits, and compensate by "taking a pill."

ADOPTING THE SAVANNA MODEL IN THREE STAGES

Put in place the new, healthy eating habits of the Savanna Model in Stage 1 and then move on to the other stages. Step by step, you will gradually modify your habits in the right direction, substituting healthy choices for your current unhealthy one. Over the course of the three stages, you will slowly wean yourself from the foods that are not good for you and start to incorporate more and more of the Savanna Model.

Take it at a pace that is comfortable for you. You can even decide to stop at some intermediate stage. Each stage is a summary of the more detailed advice already given in the book. If in doubt, refer back to the earlier chapters. For each stage, there follows examples of foodstuffs in the various categories used in the Owner's Manual.

Note: Earlier in this chapter, we gave an example of how we might eat during the day. Typically, we would eat less at a time but more often. Some might be light meals taken at regular mealtimes like lunch or dinner, others are light meals taken between them, like afternoon tea and supper. In the following segment, we talk about these eating occasions as "sessions."

Stage 1: The Lift Off

This stage is the most important—you have opened the portal to a new world, one that will change your life. Most of the changes are not difficult: much of it is the simple exchange of one food for an equal substitute. Other changes have to do with the order in which foods are eaten. None of it demands a lot of willpower.

Cooking and Food Preparation

- Avoid deep-frying.

- Reduce consumption of processed foods, fast foods, ready meals, etc., to no more than 1 serving per day (none is best).

Dietary Tips

- Eat fruit on an empty stomach.

- Avoid protein/starch combinations—Group 6 foods (Meat, Poultry, Eggs, and Fish) with Group 2 foods (Grains) and/or Group 3 foods (Vegetables, Starchy).

Accumulation of Lapses

- "Red" foods—limit to no more than 4 per day (none is best).

- "Red-Amber" foods—limit to no more than 6 per day (none is best).

- "Amber" foods—limit to no more than 8 per day (none is best).

STAGE 1
FOOD GROUP 1: GRAINS *(Bread, Cereals, Rice, and Pasta)*
Bread—have one day per week bread-free (none is best).   Pizza—have three days per week free of pizza (none is best).   Breakfast cereals—have three days a week free of breakfast cereals (none is best).   Pasta—have three days a week free of pasta (none is best).
FOOD GROUP 2: VEGETABLES, STARCHY
Restrict french fries to no more than 3 servings per week (none is best).   "Red" foods—have one day per week free of "Red" products.

STAGE 1 *(continued)*

FOOD GROUP 2: VEGETABLES, STARCHY *(continued)*

Limit "Red" products to 1 serving per day (none is best).

"Amber-Red" foods—have one day per week free of "Amber-Red" products.

Limit "Amber-Red" products to 2 servings per day (none is best).

FOOD GROUP 3: VEGETABLES, NON-STARCHY

Eat at least $1/2$ lb. mixed salad per day, "Green-Green" and "Green."

Eat at least $1/2$ lb. vegetables (cooked) per day, "Green-Green" and "Green."

FOOD GROUP 4: FRUIT

Eat at least 1 piece (serving) of fruit per day.

Focus on "Green" and "Green-Amber" fruits.

Avoid "Amber-Red" fruits (none is best).

Restrict total of "Amber" fruits per session to 1 serving.

Restrict total of Food Group 4 per session to 3 servings.

FOOD GROUP 5: DAIRY *(Milk, Yogurt, and Cheese)*

Replace whole milk by skimmed—no more than 1 cup per day (none is best).

Limit ice cream to 3 servings per week (none is best).

"Amber-Red" foods—limit cheese to 1 serving per day (none is best).

FOOD GROUP 6: MEAT, POULTRY, EGGS, AND FISH

"Green-Green" foods—consume at least 3 servings a week.

"Green" foods—can consume 2 servings a day.

"Amber" foods—limit to 3 servings a week (none is best).

"Amber-Red" foods—limit to 3 servings per week (none is best).

"Red" foods—restrict to no more than 3 servings per week (none is best).

Hens' eggs—use only omega-3-rich, free range varieties.

Restrict total of Food Group 6 servings per session to 1.

Restrict total of Food Group 6 servings per day to 2.

FOOD GROUP 7: LEGUMES—DRY BEANS, PEAS *(includes peanuts and soy products)*

"Red" foods—no more than 3 servings per week (none is best).

"Red-Amber" foods—no more than 7 servings per week (none is best).

FOOD GROUP 8: NUTS

"Green" foods—consume at least 3 servings per week

"Green-Green" foods—consume at least 3 servings per week.

Restrict total of Food Group 8 servings per session to 1.

Restrict total of Food Group 8 servings per day to 2.

STAGE 1 *(continued)*

FOOD GROUP 9: FATS AND OILS *(includes cream, ice cream, butter, and spreads)*

"Green-Green" oils—use 1 tbsp. at least 3 times a week.
"Amber-Red" fats and oils—limit to 5 tbsp. per week (none is best).
"Red" Fats and Oils—avoid altogether.
Replace butter and margarine with "Green" spreads.
Replace cream with almond cream.
Restrict total of Food Group 9 consumed to 5 tbsp. (80 ml) per day.

FOOD GROUP 10: SUGARS AND SWEETENERS

Replace "Red" table sugar with "Green-Amber" sugars (none is best).
Limit intake of "Red" sugars and sweeteners to 2 oz. (60 g) per day.
Avoid overdosing on fructose, agave syrup, and sugar replacements.
Limit intake of "Green-Amber" confectionary to 1.5 oz. (50 mg, $\frac{1}{2}$ bar) per day.
Limit intake of "Green" confectionary to 1 oz. (30 mg, 1/3 bar) per session.

FOOD GROUP 11: SALT AND SODIUM

Replace "Red" seasonings with "Amber" seasonings (none is best).

FOOD GROUP 12: BEVERAGES

Replace regular colas and soft drinks with "diet" versions (none is best).
Eliminate sweetened fruit juices.
Focus on "Green" and "Green-Amber" beverages.
Restrict "Amber" beverages to 5 servings (12 oz. mug/can) per day (none is best).
Restrict "Amber-Red" beverages to 2 servings (12 oz. mug/can) per day (none is best).
Restrict "Red" beverages to 1 serving (12 oz. mug/can) per day (none is best).

Stage 2: Escape Velocity

In this stage, we turn the screw a little tighter, but when you have mastered it, you will have escaped the gravity of your old earth-bound ways. You are "over the hump" and already fueling your body in ways that it recognizes and responds to.

Cooking and Food Preparation

- Avoid deep-frying.
- Reduce boiling and roasting.
- Prefer stir-frying, steaming, and microwave steaming.
- Reduce consumption of processed foods to no more than 3 servings per week.
- Keep meals simple.

- Eat little but often.
- Spend at least 30 minutes, once per day, feeling slightly hungry.

Dietary Tips

- Eat fruit on its own.
- Avoid combining Group 6 foods (Meat, Poultry, Eggs, and Fish) with Group 2 foods (Grains); that is, protein/starch combinations.

Accumulation of Lapses

- "Red" foods—limit to no more than 1 per day (none is best).
- "Red-Amber" foods—limit to no more than 2 per day (none is best).
- "Amber" foods—limit to no more than 3 per day (none is best).

STAGE 2
FOOD GROUP 1: GRAINS *(Bread, Cereals, Rice, and Pasta)*
"Red" foods—have four days per week free of "Red" products.
Limit "Red" products to 1 serving per day (none is best).
"Amber-Red" foods—have three days per week free of "Amber-Red" products.
Limit "Amber-Red" products to 1 serving per day (none is best).
FOOD GROUP 2: VEGETABLES, STARCHY
French fries—eliminate.
"Red" foods—have four days per week free of "Red" products.
Limit "Red" products to 1 serving per day (none is best).
"Amber-Red" foods—have three days per week free of "Amber-Red" products.
Limit "Amber-Red" products to 1 serving per day (none is best).
FOOD GROUP 3: VEGETABLES, NON-STARCHY
Eat at least 1/2 lb. mixed salad per day, "Green-Green" and "Green."
"Green-Green" foods—eat at least 3 servings per week.
Eat at least 1.5 lb. of salads and vegetables per day, "Green-Green" and "Green."
FOOD GROUP 4: FRUIT
Eat at least 3 pieces (servings) of fruit per day.
Focus on "Green" and "Green-Amber" fruits.
Avoid "Amber-Red" fruits.
Restrict total of "Amber" fruits per session to 1 serving.
Restrict total of Food Group 4 per session to 3 servings.

STAGE 2 *(continued)*

FOOD GROUP 5: DAIRY *(Milk, Yogurt, and Cheese)*

Replace skim milk with unsweetened almond milk.

"Red" products—eliminate

"Amber-Red" cheese—limit to no more than 3 oz. three times a week (none is best).

FOOD GROUP 6: MEAT, POULTRY, EGGS, AND FISH

"Green-Green" foods—preferably consume 2 servings a day.

"Green" foods—can consume 2 servings a day.

"Amber" foods—limit to 1 serving a week (none is best).

"Amber-Red" foods—limit to 1 serving per month (none is best).

"Red" foods—eliminate.

Hens' eggs—use only omega-3-rich, free range varieties.

Restrict total of Food Group 6 servings per session to 1.

Restrict total of Food Group 6 servings per day to 2.

FOOD GROUP 7: LEGUMES—DRY BEANS, PEAS *(includes peanuts and soy products)*

"Red" foods—eliminate.

"Red-Amber" foods—no more than 1 serving per week (none is best).

FOOD GROUP 8: NUTS

"Green" foods—consume at least 3 servings per week.

"Green-Green" foods—consume at least 5 servings per week.

Restrict total of Food Group 8 servings per session to 1.

Restrict total of Food Group 8 servings per day to 2.

FOOD GROUP 9: FATS AND OILS *(includes cream, ice cream, butter, and spreads)*

"Green-Green" oils—use 1 tbsp. at least seven times a week.

"Amber-Red" and "Red" fats and oils—avoid altogether.

Replace butter and margarine with "Green" spreads.

Replace cream with almond cream.

Restrict total of Food Group 9 consumed to 5 tbsp. (80 ml) per day.

FOOD GROUP 10: SUGARS AND SWEETENERS

Replace "Red" table sugar with "Green-Amber."

"Red" sugars and sweeteners—avoid altogether.

"Amber" foods—limit to 2 oz. (60 g) per day.

Avoid overdosing on "Green-Amber" sweeteners.

Limit intake of "Green-Amber" confectionary to 1 oz. (30 mg, $1/3$ bar) per day.

Limit intake of "Green" confectionary to 1 oz. (30 mg, $1/3$ bar) per session.

STAGE 2 *(continued)*

FOOD GROUP 11: SALT AND SODIUM

"Red" seasonings—avoid altogether.

Replace "Red" seasonings with "Amber" seasonings (none is best).

"Amber-Red" seasonings—avoid altogether.

Reduce "Amber" seasonings to bare minimum.

Eliminate salt added in cooking; replace with herbs and flavorings like lemon juice.

FOOD GROUP 12: BEVERAGES

Sweetened fruit juices—eliminate.

Freshly pressed fruit juices—reduce to 3 servings a week (none is best).

Focus on "Green" and "Green-Amber" beverages.

"Amber" beverages—no more than 3 servings (12 oz. mug/can) per week (none is best).

"Amber-Red" beverages: no more than 2 servings (12 oz. mug/can) per week (none is best).

"Red" beverages—avoid altogether.

Maximum total of "Amber," "Amber-Red," and "Red" beverages—4 servings
   (12 oz. mug/can) per week (none is best).

Stage 3: Infinity and Beyond

By the time you have completed this stage, you will be in conformity with the Savanna Model and you will be feeding your body in its comfort zone. You will discover the good things that happen when your biochemistry and digestive system are functioning as nature intended. Fighting a life-threatening degenerative disease? Then this stage is for you. Get to the center of the comfort zone, where your body is not just coping, it is positively rejoicing with its newfound ability to hum along like a perfectly adjusted machine.

Cooking and Food Preparation

- Reduce consumption of processed foods to no more than 3 servings per month.

- Prefer organic foods wherever available.

- Avoid deep-frying

- Reduce boiling and roasting.

- Prefer stir-frying, steaming, and microwave steaming.

- Keep meals simple.

- Eat little but often.

- Spend at least 30 minutes, three times per day, feeling slightly hungry.

Dietary Tips

- Eat fruit on its own.

- Avoid combining Group 6 foods (Meat, Poultry, Eggs, and Fish) with Group 2 foods (Grains); that is, protein/starch combinations.

Accumulation of Lapses

- "Red" foods—limit to no more than 1 per week (none is best).

- "Red-Amber" foods—limit to no more than 2 per week (none is best).

- "Amber" foods—limit to no more than 3 per week (none is best).

STAGE 3
FOOD GROUP 1: GRAINS *(Bread, Cereals, Rice, and Pasta)*
"Red" and "Amber-Red" products—eliminate.
FOOD GROUP 2: VEGETABLES, STARCHY
"Red" and "Amber-Red" foods—eliminate. "Amber" foods—limit to 3 servings per week, no more than 1 serving per day.
FOOD GROUP 3: VEGETABLES, NON-STARCHY
Eat at least 3/4 lb. mixed salad per day, "Green-Green" and "Green." Eat at least 2 lb. of salads and vegetables per day, "Green-Green" and "Green." "Green-Green" foods—eat at least 5 servings per week. "Amber-Red" foods—limit to 1 serving a week (none is best). "Amber" foods—limit to 5 servings per week, no more than 1 serving per day (none is best).
FOOD GROUP 4: FRUIT
Eat at least 6 pieces (servings) of fruit per day. Focus on "Green" and "Green-Amber" fruits. Eliminate "Amber-Red" fruits. Restrict total of "Amber" fruits per session to 1 serving. Restrict total of Food Group 4 per session to 3 servings.
FOOD GROUP 5: DAIRY *(Milk, Yogurt, and Cheese)*
"Red" and "Amber-Red" products—eliminate.

STAGE 3 *(continued)*

FOOD GROUP 6: MEAT, POULTRY, EGGS, AND FISH

"Green-Green" foods—preferably consume 2 servings a day.
"Green" foods—can consume 2 servings a day.
"Amber" foods—limit to 1 serving per month (none is best).
"Amber-Red" foods—eliminate .
"Red" foods—eliminate.
Hens' eggs—use only omega-3-rich, free range, organic varieties.
Restrict total of Food Group 6 servings per session to 1.
Restrict total of Food Group 6 servings per day to 2.

FOOD GROUP 7: LEGUMES—DRY BEANS, PEAS *(includes peanuts and soy products)*

"Red" and "Red-Amber" foods—eliminate.

FOOD GROUP 8: NUTS

"Green" foods—consume at least 3 servings per week.
"Green-Green" foods—consume at least 7 servings per week.
Restrict total of Food Group 8 servings per session to 1.
Restrict total of Food Group 8 servings per day to 2.

FOOD GROUP 9: FATS AND OILS *(includes cream, ice cream, butter, and spreads)*

"Green-Green" oils—use 1 tbsp. at least 7 times a week.
"Amber-Red" and "Red" fats and oils—avoid altogether.
Replace butter and margarine with "Green" spreads.
Replace cream with almond cream.
Restrict total of Food Group 9 consumed to 5 tbsp. (80 ml) per day.

FOOD GROUP 10: SUGARS AND SWEETENERS

"Red" sugars and sweeteners—avoid altogether.
"Amber" foods—limit to 2 oz. (60 g) per week.
Avoid overdosing on "Green-Amber" sweeteners.
Limit intake of "Green-Amber" confectionary to 1 oz. (30 mg, $1/_3$ bar) per day.
Limit intake of "Green" confectionary to 1 oz. (30 mg, $1/_3$ bar) per session.

FOOD GROUP 11: SALT AND SODIUM

"Red," "Amber-Red," and "Amber" seasonings—avoid altogether.
When cooking, use herbs and flavorings like lemon juice.
At table, use herbs and flavorings like lemon juice.

FOOD GROUP 12: BEVERAGES

Focus on "Green" and "Green-Amber" beverages.
"Red," "Amber-Red," and "Amber" beverages—avoid altogether.

WHAT TO EXPECT AS YOU CHANGE YOUR DIET

When you start to eat naturally, you are making major changes in the structure of how and what you eat. These changes have repercussions and during the transition phase may be uncomfortable. That is why it is wise to introduce the changes gradually.

Your digestive system will be in a state of shock, at least temporarily. For years, you have, probably unwittingly, been abusing and mistreating it. Many of its functions will have shut down. Your new way of eating will bring some immediate benefits: for example, elimination of bad food combining will dramatically reduce digestive problems. The increase in soluble fiber from fruits and vegetables will force lazy and atrophied intestinal muscles to limber up and become operational again. But be prepared for bouts of diarrhea or constipation for several weeks—this is normal during the transition period.

You will also start to lose excess fat from your body—that is the good news. However, as the glucagon machinery swings into action, fat will dissolve into your bloodstream, delivering its cargo of unpleasant chemicals. While the body eliminates them, you may suffer discomfort from their presence in the blood. Be prepared for symptoms, such as increased allergy activity, headaches, and feeling "one degree under," during the transition period.

Food is a potent factor for modifying the hormones in the body. As you shift the emphasis on what you eat, particularly from "bad" carbohydrates to "good" carbohydrates, you will be modifying your hormonal balance. During the transition period, you may feel the effects: mood swings, sugar cravings, and headaches, for example. This is normal.

Once you have restructured your way of eating, you will find that bowel movements will occur once or twice a day. They are soft and easy to expel, do not have a noxious odor, and are copious in quantity. Food will have a rapid transit time through the digestive tract. When you get to this point, you will know for sure that you are eating correctly. Rejoice at the wholesome feeling of health and tone in your intestines. The friendly flora and fauna will flourish, providing most of the bulk in the feces. Instead of having a clogged-up sewer system for a gut, your digestive system becomes an efficient toxic waste disposal unit.

When you eat in accordance with the Savanna Model, mouth hygiene is also vastly improved. The mechanical action of chewing a high volume of raw vegetable matter stimulates and hardens (keratinizes) the gums. Saliva quality is also improved; most people on a Western diet have a deregulated saliva composition. The saliva should contain a balanced cocktail of enzymes and antibacterial agents. Once you are eating in accordance with the Savanna Model, the saliva finds its equilibrium and fulfills a major role: keeping the mouth sterile, wholesome, and sweet-smelling. If you have poor tooth and gum health, do the best you can to get it fixed: often people are pushed into poor food choices just because they cannot chew the right foods comfortably.

HOW DOES THE SAVANNA MODEL APPLY TO ME?

The Savanna Model applies to everybody, but here we look at the specific implications for various groups. Everyone should read the next section on
babies/toddlers—not only does it set the tone for everything that follows, it will
guide you in your relations with those who have infants even if you do not have
any of your own.

Babies/Toddlers

Up to the age of about four years, human babies are "lactivores" or milk drinkers.
Nature designed them to nourish themselves on human breast milk. In primitive
societies, babies are not fully weaned until they are about four years old, although
solid foods, sometimes partially pre-masticated by their mothers, are introduced
slowly from about 12 months of age. That is the ideal, but what to do in the modern world? Mercifully, the breastfeeding movement has made this practice not
only acceptable but also practical. Today, mothers can give breast to their child in
public places, something unthinkable as recently as the 1960s. The vast majority
of mothers in the industrialized world, nevertheless, find it hard to breastfeed
after about 12 months, let alone to pre-masticate pap for a two-year-old.

Fortunately, the companies that make formula milk are getting very good at
making a product that imitates human milk as closely as possible. Reminder: in
America, you have to avoid soy-based formula milks. Most other countries ban
them because their antinutrients harm babies' health.[5] In other respects, formula
milks have come a long way in the last 50 years: no more cow's milk allergens, a
healthier ratio of fats to proteins, and a much better composition of vitamins, minerals, and essential fatty acids. They now have products that mimic the fact that
the composition of mother's milk changes as the baby gets older. For example, in
the first weeks of life, a baby's biochemistry cannot use the essential fatty acids
linoleic acid and alpha-linolenic acid. During this time, the mother's milk (and
now specialized formula milks) contain compounds that compensate for this.

However, mother's milk contains antibodies and other compounds that protect the baby from disease early in life; formula milk cannot provide these. So,
breastfeed if you can and for as long as you can, then move onto, and supplement with, the best formula milk you can find.

What about solid foods? The first principle is to follow the Savanna Model. The
more the baby eats in accordance with the general principles formulated in this book,
the better. Second, since people like to eat what they have always eaten, the best start
in life for your baby is to give him or her the taste for healthy foods. When they are
used to eating healthy foods at this stage, that liking will stay with them for life.

The first good habit to instill is the eating of plant food. No need to make special arrangements: just take what you, as a Bond Effect practitioner, eat every day
and reduce it down to a form appropriate to the child's stage of development.
Today's food blenders are a good substitute for the masticating jaws of the mother.

The next solid to be introduced should be fruit. However, take the precautions that we make for everybody: focus on the lower-sugar, lower-glycemic fruits (the "Green" category). Do not give too much at one time and give it on an empty stomach. No point in making your baby's life a misery by bad food combining. Give fruits to your baby every day.

What about animal matter? Of course, many people bring up their children successfully as vegetarians. However, staying with the Savanna Model, fish and fowl are fine. Free-range, omega-3-rich eggs are always good in any quantity. Just remember, you don't have to give your child anything that, as a Bond Effect practitioner, you would not eat yourself.

In addition, a baby has a bigger need for the essential fatty acids (in a ratio of 1:1 for omega-3s and omega-6s) than an adult. There are at least two other fatty acids that their immature bodies are not capable of manufacturing for themselves: DHA (docosahexaenoic acid) and ARA (arachidonic acid). However, don't worry about them too much because the infant fed in accordance with the Savanna Model will not be deficient in either DHA or ARA.

There will certainly be times when it is just not possible to prepare your own baby food. What about the commercially available products? Here, again, food manufacturers have gotten a lot more clever about formulating reasonably healthy substitutes. When you go shopping, the same rules apply—take your reading glasses and scrutinize the ingredient labels. Don't be misled by the attractive marketing labels proclaiming "healthy," "low-fat," "no artificial additives," etc. The food manufacturers always put the advantages of their product in large lettering, while the truth is grudgingly portrayed in small print in a corner of the label. This time you are reading the ingredient list for a dependent baby, so be conscientious. Don't buy anything that contains ingredients that you would not want for yourself: salt, sugar, glucose syrup, vegetable oil, fat, starch, and so on.

Finally, if your infant is not drinking mother's milk or formula milk, then the only other beverage he or she should have is plain water. Will any kind of water do? Tap water, unjustly, is much maligned and is quite safe to use when boiled. For all young babies, you should boil the water anyway. For the cautious, by all means buy bottled water. Avoid the high-sodium brands, and distilled water is the safest. Juiced "Green" vegetables from Group 3 are fine, but avoid carrot juice and fruit juices—they give a sugar rush and help rot teeth. As for packaged drinks, be ultra-suspicious. Read the fine print, as they are almost always loaded with sugar and other harmful substances. Don't even think of giving your child colas and other carbonated drinks. Get your child to accept water as the normal thirst-quencher.

Don't forget, this is one phase in your child's life when he or she is most open to influence from adults. It is now that you have to indoctrinate good consumption reflexes. This is not the time to introduce your child to pizzas, hamburgers, take-out chicken, or hot dogs. Even less is it the time to introduce your child to candies, cookies, ice cream, and confectionary. If you can get him or her through this phase without ever having tasted them, then you are well on the way to insulating your child from addiction later on.

Many adult health problems are established in these formative years. Perhaps the most significant is obesity. If your baby is allowed to get overweight, then the chances are that he or she will be overweight, or even obese, for the rest of their life. Worse, if your baby is overweight, he or she is already laying down plaque in the arteries and storing up a mid-life heart attack, as well as laying the foundations for cancer, arthritis, and a host of degenerative diseases.

Children/Adolescents

The special needs of children and adolescents are often exaggerated. They will be eating a lot for their size, but they do not need any particular divergence from the Savanna Model. By far the greatest problem is to stop them from eating harmful foods. It is too much to expect that you can, like the little Dutch boy with his finger in the dike, hold back the floodwaters of the junk food society. Accept with good grace that your child will eat junk food from time to time, but don't be defeatist. Make sure that at home he or she is following the Savanna Model. If that is assured, then your child will survive the storms of junk food relatively unscathed.

Avoid using junk food as a treat, much less as a reward. Rather, you need to indoctrinate children with the idea that junk food is shoddy, tacky, malignant, even hazardous, toxic, and poisonous. Children will accept that they are different from their peers if you present it as their particular belief system. You need to give them the arguments and words to use when well-meaning friends and relatives question their eating habits. Let them understand that they are eating in a way that avoids the deficiency diseases of their peers.

Play hardball. If necessary, discreetly draw attention to the signs in their friends of deficiency disease, malnutrition, and over-indulgence. Point out their poor complexion, constant colds and flu, listless eyes, allergies and eczema, bad breath, lack of physical fitness, and grossness of obesity. You may have scruples against this approach, but be aware that your child is being peddled temptations even more prevalent than those offered by the neighborhood drug dealer.

Does this mean that your children should never have a hamburger, cola, ice cream, or candy? No. If you have done your job well, your children will be sensible and be able to handle social situations adroitly. They will still want to go to birthday parties and proms, and hang out at the local burger joint. But this is where they will need the self-discipline, confidence, and social skills to limit the potential damage.

At home, you have an iron responsibility to ensure that the right foodstuffs are constantly available. Always have a supply of ready-to-eat fruit, vegetables, and salads. Have homemade dishes like vegetable hot-pot and ratatouille available in the fridge and freezer. Have stocks of oily fish like canned salmon, sardines, and tuna. In other words, have a larder well-stocked for the Bond Effect. Water should still be the main drink; try carbonated water with a twist of lemon. Tea, iced or otherwise, is also okay. Finally, remind yourself that a child needs a role model. From the youngest age, your child will want to emulate the feeding patterns of the adults in the house.

Get your child into the habit of filling up with food at home, and preparing and taking food supplies with her when she goes out. Never have junk foods in the house. Never buy cookies, cakes, pastries, candies, hamburgers, hot dogs, ice cream, pizzas, or ready-made meals. Never have colas, fruit juices, or carbonated drinks in the house.

What about condiments? It's been said that the only way to get a kid to eat his vegetables is to smother them in ketchup. Strangely, if that is what works, then it is tolerable. A good quality ketchup is not such a bad condiment. The main drawback is the sugar content. But, for a Bond Effect practitioner, ketchup used in modest quantities is a small and tolerable lapse. Don't forget herbs and spices. They are full of healthful micronutrients (hence their pungent taste and aroma). Get into the habit of using copious quantities of "Green" natural herbs and spices in all your dishes. Wean yourself and your family off processed and junk sauces.

We cannot emphasize enough the importance of a healthy adolescence. Ensure that your children follow the Savanna Model, lock into place healthy habits for them, and they will be grateful to you for the rest of their long, disease-free lives.

Pregnant and Nursing Women

All we know about how our bodies work, and how our prehistoric ancestors evolved, shows that no special departure from the Savanna Model is indicated during pregnancy. Sometimes women are, mistakenly, advised to load up on calcium tablets. However, our ancestors never knew anything about calcium. Certainly, we have no instincts to search out calcium-rich foods. But if that doesn't convince you, studies show that calcium supplementation does not make any difference to calcium metabolism.

The mother's body naturally meets the demand for extra calcium by three hormonal activities. First, the intestines absorb a higher percentage of calcium from everyday foods. Also, the kidneys become more efficient at recycling calcium recovered from the urine. Finally, some calcium is borrowed from the bones. Nothing that the mother eats, supplements, or does changes this process.[6] As soon as menstruation restarts, bone density steadily recovers all by itself.

Our forager ancestors had pregnancies spaced about every four years. This happened mainly through biological machinery: a woman is much less likely to conceive when breastfeeding, and she is less fertile when her body's food stores are low. The main lesson to draw from this is to space pregnancies by about four years, just like our ancient ancestors, so that the bones can recover their full health before the next pregnancy.

Your doctor will probably prescribe all kinds of dietary supplements. There is not the space in this book to explain, one by one, why these supplements are not necessary, so you will dutifully take them. Just know that the pregnant Bond Effect practitioner need have no fear of dietary deficiencies. For example, one of the latest vitamins to be recommended for pregnant women is folic acid because the diet of the average American woman is deficient in it. But where is folic acid found? In foliage! The Bond Effect mother will be absorbing high levels of folic acid in salads and other vegetables, as well as all the other essential nutrients for her baby.

On the contrary, it is ever more important to not consume the non-conforming foods like bad fats and bad carbohydrates. The bad fats will reappear in the fetus and in breast milk. The excess insulin levels will upset the baby's metabolism.

Finally, what about the cravings and nausea of morning sickness? This is definitely a tough time for the pregnant woman. According to evolutionary biologist Dr. Margie Profet, this sickness is nature's way of preventing women from consuming plants whose antinutrients might harm the fetus.[7] In addition, the fetus is already manipulating the woman's hormones to serve its own purposes, making her feel bad. What should she do? The truth is, not a lot. This is a time for going with the flow. She eats when she can and what she can bear to eat. Just relax and wait for this phase to pass. The fetus will make sure it gets all it needs, robbing if need be, the mother's own stores.

Thirty-Something-Year-Old People

This is likely to be a phase of life when health will seem good and there is no need to concern yourself about the future. The reality is that it is this period of life when you need to set the scene for your later years. Bad eating habits now will lead inexorably to obesity, heart disease, and diabetes. They lay the foundation for the degenerative diseases of middle and old age—cancer, arthritis, osteoporosis, rheumatism, and even Alzheimer's.

It is at this age that the blood sugar control mechanism starts to show its age. It copes less well with the stress that we put on it. It is now that "middle-age spread" begins to show. This is your warning that you are pre-diabetic—take it seriously. Change your eating pattern and relieve your body of that sugar-stress by following the guidelines in this book. But, most importantly, this is the end of the phase where your body easily builds up bone density. Now is the time to ensure that your bone capital is at a maximum.

The Menopausal Woman

Menopausal changes start in the early forties and build up to a finality in the fifties. As with pregnancy, this is a time when a woman's hormones are undergoing a major reshuffle. It is potentially a period when Western women will have those familiar symptoms of hot flashes, irritability, hypersensitivity, depression, tension headaches, and night sweats. However, in most simple societies, these symptoms are almost unknown. Indeed, many women in the West do not suffer them either. What makes the difference?

Not surprisingly, the main thing influencing hormonal balance is food. The bodily dysfunctions caused by dietary errors will be amplified during menopause. Controlled studies show that a diet rich in bioflavonoids and vitamin C provides relief of menopausal symptoms for many women. Where are bioflavonoids and vitamin C found? In fruits and vegetables! Just boosting the intake of fruits and vegetables is enough to dramatically reduce the disagreeable symptoms. And don't forget that bad carbohydrates and bad fats have a major effect on hormonal balances. Getting these right helps enormously too. Eliminate dietary errors by eating according to the Savanna Model.

There are also secondary dimensions, such as the stress of the Western way of life, the psychological finality of becoming infertile, and the tension in relationships caused by changes in libido, that affect women in menopause. There is a strong mind/body connection: managing stress and moods will also help stabilize hormonal balance.

What about the long-term effects? What about osteoporosis and heart disease? These are both major problems for post-menopausal women, but only in the West. If you get your eating patterns right and get other lifestyle factors into a conforming pattern, you can get on with life and not worry about these conditions.

Finally, what about hormone replacement therapy (HRT)? We can be fairly confident that Pleistocene grandmothers did not drink pregnant giraffe's urine to obtain estrogen-rich extracts. There is no reason from a health viewpoint why a menopausal Bond Effect practitioner should supplement with estrogen.

The Elderly

It is in the later years of life that eating in harmony with our savanna-bred natures can bring rapid relief to distressing ailments like stiff joints, arthritis, digestive upsets, and general ill-health. These are the ailments that emerge, like the wreck of a ship, as the tide recedes. For a great part of our lives, our body's biochemistry has sufficient "redundancy" built into its system to patch around errors of lifestyle. With old age, these margins of error disappear. Now more than ever, it is important to harmonize how you eat with the needs of your body. When you do so, many of these troublesome maladies disappear.

Eating in accordance with the Savanna Model is the ideal and there are no other special measures to take. Just make sure that your teeth, whether original or artificial, are working efficiently. Many old people eat badly simply because they choose foods that don't need chewing. As an older person, make sure that you are eating the proper rations of fruit, salads, and vegetables. Surveys show that older people, who tend to have less efficient digestive systems, often skimp on these foods. As a result, they, and their immune systems, are deficient in anti-oxidants and other essential micronutrients. Get that right and you'll live out your years in good shape.

Vegetarians and Vegans

By "vegetarian," we mean someone who avoids eating animals that have been killed, but consumes other foods of animal origin, such as dairy products and eggs. By "vegan," we mean someone who avoids foods from any animal source whatsoever. Many vegetarians and vegans make the mistake of simply eliminating animal matter from their normal, "eat anything" diet. As a result, some vegetarians and vegans are obese, have poor complexions, and suffer ill health simply because they are continuing with other bad habits. Notably, this is because they replace the animal food by increased consumption of cereals, bread, pasta, and other complex carbohydrates. There are other errors as well, such as the use of dairy products, lentils, beans, tofu, soy protein, and bad fats and oils.

Vegetarians and vegans will find in the pages of this book exactly the right prescription for eating healthily. All you have to do is eat in accordance with the Savanna Model, ignoring the animal products where they are mentioned, and choose the vegetable alternatives instead.

Veganism can be a healthy lifestyle, provided that you carefully follow the Savanna Model consumption pattern. The secret is to eat like the gorilla, a natural vegan: consume very high volumes of plant material, including nuts, and avoid all the bad foods that do not conform to the Savanna Model diet. Vegans need to worry about the one nutrient that is not available in their diet: vitamin B_{12}. The gorilla makes it in his intestine, but humans do not. (This suggests that veganism is not a natural human eating pattern.) Vegans should take supplements of vitamin B_{12}: it does not require much, just 2 micrograms per day will be enough. Vegetarians, on the other hand, will get all the B_{12} they need by eating eggs.

8. The Savanna Model Lifestyle

We have seen how our ancient environment conditioned our bodies—and our very natures—for life on the savannas of east Africa. We called this lifestyle the "Savanna Model" and outlined how our ancient ancestors fed themselves for thousands of generations. Now, we look at aspects of the Savanna Model lifestyle: physical activity, social well-being, and living arrangements. Our modern lives, in all their aspects, are at variance with the way nature designed us for life. The Bond Effect is learning to live in harmony with the way nature intended. This manner of looking at who we really are elegantly resolves many enigmatic lifestyle questions. It cuts through much humbug to reveal fundamental, if uncomfortable, truths.

PHYSICAL ACTIVITY

Over the millions of years of evolution, what were the patterns of physical activity practiced by our species? What will that tell us about the amount of exercise we should be getting today? Surprisingly, we can work out a lot about the physical activity of our Pleistocene ancestors. We know how they must have foraged for food, how far they traveled, how fast, and even their muscular development. Our study of contemporary forager tribes like the San shows how they organize themselves on a daily basis.

A typical African Pleistocene group would camp in one place for a few days and then move on to make another camp 10 to 20 miles away. They carried very little with them, but they still had to walk all the way. They moved, not for the fun of it, but because they had to. The terrain was open, savanna-type grassland.

While camped each day, the group would split up to forage for food. The women, children, and old men went off in one party, foraging for roots, fruits, tubers, berries, and easily caught bugs and animals. This party on average covered about 5 miles, they leisurely walked and rested from time to time, and after about 4–5 hours they were done. It is estimated that the average adult female energy expenditure on physical activity was 600 kilocalories (kcal) per day. This compares to 230 kcal for today's sedentary female office worker.

The able-bodied men went off chiefly looking for small game, but would also be collecting other edible matter on an opportunistic basis. This party would cover more ground during the day—9 to 12 miles on average. Part of the time, they would be running or jogging, to chase and trail potential game. Most of the time, they would be finished after about 4–5 hours. Less frequently, they might be away for as much as 48 hours, tracking a wounded animal. It is estimated that their daily expenditure of energy was over 1,000 kcal. Compare this to the 306 kcal of the average sedentary male office worker.

There are therefore two patterns, one for each gender. Females would pass their lives exercising to a moderate extent and with low intensity. Males started their lives with the female pattern, graduated to the male pattern (vigorous and more sustained physical activity) for most of their lives, and then tapered off to lesser levels again in old age.

How does this fit with what we know about human biology today? Evidence is that women do not need to exercise as long or as hard as men to maintain their health. Men need more vigorous physical activity to remain healthy. What happened to our ancestors in old age? What is striking is that old people stayed physically active until their very last days. They were athletes right to the end.

Exercise and Your Health

So, what are we to make of this? Everything we know about individuals who get this amount of physical activity demonstrates that, as a result, they have better health than they would otherwise have had. The big question is, are there any vital body functions that depend on physical activity? Studies, whether on bedridden people or on astronauts, all point to a number of conditions brought about by a lack of physical activity.

• **Bone Demineralization and Fractures.** The absence of exercise is one of the factors that undermines bone health. Regular physical activity improves bone structure, volume, and its resistance to fracture. Elderly women can benefit from as little as one hour per week of low-intensity activity—a 42% lower risk of hip fracture and 33% lower risk of vertebra fracture.[1] The rhythmic jolting associated with walking or jogging excites the bone-building cells (osteoblasts) into raising their tempo. In young people, the bone-builders work faster than the bone-strippers (osteoclasts) and their bone mass increases. Even in older people, the bone-builders will work harder and maintain pace with the bone-strippers.

• **Syndrome X.** Syndrome X is a metabolic disorder that represents a cocktail of "diseases of civilization" that occur simultaneously. The main conditions are high blood pressure, coronary artery disease, obesity, high cholesterol, and diabetes. They all have a common link—high insulin levels. Low exercise levels mean that more insulin has to be secreted to handle a given glucose load. The result is more insulin floating around creating mischief. Exercise is essential to maintaining optimum resistance to diabetes, obesity, hypertension, and heart disease.

The Process of Bone Remodeling

Our bones are continuously being broken down and rebuilt. It is estimated that our entire skeleton is completely rebuilt at least three times in a lifetime. Our bones are like a girder bridge whose struts are removed one by one and replaced. There are specialized cells that do the strut-removal called osteoclasts. The cells that put in new struts are called osteoblasts. The process is known as bone remodeling. The cells speed up or slow down in response to stress placed on the bones, various hormonal instructions, and the body's need for calcium. Trouble occurs when struts are removed but not replaced, leading to osteoporosis. This is a dysfunction caused by many different factors, one of which is the absence of stress (such as physical activity) placed on the bones.

• **Arthritis and Joint Stiffness.** Regular activity of the kind practiced by our Pleistocene ancestors encouraged cartilage maintenance, lubrication, and renewal of the wearing surfaces in joints. Dysfunctional joints are due in large part to not giving them enough to do. It is a cliché, but true: if you don't use it, you lose it.

• **Lower Leg Circulation.** There is an artery that passes through the ball of the foot. As you walk or run, this artery is alternately compressed and released, and the general effect is that of a pump. Walking or running helps pump blood through the lower leg. Without it, the lower leg gets poor circulation and is prone to deep vein thrombosis. Are you one of those people who, after a little while sitting at a desk or table, find their knees jogging up and down? This, too, is a natural reflex helping to maintain lower leg circulation.

• **Lymphatic Circulation.** As handmaiden to blood circulation, we have a secondary system of circulation known as the lymphatic system. This is responsible, in part, for transporting the products of digestion to other parts of the body, bringing immune system cells to parts of the body under attack, and flushing away debris and toxic matter. Unlike the blood, which is pumped around the body by the heart, the lymphatic system does not have a pump of its own. It relies on the general flexing of muscles to do the job. Lack of physical activity means sluggish lymphatic circulation and a host of potential maladies.

• **Longevity.** Studies on identical twins conducted over many years have demonstrated what many people have long suspected—that physically fit people live longer. In one study, it was found that in any given period, sedentary people were 1.3 times as likely to die as the "occasional" exercisers and nearly twice as likely to die as the "conditioning" exercisers. The figures were the same for both men and women. The use of twins, often brought up apart, was particularly useful: it meant that genetic factors could be eliminated as possible reasons.[2] We do not know the effect on longevity if we raised our physical activity to the level of our prehistoric ancestors, but it would no doubt be further improved.

• **Stress, Depression, and Mood.** Physical exercise has a beneficial effect on a whole range of hormones that regulate mood. Exercise restores the way the brain chemical serotonin functions, helping to lift depression. Physical activity puts a brake on the production of stress hormones (such as cortisol and adrenaline), which calms feelings of panic and stress and reduces damaging insulin production. Finally, endurance athletes can reach a "high," where their bodies are producing morphine-like substances, giving them a tremendous feeling of well-being.

Physical activity is not an option but a necessity. Our bodies are shaped by our ancestral environment and their proper functioning relies on a particular kind and amount of exercise. Without it, the rest of the body's systems cannot work properly.

SOCIAL WELL-BEING AND THE IDEA OF HUMAN NATURE

The way we live our lives today puts us under tremendous psychological pressure. In a great many ways, our savanna-bred natures are not made for modern, industrialized society. In the rest of this chapter, we bring forward new ways of thinking about what it means to be human in terms of our social environment. Some of these ideas might seem surprising: rather like going round the back of a Wild West film set and discovering that the saloon is just a plywood facade held up by ropes and stays.

Bear in mind that we are talking about the deep undercurrents in human nature. The purpose of the rest of this chapter is to make you aware of our deeply buried instincts. You will see how our choices, often made with the best of intentions, sometimes run counter to these savanna-bred instincts. However, bear in mind that all social interactions are highly complicated affairs: we are constantly balancing a Pandora's box of conflicting desires, postponed gratification, calculation, and social conformity. The insights in this chapter will help you make better choices within the framework of this rich and challenging context.

The social sciences deal with the social and cultural aspects of human behavior. Regrettably, these sciences were hijacked in the early part of the 20th century by academic theorists such as the German-born American anthropologist Franz Boas. They built on the romantic notions of the 18th-century French philosopher Jean-Jacques Rousseau, who asserted, without any evidence, that man is good by nature but has been corrupted by society and civilization. If only, stated Rousseau, we could return to the state of the "Noble Savage," we would all live happily ever after. Boas went further and asserted that humans have no inherited instincts, abilities, or feelings. He declared that all humans are born as a "blank slate" and behavior is purely the result of social and cultural conditioning. Thus, we are all born with identical potentials to become anything. In other words, there is no such thing as "human nature."

We now know that this is quite wrong: humans inherit, with their genes, very deeply programmed desires, feelings, and instincts. They cannot be "conditioned" out of existence. But the social sciences are still riddled with false notions. In consequence, we are under pressure to change our behaviors in ways that social theorists consider desirable. Often, these pressures cut across our savanna-bred natures, causing distress, unhappiness, and ultimately mental illness.

Social engineers wanted to believe that human behavior is "infinitely malleable." If necessary, they faked scientific studies to fit their prejudices. The most celebrated case was that of Margaret Mead. An anthropological student of Franz Boas, Mead became famous for her doctoral research in 1925 that allegedly showed that Samoa is a paradise in which sex is unrestricted; where jealousy, rape, and adolescent adjustment problems are unknown. But none of it was true. Mead never learned the Samoan language and she interviewed only two schoolgirls who, only in their old age, admitted that they had deceived her for their own amusement.[3] She wrote a book about her "research" entitled *Coming of Age in Samoa*. It became a best-seller and required reading as "a classic of universal truths" in university courses.

In the book, Mead claimed that adolescent behavior in humans could be explained only in terms of the social environment. Human nature, she declared, was "the rawest most undifferentiated of raw material." It wasn't until 70 years later, when anthropologist Derek Freeman unearthed the truth about Mead's sloppy studies, that her theories were finally debunked.[4] In the meantime, Western thinking—and societies—have been distorted for several generations. We now know that deep-seated urges and instincts underlie and direct human behavior.

Anthropologists and other researchers have studied the huge range of different cultures around the world. From these studies, they have teased out the characteristics that are common to all human cultures; they call them "human universal values."[5] In other words, they are features that are hardwired into human behavior and not affected by cultural conditioning. We will now examine the main features and show how the San shape up to these features, then we will see how they compare with common practice in our Western culture. This will throw into relief any discord with our savanna-bred natures.

Every normal human on this planet has fundamental feelings of pain, fear, happiness, and physical attraction. These are emotions that manipulate our bodies for basic survival and reproduction. Indeed, it is difficult to imagine how any species can survive if it does not have a similar impulse system to signal when, for example, to fight for vital space, to flee from danger, or to mate.

Hardwired Behavior

All creatures are born with a set of instructions wired into their brains, mostly simple "rules of thumb." For example, a newborn duckling's tiny brain is wired with the instruction, "Attach yourself to the first moving thing you see." In nature, this would be the mother duck, so this works fine. However, if the emerging duckling first sees a balloon, it bonds with that instead. Psychobiologists call this process "imprinting." This phenomenon is of the utmost importance in understanding how early experiences, if they are not what nature expects, can program our brain's computer incorrectly. Not surprisingly, today our lifestyles often program modern infant brains inappropriately.

Humans' hardwired instructions are the first level reflexes, which occur subconsciously. Typical examples are blinking, swallowing, and the knee-jerk. Others invoke emotions, which have an evolutionary and survival purpose—to make the brain give instructions to the body. A clear example is when a lion attacks. Our body's sensors, chiefly the eyes and ears, send signals to the brain. The brain speeds up the heart and puts the muscles in overdrive. We feel this cascade of activity as fear. All this happens subconsciously—it is an automatic, hardwired reflex.

Antonio Damasio, a neuroscientist at the University of Iowa College of Medicine, specializes in finding out how the brain detects emotion and feeling. The brain is receiving billions of reports every second from every cell in the body. The brain then integrates these reports and we perceive the result as an emotion.[6] "Background" emotions work at a subconscious level and only surface to our consciousness vaguely: we can feel "under the weather" or we can have an instinctive dislike of someone. "Primary" emotions are basic ones such as fear, sadness, and happiness. Yet another category concerns "social" emotions, which evolved to make us behave in appropriate ways in society and in personal relationships. They are genetically programmed feelings such as conscience, self-respect, remorse, empathy, shame, humility, dignity, rejection, humiliation, moral outrage, sorrow, mourning, and jealousy.

When we talk about "programming," "hardwiring," and "genetically programmed emotions," where do these features come from? The answer, quite simply, is in our genes. In the words of evolutionary biologist Richard Dawkins, genes "are the replicators and we are their survival machines."[7] Down through the eons, genes in bodies that failed to reproduce died out. We are all carriers of genes that succeeded in getting into the next generation—millions of times over. To do that, they had to make sure that the bodies they found themselves in were fit for survival. In this regard, we still inhabit bodies honed to perfection for successful gene transmission in the savannas of east Africa.

Genes can aid their reproduction more subtly too, by helping copies of themselves that are in other bodies. They manipulate the body they are in to help other bodies survive if they are likely to contain copies of themselves. We perceived this manipulation as instincts, emotions, and feelings. Human mothers feel more like risking their lives to save their own baby than they do for an unknown person; it is a phenomenon that we call, quite naturally and innocently, maternal instinct.

Instincts, Emotions, and Feelings

Instincts, emotions, and feelings are the genes' way of ensuring their self-preservation. There is a powerful lesson to be drawn: nature designed this mental life to work in forager groups in the African savanna. Our lives today are so far removed from these conditions that we are continuously stressed by emotional signals occurring in inappropriate ways.

For example, humans are programmed with instructions that say, "If you see tasty food, eat it until it is all gone." This worked fine in our ancestral homeland as food was not abundant, was largely bland in flavor, and required work to obtain. Today, that hardwired instruction is self-defeating. Food is abundant, food companies are experts at making it appealing and tasty, and we have lost the link between obtaining food and the work required to get it. Our emotions are crying out "eat!"

Humans, as well as many other creatures, have mechanisms that can override the hardwiring. We can still choose to not eat even if the food is there, even if we are hungry or if the food is tasty. But this requires two things: the recognition that there is a good reason to override our instinct and the exercise of willpower to carry it out. This process is unpleasant and stressful.

The culture we grow up in provides the "reason" to override our instincts. It imposes a set of behavioral values that are commonly accepted by society, often strongly bound up with religious doctrines that have developed over centuries. Frequently, cultures impose behavioral patterns that are quite at variance with human nature. *Taboo* is from a Polynesian word (*tapu*) that means a prohibition imposed by social custom against a particular behavior. Humans seem to be hardwired to adopt taboos in general. However, the *nature* of the taboo can be whatever the culture programs into the brain circuits. For example, to Western culture, cannibalism is taboo, whereas it was common practice in many peoples from the Polynesians to the Aztecs. Taboo, and especially its breaking, arouse incredibly deep, visceral emotions. There are many taboos that seem to be common to all cultures; they are "human universal values." An example is the taboo against incest, which is the result of imprinting, a device by which our genes maximize their survival into the next generation. Taboos that have arisen for this reason are good for well-being; most others are not necessarily so. We must, therefore, make fundamental distinctions among those notions that come to us because of our hardwiring, those imprinted at an early age, and those that are programmed into us as "ideas."

Ideas and Indoctrination

Ideas float around in the environment waiting for a susceptible brain to colonize. We all carry a baggage of ideas, opinions, beliefs, and prejudices that have taken up residence in our minds, usually in a haphazard way. New ideas have to fight the current incumbents for a place to be heard. If they are successful, they in turn take up residence and modify our behavior. If these ideas are really successful, they multiply by getting us to tell other people about them. Richard Dawkins has likened the behavior of ideas to that of viruses. He even coined a name for them: mind-viruses or "memes."[8]

The Vienna-based founder of psychoanalysis, Sigmund Freud, had a remarkable nephew, Edward Bernays, whose family migrated to America when he was a baby. In 1919, Bernays opened a marketing agency in New York. He offered techniques using Freud's psychological principles to "influence people to buy products they don't need or want." Bernays coined the term *public relations* for this technique. Bernays used these psycho-techniques with remarkable success; for example, in the 1920s, to persuade women that it is acceptable to smoke in public. His delighted client, the American Tobacco Company, saw cigarette sales soar. Bernays "engineered" public opinion in many other celebrated cases, including the idea that bacon is a breakfast food.

We have all been indoctrinated from the earliest age: by our family, schools, health professionals, sociologists, our cultural belief system, and much else. In matters to do with food, for example, we are under constant, sophisticated, and persuasive assault by the food industry. For generations, they have provided, free of charge, attractive yet self-serving propaganda in the form of educational materials to schools. They take charge of food supplies in schools, hospitals, and other institutions. Various lobbies, including dairy, snack-food, sugar, fast-food, processed food, and cattlemen, deploy the most sophisticated psychological techniques to seduce us into buying their products.

We have the challenge of understanding how our minds are being manipulated. When we have done that, then we have the next mental challenge—changing our habits.

LIVING ARRANGEMENTS

We have to remind ourselves that the way we live today is light years away from our naturally adapted pattern in the tropics of east Africa. Our ancient ancestors (and forager tribes like the San) slept according to the rhythms of light and dark. In the tropics, whatever the season, dusk comes around 6 P.M. and dawn around 6 a.m. For a few hours after dusk, the San huddle around the campfire talking quietly and doing tasks by the firelight. Sleep would come around 9:30 P.M. and they would wake up with the sun.

The creatures from whom we are descended, *Homo erectus,* discovered fire at least one million years ago. We can imagine the nights with strange unknown rustlings in the dark; the campfire must have been a great comfort. We all feel, even today, the fascination of a fire: gazing reflectively into the flames is a pleasure deeply anchored in our psyches. Campfires constitute a flickering island of reassurance going back to the beginning of human existence. This is our naturally adapted prelude to sleep.

Up until the beginning of the 20th century, populations, even in the West, did not have the luxury of much light after dark. They just had flickering whale-oil lamps and beef-fat candles; people still followed ancient ancestral sleep rhythms. Since 1900, light at night gradually became more common, first with gas lighting and then with electric light. The net result is that we do not prepare our brains for sleep in the way nature envisaged. Today, the average American sleeps two hours fewer than in the 1960s. He or she certainly sleeps less—and less well—than the ideal for which our naturally adapted sleeping pattern has programmed us. Some of the consequences are predictable: loss of concentration, lowered resistance to stress, and a depressed immune system. An unexpected consequence is that sleep deprivation reduces appetite-suppressing hormones such as leptin and it increases hunger-inducing hormones such as ghrelin—the less we sleep, the more we overeat.

Sunlight as Human Food

In contrast to too much light at night, we are not getting enough sunlight by day. Our African Pleistocene ancestors spent all their time unclothed and out-of-doors. With the spread of humanity to all parts of the globe, it is indicative that human skins have adapted to soak up sunlight more easily the more people distanced themselves from the tropics.

Years ago, we never used to worry about how much sun we got. Parents would even urge their children to play outside and "make some vitamin D." This was a key insight: sunlight is an essential piece of nutrition for humans. The scares over sunburn-induced skin cancers have caused a hysterical overreaction. The modern denial of sunshine has led to a surge of diseases that are connected to sunlight deficiency, including cancers, rickets, and depression.

Cancer researcher E.M. John found that cancers are much more prevalent in the northern cities of the U.S. than in the southern rural states. In particular, the risk of breast cancer is increased by three times.[9] Researcher William Grant estimates the yearly toll from cancers caused by lack of sunshine at 100,000 cases and 40,000 deaths; this is four times the mortality from skin cancer.[10] The vitamin D deficiency disease, rickets, thought to be vanquished long ago, is resurging in cities. We all need to get adequate sunshine; just be sensible and avoid burning.

Population Density

Pleistocene humans had a very low population density. While 50 persons comprising a band of foragers lived in close proximity to each other, the nearest neighboring band would be 20 to 30 miles away. At various times of the year, groups would meet up for a festival. It was the occasion to find mates, trade artifacts, overeat, and have a good time. Even so, those humans did not meet more than a few hundred different people in a lifetime. There is no doubt that, in the wandering band of 50 or so people, life could seem dull compared to the excitement of the festival. Today, the excitement, anonymity, and opportunities of living in crowded cities operates on our minds like a recreational drug. Is there a downside to living in such crowding?

Researcher John Calhoun published a pioneering animal study 40 years ago and found that crowded female rats had low fertility rates and high rates of miscarriage and death in childbirth; they also had poor nesting and poor parenting behaviors. Male rats had high rates of sexual deviation, homosexuality, aggression, violence, cannibalism, pathological depression, and withdrawal. There were high rates of social disorientation, infanticide, and infant mortality. Calhoun finished his report with the observation that we might advance our understanding "about analogous problems confronting the human species."[11]

Does this have the ring of truth to it? Today's high population densities have put us on a treadmill requiring industrialized, intensive forms of society. Many of us are worn down by congestion, crowds, and lack of time to even think. We dream of lives in closer contact with natural surroundings. There is no doubt that our mentalities are best adapted to much lower population densities.

TERRITORIALITY

Human beings have evolved, over a very long time, to live in bands of 40 to 50 people. All band members are close relatives by marriage or birth—in other words, each band forms one extended family. This was the pattern for millions of years of human evolutionary history, with the extended family as the basic survival unit. It is only in the last few thousand years that we have broken with this deeply programmed existence.

Each band had its vital space or territory of some 200 square miles. We use the term *vital space* deliberately: this territory provided everything vital for survival, especially food. But it was also the land where their gods, heroes, and spirits dwelt, where their dearest dead were laid. Even though they were nomadic within this territory, every nook and cranny of it was familiar to them—it was "theirs" and the feeling of ownership is desperately important. In contrast, should they venture onto adjacent territory, they would feel uncomfortable and out of place because they were trespassers. The band had to hang together for survival and to protect their vital space from adjacent bands. This pattern of existence has molded deep characteristics into the human psyche.

In particular, band members strongly identify with, and give their loyalty to, their own band. In other words, humans have a strong genetic predisposition to identify with their own "in-group" and to be suspicious of "out-groups." The need to have a feeling of "belonging" to a group is a human universal value.

In-Group, Out-Group

A stranger (by definition, from an "out-group") is a threat. If a stranger is on your territory, he is probably up to no good. He might be out to capture a mate, steal honey, or take murderous revenge in a long-running vendetta. Primal societies around the world demonstrate a similar mistrust of strangers. Jared Diamond describes in *Guns, Germs, and Steel* how when New Guinea tribesmen meet, they strive to discover "some reason why the two should not attempt to kill each other."[12] In Polynesia, two strangers recited their memorized genealogies in order to find a common ancestor.[13] The San Bushmen would stop 40 feet from a stranger, both sides would lay down their arms, and then they would approach each other with caution to find common purpose.[14] Of course, often the stranger was not well-intentioned and a battle would ensue.

Genes, Relationships, and Conflict

The biologist Robert Trivers derived an elegant explanation of the way human relationships operate. It explains how we feel toward our parents and children, siblings, lovers and friends, and in-group and out-groups.[15] The answer lies in our genes.

We all possess genes that work to help copies of themselves lying in other bodies. Of course, we cannot know precisely which bodies contain copies of our genes. Trivers insight was to see that creatures help other members of their species in proportion to their degree of relatedness. In this way, a child gets 50% of his or her genes from the mother and 50% from the father. A mother has 50% of her genes in each child, and 25% with each grandchild. By the same token, a child shares 50% of his or her genes with siblings and 25% with maternal aunts and uncles.

In the forager society, everyone was related to one another in some way, so there would be "gene pressure" to help and cooperate with each other and to refrain from feuding with and killing each other.[16] Even in modern societies, the more closely people are genetically related, the more likely they are to come to one another's aid, especially in life-or-death situations—"blood is thicker than water." Genetic relatedness feeds directly into in-group/out-group conflict: such conflicts are really battles between gene groups manipulating their host bodies for supremacy in the struggle for life.

Humans are not the only creatures to be hostile to out-group members. Male chimpanzees patrol the borders of their territory, and if they find a strange male, they kill him.[17] According to Frans de Waal, a leading authority on the social intelligence of apes, "Sometimes a small group of chimpanzee males stealthily enters a neighboring territory to overwhelm a single male that they viciously beat and leave to die."[18] Likewise, if a lone chimpanzee becomes aware of out-group males intruding on his territory, he becomes worried and his hair stands on end.[19]

Buried in these accounts is the assumption that out-group hostility is a male phenomenon. However, females had every reason to fear strangers too: they could be raped, abducted, or murdered, and the same fate could happen to their children. Women who allowed that to happen did not pass on their genes to the next generation. Women who survived are therefore those programmed with successful survival responses.

A landmark study led by Shelley Taylor shows that women respond to extreme danger with a cascade of brain chemicals, including one called oxytocin. These hormones drive women to tend children and gather with other women. Dr. Taylor dubs this the "tend and befriend" response.[20] This is in opposition to the men's "fight-or-flight" response. It is interesting to reflect that, in an emergency on the African savanna, the women were programmed to round up the kids and get everyone into a huddle, while the men, pumped up on testosterone and adrenaline, battled off the danger.

We all, therefore, are deeply programmed to mistrust strangers. However, with the rise of farming and the concentration of multitudes of humans into cities, how is this mistrust managed? In the words of Jared Diamond, "People had to learn, for the first time in history, how to encounter strangers regularly without attempting to kill them."[21] Every person in the world has to learn how to manage relationships with strangers. This is a process of indoctrination designed to paper a veneer of "civilized" behavior over innate, mistrustful insecurities. Society manages this at two levels: as individuals, we are taught to suppress our natural tendencies and become self-effacing. We avoid eye contact, we stoop our shoulders, we look at the ground, we scurry along with small steps, we avoid confrontation, we are taught "courtesy" and polite manners. At the level of the state—through institutions such as the police, military, and the legal system—it alone enacts laws and it is the final arbiter in the settlement of disputes. Social idealists add a third pressure: the theory that humans ought to want to live in "diverse" communities.

Here we see a number of divergences from our naturally adapted instincts. Our human natures are telling us that we are most comfortable when we are living and working with people "like us"; that we need to "belong" to a group, give it our loyalty, and reject outsiders; that we should take personal responsibility for protecting our in-group, and its territory, from out-groups; and that males have different reactions to females when danger threatens. However, all these deep instincts are frustrated by modern living arrangements.

From these insights, we can predict that multicultural societies are likely to be more neurotic and stressful. By suppressing, even denigrating, normal roles for male aggression, societies will suffer increased levels of unorthodox activity: violence, hooliganism, gang warfare, and criminality. The frontier defenses of Western countries, protected with razor wire, harsh deserts, and armed patrols, are an open invitation to a Third-World youth to test his mettle. It is normal for the defenders to feel viscerally opposed to the invasion of their in-group territory by such outsiders.

We have given the impression that each forager band operates in hostile isolation from its neighbors, but this is not entirely true. Neighboring bands also needed to cooperate at many levels. Wives would almost always be brought in from an out-group. Potential husbands from one group had to visit the other group to find mates and negotiate terms. There would be exchanges of gifts and other obligations. Everyone thus had uncles, aunts, cousins, and other family members in nearby bands whom they would visit on occasion. In extreme situations, such as those of the San who live in a particularly hostile natural environment, bands contracted understandings for emergency access to resources, notably water, in times of distress.

The "natural" size of an in-group is therefore the extended family as denoted by the forager band. With the rise of agriculture and the concentration of populations into larger units such as towns and cities, the size of the in-group had to increase. This was not always easy—somehow people had to sink their differences and invest their loyalty into a grouping that included other extended families. The rise of a charismatic leader who inspired everyone's loyalty was part of the answer. Another part of the answer is provided by the need to cooperate to fight off an external threat.

As George Washington said to his fractious and jealous state-loyal armies, "Either we hang together or we shall surely hang apart." The Normans welded together the Anglo-Saxon kingdoms of England by deploying another, long-term strategy—that of instilling a sense of national patriotism. They used the tools of pageantry, flags and foreign wars. In this way, one of the earliest nation-states was born. It grouped together peoples who had the same language, culture, and religion and gave them a national identity. This, it seems, is about as good as it gets.

Political entities that group together peoples of different languages, religions, or sharp cultural differences are inherently unstable. We see this all over the modern world. Yugoslavia and Somalia broke up in bloody conflict. Rwanda, Congo, and Sudan suffered genocidal massacres of one ethnic community by another. In yet others, low-level conflict continues like a running sore: India (religious conflict), Sri Lanka (out-group Tamil settlers against indigenous peoples), Chechnya (indigenous peoples against out-group Russian occupiers), Northern Ireland (indigenous Irish against out-group occupiers), Spain (Indigenous Basques against out-group occupiers), and Palestine/Israel (indigenous people against out-group occupiers). We draw the uncomfortable conclusion that the notion of a multicultural society is a contradiction in terms.

Warfare

> *"The story of the human race is war. Except for brief and precarious interludes there has never been peace in the world; and long before history began, murderous strife was universal and unending."* —WINSTON CHURCHILL

At the time Churchill wrote that (1925), the world was still reeling from the carnage of World War I. It had been so traumatic that politicians (but not Churchill) billed it as "the war to end all wars." Churchill had a layman's pragmatic and unromantic opinion of human nature. Meanwhile, the experts—social anthropologists—were turning their misty eyes to the ideal of the Noble Savage. They thought that warfare was the result of bad upbringing.

So, is there any truth in the idea that humans are naturally warlike? We have the archaeological remains of Stone Age battlefields and everywhere we look are signs of humans killing humans in murderous conflicts. The American anthropologist Napoleon Chagnon extensively studied the Yanomamo, a tribe of the Amazon rainforest, for over 30 years and he estimated that 30% of males died violent deaths from warfare.

Our model forager tribe, the San, frequently warred with neighboring groups: they had a murder rate greater than America's inner cities. In one account, one band avenged a killing by sneaking into the killer's camp and murdering every man, woman, and child as they slept.[22] The Australian Aborigines had a similar pattern—jealousies, vendettas, and revenge killings were frequent features of aboriginal life. Neighboring camps would be raided and bitter fights would be fought to the death. American anthropologist W. Lloyd Warner lived among the Aborigines of Arnhem Land from 1909 to 1929. He estimated that 200 men died in organized warfare during that period.[23] The total population was only 3,000, so this was a colossal rate of casualties.

Archaeologist Lawrence Keeley has summarized the proportion of male deaths caused by war, even today, in a number of primal societies.[24] The proudly independent Jivaro tribe in Peru is notorious for their use of poison-dart blow-pipes and head-hunting. Keeley estimates that some 60% of Jivaro males die in battle. Half a world away, the Mae Enga of the New Guinea highlands lose 35% of males in murderous conflicts. In contrast, European and American male battlefield deaths in the 20th century (which included two world wars) averaged less than 1% per year.

It seems, then, that for most of human evolutionary history, human males have been involved in bloody conflict. There are a few other species that also do this—chimpanzees, gorillas, and wolves are examples. A common thread is this: the killing is of "them," the out-group. The fact that there are indeed other species that seek to exterminate their own kind, albeit from an out-group, forces us to recognize the possibility that this trait is, in some way, evolutionarily advantageous. Richard Wrangham, professor of anthropology at Harvard University, says that evolution favored humans and chimps who warred because "this makes grisly sense in terms of natural selection." Successful males, the ones that survive, enjoy high status among other males. High-status males are strongly attractive to females and have more matings, so they generate more offspring. The genes sitting in successful warriors become more common, while the genes in wimps don't get into the next generation in the same numbers. We are all descended, on average, from males who were better-than-average murderous warriors.

A second consequence of early male death in battle is highly important yet little remarked: adult males were in a minority. Females sometimes outnumbered them by two to one. Most men had at least one "wife" and many had two or more. There was competition among women to "get a man." Warfare, then, was a way for males to get rid of some of the competition. Genes in males who promoted warfare *and* who were successful warriors spread throughout the population.

We cannot hope to deal with modern conflict if we do not recognize the hardwiring in young males that drives them to risky activities and violence. Of course, the violence is only a means to an end. It leads to high status, which is an important staging post on the way to the end. However, the only end that counts is getting the genes into the next generation.

WORKING PATTERNS

In Chapter 1, we talked about "women's work" and "men's work." The women would go off in a group with the small children on their backs and forage for food. For safety, they stayed within "hailing distance." To do this, they kept up a steady chatter. If they sensed silence, they got uneasy and tried to reestablish verbal contact. The women were foraging in a largely cooperative way; they would be giving constant advice to each other. They would call each other over if they found a particularly rich resource. They had a fine eye for the little signs of food and a delicacy in harvesting it. The women moved in a group, slowly and along familiar paths. They decided where to go and knew the way back.

The men, meanwhile, would go off in ones and twos on their hunting trips. Stealth was of the essence and so talking was kept to a strict minimum, just enough to convey facts about their quarry. Often, communication was simple signs. The men would follow prey along all kinds of unpredictable paths. The prey decided "where to go" and the men had to somehow keep track of where they were.

Laurens van der Post describes how he followed a band of Bushmen while they chased an eland for several days: "The trail twisted and turned so much that I had no idea where we were or in which direction our camp lay. But Nxou [chief hunter] and his companions had no doubt. That was one of the many impressive things about them. They were always centered. They knew, without conscious effort, where their home was, as we have seen proved on many other more than baffling occasions."[25] He should not have been so surprised. Many studies have shown that men today still have remarkable powers of "way-finding" compared to women.[26]

The men had a fine eye for the signs of suitable quarry—they were expert trackers. When they hunted down a quarry, the result was brutal: it was bludgeoned or stabbed to death. The spoils were hacked up as necessary and carried back to the camp. The men's occupation was largely competitive and their status with other males depended on their success.

When there was the chance of a really big kill, like a one-ton eland or a giraffe, all the men would go off in a hunting party. They might even team up with men from an adjacent band, especially if the quarry was roaming over both territories. In this case, the men would temporarily settle their differences in the interests of the wider objective. In either case, there were complex rules about who got credit for a kill and who received what portion of it afterwards.

On return to the camp, each hunter would distribute the spoils in a particular way: his wives and children received the largest part and other portions were distributed to more remote relatives and people who were owed debts. The actual details might vary with circumstance and from tribe to tribe. However, there is one aspect that is a human universal value and of fundamental importance: wives, and sometimes other recipients, would receive more than they could consume, so they would have a surplus they could use to endow gifts and return favors. The wives and the rest of the man's entourage would therefore derive status from the exploits of "their" man.

The women could easily collect enough food to feed the whole family. However, a woman is vulnerable to someone stealing that food. Higher-status women and other men were lying in wait to bully and browbeat that woman out of her hard-won resources. The reason that this rarely happened is simple: she had "her man" who would protect her against any aggression. In Chapter 1, we asked "Why would a woman need a man?" Here, we have most of the answer: without a man committed to her physical protection, the chances that she and her children would survive were reduced. On average, women who were not driven to seek a male bodyguard were less likely to get their genes into the next generation.

So, the women went out foraging every day and they took their babes-in-arms (up to 4 years old) with them. Men were not invited to, and did not volunteer for, the working party. The total working day was 4–5 hours and a woman could find enough food to feed the family. What pointers are there for us today? We might tentatively suggest that it is normal for a woman to go out to work, but that she has her small children with her. It would be normal for a woman to work with other women and not with men. It is probable that women have different inborn talents and ways of working compared to men. They probably find comfort if their working environment allows them to talk freely.

In contrast, the men went hunting at irregular but frequent intervals. Their activity was often dangerous, required strength, violence, subtle reading of animal tracks, and ingenuity. They were excited by the challenge and tended to underrate the risks. Mostly, they worked alone and in silence and often their efforts were unsuccessful. Sometimes, they formed teams that worked closely together to achieve a kill. It was work that women could not do. The results of a man's work would decide his status with other men. If done well, it would buy him gift-giving power and bring admiration and appreciation from his womenfolk. What lessons might there be for us today? Again, this is sensitive territory. However, we might tentatively suggest that men have innate talents different from women's talents. They prefer to work alone or in a project-focused team with other men. Their way of working would clash with women's way of working if they had to work together. A man needs to feel that his work is important and something women could not do. He works hard for success, proudly anticipating the admiration of his womenfolk.

Until recent times, working patterns often fit quite closely to this specification. Even in the upheaval of industrialization, most occupations were segregat-

Male Hierarchy

The concepts of status and status-seeking are human universal values. For men, and particularly the genes they carry, status is of prime importance. In our Pleistocene past, genes that found themselves trapped in a low-status body were condemned to oblivion. Hence, the gene-driven competition to make "their" body the dominant male. By a mixture of strength, hunting skills, and force of personality, one male would emerge in the forager band as "chieftain," "headman," or "honcho." Whether it is humans or some other species, biologists refer to this individual as the "alpha male." All the other males are lower status.

By the very nature of things, very few men make it to the top. A few others are candidates on the way up, others are on the way down. In the forager tribe, many men are none of the above: they are "low status." Modern "Blank Slate" policy directs that there should be more women in top positions, but it does not admit that there is no genetic, status-seeking drive to be there. The irony is that while males do indeed predominate in boardrooms, politics, and so forth, the vast majority of men are not in top positions. In today's society, most men are nobodies.

ed. The women worked in large groups in factories, concentrating on the finer work such as cotton and lace-making. The men did the perilous and dirty jobs such as those in coal mines, shipbuilding, or blast furnaces. The men took pride in their daily wrestle with danger; they had a sense of fulfillment, of purpose, and of camaraderie.

The Modern Workplace for Men and Women

For several generations now, the "Blank Slate" philosophy has permeated policy-making in the workplace. The attack has been on at least three fronts. The first is the theory that any work that men can do, women should do too. The second is the drive for women to get the same pay as a man for the same work. The third is that women should be educated to the same level as men. All these proposals seem reasonable on the face of it. However, they cut across some fundamental, genetically programmed, gender drives and needs. As we saw earlier, women have different personalities and work in a different way. When both genders are expected to work together, the result is rather like a badly coordinated pair in a three-legged race. Each has much to contribute, but each is frustrated by the stumbling induced by being out of sorts with the other.

There is, however, a deeper and more potent source of distress. A man's work (hunting) was where he went to get his sense of identity, where he found prestige and a sense of self-worth. A woman did not go to work (foraging) to find her identity—she got that by being a mother to her children. Modern ideas of work destabilize this major asymmetry. We can expect a man to feel diminished if a woman does the same job; at the least, he will not feel special or important. Here, we lose an important prop to self-esteem, especially for a male of low status. The situation gets even worse if, in the hierarchy, he is subordinate to a woman. In these circumstances, the man's workplace, instead of being his main source of self-respect and status-enhancement, will be the opposite—an unhappy place that reminds him daily of his mediocrity. An unplanned consequence is that such men will seek their identity, status, and prestige outside the workplace. Some might do it in innocent ways, through pastimes, hobbies, and sports. Many others will find it in street gangs, violence, and organized crime.

A similar problem arises with equal pay. Until recent times, men and women mostly worked in different occupations, so there was nothing to compare. It gave a sense of responsibility and purpose for the man to be the "breadwinner"—he took pride in it. He brought home more pay than his wife and this gave him status. He was important to the prestige of the family and the sharing out of his wages had direct parallels with his forebears' sharing out of meat. In recent years, the workplace has become feminized. Coal miners, steelworkers, and ship's stokers have had to learn how to stack supermarket shelves and flip hamburgers. Most occupations have women doing the same work as men and they expect the same pay. This has an unexpected consequence: men's pay trended down to the level of women's pay. The man's salary is no longer special. Indeed, in many situations, the woman can support herself and her children on her own.

As a hunter, a man would take pride in being quick-witted, ingenious, and a master of solving the clues left by his quarry. A man would feel his self-esteem swell as he recounted his exploits to the other men. These exploits deployed a combination of hardwired talent and intelligence. It was the kind of smartness that had no parallel in the world of women. In our modern society, this aspect of human endeavor has morphed into the process called "education." Authorities have made an immense effort to promote female scholarship: they bias teaching methods to favor the way girls learn best. Boisterous boys are treated as behavior problems and, under pressure from the schools, their parents dope them with Ritalin to make them docile.[27]

The policy has worked. By the year 2003, 60% of American college graduates were women. This sounds good, but it means that, for every four women with a degree, there are only three men. One man in four will find himself paired with a woman who is more educated than he is. This is a third area where a low status male will be reminded daily of his inadequacies.[28]

The "natural" order of things in the workplace has been upset by social engineering. The irony is that most women will not see any problem. If they earn more than their man, they will say, "I don't mind. What I earn is for both of us and I am happy to share it." If they are more educated than their man, it is a similar reaction. Women in this situation are puzzled that their man is not consoled by such generosity. For women, these matters are not central to their identity and they cannot imagine the devastating feelings of inadequacy that a man experiences.

Many women today can now have their cake and eat it too. A woman's chief source of self-esteem and identity—her ability to have a family—will never go away. At the same time, she can pursue an occupation in ways that were unimaginable just a generation ago. Her problems are the mirror image of the man's. She will find it harder to find a suitable man and when she does, her relationship with him will be bedeviled by his crises of esteem and identity. If indeed she pursues a high-powered, all-consuming career at the expense of developing a family life, she might find that the harvest is bitter.

Genes never let the majority of women ignore their true priority: family and quality of life. This translates through to the money-earning scores of women. If there is a sex-gap in pay, it is because women make a clear trade-off between career and family. Social economist Satoshi Kanazawa, who has carried out pioneering and detailed scientific analyses in this field, states, "My conclusion is that the sex gap in pay exists because women have better things to do than to earn money, *reproductively speaking*. (my italics)"[29] He makes the point that money-earning for men is the route to getting more genes into the next generation. This is not the case for women—their route is through nurturing their offspring.

TRIBAL RELATIONSHIPS

Within the band, everyone had a basic understanding that they must all pull together to survive. That is to say, the balance was tipped in favor of cooperation with other members of the band. Conflict and rivalry, while always present under the surface, were kept within tight limits.

The forager band had a body of unspoken laws, some of them human universal values and others particular to their culture. The band members constantly juggled self-interest, gift-giving, obligation, jealous watchfulness, and anger with a fear of hostility and rejection. In modern foragers, the San have not been observed to show much altruism, gratuitous kindness, sympathy, or gen-

Suckers, Cheats, and Grudgers

Evolutionary biologists have found that almost any population, whether pigeons, puffer fish, or chimpanzees, is composed of three main personalities. There are those that abide by the rules, but have no instinct to protect themselves against rule-breakers. Evolutionary biologists call these "sucker" populations. There are those who find it easier to scrounge off the suckers—these are known as "cheats." This type of asymmetric situation is neatly summed up by the American writer of humorous poetry, Ogden Nash:

Pale Ebenezer thought it wrong to fight,
But Roaring Bill—who killed him—thought it right!

There is also a third category dubbed "grudgers." These are the ones who see the cheating, or have been cheated once, but refuse to be cheated a second time. They still have the other qualities of the suckers, but this time they learn to resist the cheats and carry a grudge against them for having been cheated.

The proportions of grudgers, cheats, and suckers is constantly changing. Professor Richard Dawkins had this to say about it:

"The first thing that happens is a dramatic crash in the population of suckers as the cheats ruthlessly exploit them. The cheats enjoy a soaring population explosion, reaching their peak just as the last sucker perishes. But the cheats still have the grudgers to reckon with. During the precipitous decline of the suckers, the grudgers have been slowly decreasing in numbers, taking a battering from the prospering cheats, but just managing to hold their own. After the last sucker has gone and the cheats can no longer get away with selfish exploitation so easily, the grudgers slowly begin to increase at the cheats' expense. In due course, the proportion of suckers increases and the cycle starts all over again."

This is a lurid analysis of the social dynamics in many species, including humans. Forager society was organized with checks and balances such that the tendency to cheating was swiftly recognized and then punished.

uine generosity.[30] The San band members give, receive, and exchange gifts in a way that has strict unspoken rules: a gift must never be refused, even if the recipient doesn't want to be beholden to the donor; and a gift must always be reciprocated, not the same object but one of equal value. The reciprocal gift should be made only after a "decent" interval, which can be from a couple of weeks up to several years.

Wrongdoing to the San is not always what might be expected. They don't think lying is particularly bad and stealing is so certain of discovery that it rarely happened ("it would only lead to trouble").[31] On the other hand, breaking of respect for ownership of a resource is severely sanctioned. The furious "owner" killed the man who took honey from the tree where he, as "finder," had made his mark. Other disputes arise over the share of a major kill. There are no formal institutions for enforcing rules, contracts, or obligations, so individuals or little groups have to take matters into their own hands. Squabbles break out for all kinds of reasons but, unlike those with neighboring tribes, they have to find ways to resolve them internally.

We now understand that human society (and even chimpanzee society) operates on a transactional basis. Favors are given and received, deals are done—society can only function if these understandings operate properly. In this way, humans (and chimpanzees) are programmed with social feelings: of obligation to someone for a favor received, of rightful dues for favors given, of outrage against cheating and injustice, of revenge against cheaters, and of retribution to redress a wrong. People who are emotionally driven to retaliate against those who cross them, even at a cost to themselves, are more credible adversaries and less likely to be exploited.

One of the most powerful drives is the feeling of loyalty to the band and to its members. The feeling of "us" and "them" is a deeply programmed emotion. One of the worst fates that can befall an individual is to lose the support of other members of the band, so it is normal to be sensitive to the feeling of rejection and want to do whatever is necessary to avoid it. Today, we live in a world where each of us is a member of a number of in-groups: our family, our world of work, and our co-adherents in a belief-system. Overarching all these are our countrymen and our country, the final conditioner of our lives.

One of the curses of human nature is the vendetta: a grudge by one group is avenged, which in turn provokes a new revenge. The cycle continues seemingly without end. The 16th-century English philosopher Thomas Hobbes recognized that to break the cycle an independent law enforcer was needed. In his major work, *Leviathan*, Hobbes proposed that people should be prevented from taking the law into their own hands. Rather, they should entrust the redressing of grievances to a third party, the state, that would impartially decide the case and carry out any retribution. The state acts as intermediary, prevents revenge, and makes punishment a neutral act. In this spirit, states around the world have instituted systems of justice and punishment on which they have the monopoly. This system has proved to be remarkably successful in reducing tit-for-tat punishments and the overall level of violence in society.

MALE-FEMALE RELATIONS

In most mammal species, males are bigger than females. This is true of elephants, reindeer, lions, and elephant seals. Of our close cousins, the gorilla is at one extreme: the male is twice the size of the female. At the other extreme, chimpanzee males are about the same size as females. Biologists have discovered that this difference between male and female (known as "dimorphism") is a reliable indication of the amount of physical male competition for females. The biggest gorilla (or reindeer stag) is the one that fights off the male opposition to mate with females. In this way, genes that build large males in these species are more likely to multiply into the next generation.

In humans, males are, on average, 20% bigger than females. This is a strong indication that human males have been hardwired over millennia to physically compete with other males for access to females. This competition has a number of consequences. Males who are not up to success in physical combat might use other strategies. They will form alliances with other males who act as their sidekicks. (Chimpanzees, who do not benefit from physical superiority, deploy this strategy frequently.) So, some males get to their objective by being good at doing deals with other males. All males will be careful to avoid revealing their weaknesses. In this way, males that are genetically programmed to avoid showing their emotions, to avoid signs of distress (such as crying), and to not talk about their feelings will all do better in competition with other males. When males do talk, it will be mainly to convey factual information that reveals nothing about their degree of insecurity.

In contrast, the female of our species is generally physically weaker, less violent, and programmed to cooperate with other females in the foraging workplace. However, they were also in competition with others for resources and favors from "their man." In this regard, human females have developed two strategies: the first is physical and aggressive, but the second is more prevalent and subtle. This is the use of indirect means to obtain their objective—females who are good at reading moods, analyzing motives, and probing for weakness, and who can use these skills to undermine their rivals, will do best. More of their genes will get into the next generation. Girls begin to show these traits as young as three years old.[32]

There is a fundamental, and decisive, biological difference between the sexes. The female can only have one pregnancy at a time, while males can impregnate many females at a time. This asymmetry applies throughout the animal kingdom. In the numbers game, genes that get their host male to mate with many females rather than just one will spread faster. There is, therefore, a strong selection pressure for males to mate with as many females as possible. In contrast, there is no selection pressure for females to mate with more than one male. She can still have only one pregnancy at a time and the number of partners makes no difference. In humans, a female's success in child rearing depends on the commitment of a male to protect her, so she will do even better if she can stop the male from diluting his commitment with other females.

We are all descended from males who, on average, impregnated many different women. Geneticists estimate that an astonishing 8% of the Mongol population is descended from Genghis Khan, who had many concubines.[33] In contrast, we are all descended from females who were good at getting male commitment, were clever at stopping the male from committing to other women, and ruthlessly fought other women for a major share of the male's resources. Herein lies a strong source of male/female conflict—the genetically programmed male agenda is diametrically opposed to the female one.

Sexual Selection

We have seen that women are attracted to mate with high-status men. How is this status perceived? One powerful criterion is the status that the man has with other men. Other men will accord high status on qualities that appeal to them, not what appeals to women. One of these qualities is futile risk-taking: men will admire another man who indulges in reckless or dangerous behavior. Women are not impressed by the exploits in themselves, but in the importance other men give to them.[34] A second criterion is choosing a male who will give them sons who, in their turn, will be attractive mates and provide lots of grandchildren. That means mating, if possible, with a male who is attractive to other females right now. In other words, she might only find him attractive because other females do.

Males are in strong competition to attract a woman. Those who are not naturally endowed might try another tactic—bluff. A man might give outward appearances of being strong and with good commitment potential, but how is the female to be sure? How many of his stories about his exploits are really true? Some males might be good at deception on this score, so the female has to develop finely tuned antennae to detect it.

How do truly meritorious males convince a female that they are not bluffers? One interesting evolutionary strategy is handicapping. The peacock trails a long cumbersome tail behind him, which makes him more vulnerable to predators. So, why do cumbersome-tailed peacock genes persist in the gene pool? The probable answer was first formulated by Israeli researcher Amotz Zahavi.[35] It is a way for a peacock to show a peahen that he really is strong: he can carry this burden around and still survive. In modern terms, it is like the man who drives a Hummer rather than a sensible car—he is showing to the females that, in spite of the immense burden of monthly payments and gas costs, he is fully functional and a magnificent source of good genes.

Here, we have a powerful mechanism to explain why "keeping up with the Jones's" is a ubiquitous preoccupation: status is relative. As soon as Hummers become common, males are driven to take on yet more onerous commitments and habits. They must progressively strive for a higher-status job, move to a better neighborhood, eat at expensive restaurants, and wear pricey designer clothes. Even if the man is married, he cannot step off the treadmill: his wife gets her status from her husband and she will be pushing him just the same.

There is a huge irony in all of this. Evolutionarily speaking, the only purpose of a male striving for high status is to get more matings than average and so more genes into the next generation. In modern Western society, the process of acquiring status symbols becomes the end in itself. The reason? The Western concept of marriage.

Marriage

Just about every tribal society on Earth practices an arrangement where a man and a woman become contractually bound to each other. The fundamental terms of the contract are straightforward: the woman provides sex for the husband; food for herself, her husband, and their children; and nurturing for the offspring. The man provides commitment, protection, status, security, and hunted status-food for gift-giving and sharing; he accepts any offspring of the woman's previous marriages. San women enjoyed the "sweetness" of the sexual dimension just as women do today.[36] The contract is cemented by rituals and oaths made in front of witnesses, notably close relatives.

How do the man and woman find each other? The woman's first marriage is usually when she is very young. In San society, a girl's first marriage is between 13 and 15 years of age, before she has reached puberty.[38] The parents will negotiate a marriage with a carefully selected man. They try for the best status they can find—someone who will bring security, reflected glory, and some

Female Puberty and Fertility

In forager populations, a girl's first period (known as menarche), on average, occurs between the ages of 15 and 17. This is followed by two or three years of "adolescent sterility" before she begins ovulating and can therefore conceive. Thus, a woman does not bear her first child until she is between 18 and 22 years of age. The first pregnancy is followed by four to eight others spaced 3–5 years apart, until menopause occurs sometime after age 40. In today's Western society, girls reach menarche three years earlier and have only 12 to 18 months of adolescent sterility.[37] Seemingly, this is not how nature intended. A number of factors contribute to this abnormality, including lack of hard physical work, lack of feeling hungry, and too much body fat.

meat-sharing for the parents too. In the words of developmental psychology professor David Geary, "Culturally successful men have more reproductive potential than other men, and women's mating and marriage preferences suggest that they are motivated to capture and use this potential for their own reproductive ends."[39] The husband will usually be much older, by 7 to 15 years. Often the daughter's preferences, feelings of attraction, and affection might be taken into account. First marriages in the San are unstable and many break up within a short period.[40]

In forager societies, women get married several times in a lifetime. By the time she is a little older, and maybe already a mother, parental influences diminish and emotional preferences play a greater role. Often, it is the woman who puts an end to an unsatisfactory marriage. Even though women outnumber men, there is still fierce male competition for access to females, so she is unlikely to remain without a protector.

Almost always, the man stays in his own band and seeks a bride in an outgroup, a nearby band. In this respect, the human species is what anthropologists call "patrilocal"—that is, the woman marries into the husband's family. This is a strong source of asymmetry in the relationship. The man is on home territory, among his close family and allies. In contrast, the bride is entering a world of people with whom she has little prior affinity and she is ignorant of "their ways." The successful wife is one who learns quickly how to assimilate into this culture. She must be skillful at detecting the dynamics in relationships, be good at adapting her behavior to "fit in," and transfer her loyalty to the new group.

Over the eons of evolution, we might expect that genes would evolve to make such skills instinctive, and indeed this is the case. We find that women (compared to men) have greater ability to sense atmospheres, to feel undercurrents, to detect ulterior motives, to conduct intrigue, to ingratiate themselves, and to manipulate their new environment. They will be especially sensitive to rejection by the new family and group. They are good with words and know how to use them to trigger powerful reactions. Women more easily move their allegiance to different groups, often several times in a lifetime.

Polygamy

Earlier, we saw how women outnumbered men and that some men were attractive partners and some were not. It all adds up to some men having several wives and some getting only one or even none. This was a source of strife. Mateless males would be constantly on the prowl: they might be "losers," but they still had the mating drive. That is why the mated males had to be both powerful and vigilant. They had to protect their women from rape by out-group males or from the discreet attentions of an in-group male.[41]

In our discussion so far, we have avoided stating the obvious: that human societies are by nature polygamous, or more precisely "polygynous." That is, they are societies where males (but not females) have more than one mate at a time. In other words, polygyny is a human universal value. Most populations of the world today practice it—the only major exception is Western culture, where monogamy is the socially imposed rule.

This was not always the case. The doctrines associated with monogamy were adopted by the Christian church in the early Middle Ages. Up until that time, even popes and priests had wives and concubines. Then, an ancient Greek mind-virus known as "asceticism" took hold. Asceticism takes the view that true spirituality can only be obtained through abstinence of earthly needs, including sex. According to the ascetic doctrine, celibacy is the ideal that we should all strive for. However, being practical, the church recognized that humans need to reproduce. It adopted a compromise doctrine that allowed ordinary folk to make babies but kept the sexuality to a minimum. A man could marry just one woman, provided he entered an indissoluble contract to stay with her for life. The Christian sect was determined to regulate the marital and sex lives of its adherents. By various means, it got kings and parliaments to adopt monogamy into law and make it virtually impossible to divorce.

However, the instituting of monogamy has some interesting consequences. It intervenes massively in a delicate balance, the one where men strive for several mates and women strive for an exclusive deal. This intervention hands women the exclusive deal. To make sure that there is no back-sliding, the marriage contract is shored up with legally enforced sanctions. In practical terms, the male's evolutionary drive is subordinated to the satisfaction of the female's evolutionary drive.

Secondly, it has the effect of distributing the females almost equally among the men. This is good for low-status males, for even they will find someone to pair up with. It is even more important in modern societies, where the proportion of males is equal to females. The limits to this were illustrated in the aftermath of World War I. During that time, the major combatants, France, England, and Germany, lost young men at the same rate as in hunter-gatherer times. As a result, there was a dearth of young men after the war. With the rigidities of monogamy, many young women stayed in spinsterhood for the rest of their lives.

We saw earlier that in Pleistocene times, high-status men would have many offspring and low-status men few or none. The kinds of genes that make for high status in Pleistocene times included those for risk-taking, bravery, strength, aggressivity, heroism, female protection, ingenuity, and hunting skills. In the Western world, for over 1,000 years now, genes in low-status men have been spread at the same rate as those for high-status men. No one knows what this means for the future.

Mating Games

We mentioned earlier that women could rightfully fear a husband's involvement with another woman. But why would a woman be interested in taking a lover? After all, she only needs one man at a time: a second man contributes nothing to the number of children she can have or the protection that the husband provides. The main answer, unsurprisingly, lies in the genes. A woman might be attracted to another man if her genes sense that he will give her offspring a better start in life. A woman may well have a husband, but does he have the best genes in the barnyard? If she has a low-status husband, her current genes will do better if she can mate with a man whose genes are better than her husband's. She will be attracted to mate discreetly with high-status males. Whence the excessive insecurity of a low-status male when a high-status male is hovering around his wife.

Conformity of individual members to the norms of the group is shored up by social emotions such as moral outrage, revenge, remorse, and guilt. The emotions themselves are human universal values, but the norms to which they are applied are not. In the West, we are conditioned to the idea that monogamy is the social norm. It is interesting to notice how the social emotions are expressed when confronted with norm-breakers, particularly males. The full weight of moral outrage is unleashed against them: they are called "cheats," "two-timers," "home-breakers," and "cads."

The husband has only given his commitment to the raising of his own genes. One of the worst things that can happen to a gene is that it finds itself in a body which, instead of promoting further copies of itself, is promoting someone else's copies. Such a case can occur if the wife has been sexually active with some other male. The husband could find himself raising another male's genes. Males are therefore descended from a line of males who did a better than average job of ensuring that they were raising their own genes. How did they do this? There are several gene strategies and the most powerful is that the gene is coded to provoke feelings of sexual jealousy. The male, once he has made a commitment to the female, will be jealous, almost insanely so. He will get violent if he senses that his woman is attracted to another man and if higher-status men are interested in her. Jealous violence also has a preemptive role in deterring infidelity. These effects are strongest if the woman is in her prime for childbearing and if the male is low status.[42] Even so, no man is exempt from these emotions— they are part of the hardwiring.

This brings us to one of the fundamental worries for a woman, an emotion deeply programmed from our Pleistocene past—fear of neglect and abandonment. On average, the genes of women who allowed themselves to be neglected or abandoned did not survive so well. She will be constantly seeking reassurance that her man is not planning any changes. She has sensitive antennae trying to second-guess his thoughts. A woman will be jealous of a rival mainly because she fears dilution of her man's commitment, resources, and status, even abandonment.

So far, we have been talking rather mechanistically, but what about love and affection? These are powerful emotions, a kind of madness even. Nevertheless, it is a human universal value that, in the matter of marriage, they take a secondary role. The vast majority of societies (outside the Western middle class) see marriage as a contract, best arranged by those who have a cool understanding of the issues. They see the addled states of lust and romantic love as an unreliable basis for such an important commitment.

In forager societies, women are more focused on keeping their children alive than on developing intimacy with their husbands.[43] Love is the icing on the cake: all other things being equal, women still prefer men with whom they can develop an intimate and emotionally satisfying relationship,[44] although this appears to be more of a luxury than a necessity.[45] Women also prefer men with whom they feel physically safe and who are physically capable of protecting them should the need arise.[46]

Sexual jealousy is not the only reason why domestic situations turn to violence. We have seen that there is asymmetry in the way women and men handle problems. Women are good at using words and they use this ability to pursue their argument by indirect means with elaborate emotional verbal tactics. Men, on average, are not good at handling emotional verbal cut-and-thrust. The female ability to exquisitely torment their dignity and self-esteem maddens them. They feel impotent, frustrated, and outmaneuvered, faced with the seeming irrational, unjust, and slippery nature of the argument. In contrast, men are made to pursue their arguments by simple, direct means: physically. In other words, men are best at physical warfare, while women are best at psychological warfare.

There are several reasons why domestic conflict in forager societies was low. First, women and men were thrown together less—they simply did not interact in areas where they were psychologically unsuited. Also, in modern society, both women and men have heightened expectations of the other, expectations that are unrealistic and frustratingly unrealizable. Finally, should a dispute arise in a forager society, the man had no hesitation parrying the woman's psychological aggression with some low-level physical aggression. In the modern world, the use of physical aggression is thoroughly condemned, which has the interesting consequence of disarming men in domestic disputes, leaving the female verbal and psychological weaponry intact. Many men can cope with this, but all have to suppress their natural inclinations.

PARENTING

In 95% to 97% of mammal species, the males take no part whatsoever in parenting.[47] This includes our closest cousins, the chimpanzee and gorilla. (Chimpanzees never even know who their father is: the female mates with all males in the group.) In the remaining 3% to 5% of mammal species, male parenting exists but in a weak form. Seemingly, the human species falls into this second category.

Fertility Assessment

Evolutionary psychologists and biologists are painstakingly demolishing the Blank Slate doctrine that beauty is purely a matter of cultural upbringing. Men down through the ages who were not good at selecting fertile women had fewer offspring on average. It follows that today's men are descended from a long line of men who were good at picking fertile women.

How does a man tell if a woman is fertile? He has no way of directly measuring it, however, his genes have an indirect way—he detects "attractiveness." Women rated attractive by men consistently have higher levels of reproductive hormones and fertility. On average, a woman who looks young, has a curvy hourglass shape,[48] taut and vibrant skin,[49] good muscle tone, a pleasing voice,[50] and exudes a mysterious aura of sexuality[51] is probably fertile. These signals might only be a crude guide, but on average a man would do better to mate with a woman like that than one who did not display these signs.

In forager societies, direct male involvement with their small offspring is minor. Indirect involvement has to do with the "social" context, for example, meat-sharing to enhance status and forceful protection from bullying and aggression.

A male can never be totally sure if he is the father of the children borne by his wives. This uncertainty plays itself out in many ways. One of them has to do with nephews and nieces. In many societies, men develop stronger relationships with their sister's offspring than with the ones that purport to be theirs. He and his sister have the same mother with total certainty. In other words, he is bound to share some genes with his nephews and nieces by his sister. Many societies such as the Romans and Anglo-Saxons worked this out, even if they did not know about genes—they talked about being "blood relations" and sharing "bloodlines."

All this is not to say that forager fathers ignored children totally. He will happily dandle a small child on his knee for a bit, but the child is part of the women's world and his role, at this stage, is to be protective of his child's safety and interests. Only when a boy is approaching his rite of passage to manhood does the father take on a responsibility for his daily instruction—he becomes his buddy. In modern times, do not expect a father to change a diaper with any sense of warm, nurturing love. In contrast, expect him to intervene forcefully if his child is bullied in the park, and he will be right there when it is time to take his son to a ballgame.

Child Rearing

We will first look at what happens in our typical hunter-gatherer society, the San Bushmen. It is highly likely that our Pleistocene ancestors practiced their form of child rearing for all of our evolutionary past. It is therefore likely that parents and children are genetically programmed for this child-rearing pattern even today.

In forager populations (typified by the San), on average, women had their first child at 19 years old and the last by the age of 49. The mother usually goes off into the bush alone to give birth.[52] Australian Aborigines followed a similar pattern. If the group is on the move, the woman pulls off to the side to give birth, tie the umbilical cord, and wash the baby if there is water nearby. If she is in camp, she will go off into the bush with another woman for companionship.[53] It is a human universal value that childbirth is treated as an entirely female and private matter. Men are not invited to, and show no interest in, its mysteries.

Infant mortality is high: 20% die within the first year of life. On occasion, the mother practiced infanticide on the newborn for one or more reasons: if the child is born too soon after an earlier one; if it is physically defective; if twins are born (in which case one is killed); or if the woman feels too old to breastfeed another baby.[54] The Aboriginal women gave birth to six to eight children in a lifetime, of which estimates suggest that nearly half were killed at birth.[55] There is no suggestion that there is any gender choice in these life-and-death decisions.

Babies and toddlers are breastfed until about three to four years old. The mother then introduces easily chewed, solid foods after the first teeth have broken through. Children tended to be spaced at least four years apart. That is, a new child is not allowed to compete with an older child for the mother's breast milk.

The San believed that breast milk was for the fetus, so a woman stopped breastfeeding a child as soon as she became pregnant again, not when the new baby was born. At this point, the current child is weaned and has to manage entirely on solid foods. Weaning is never an easy time and children often suffer depression that lasts a long time.

During the day, the mother carries her baby in a light sling on her hip. The baby is facing forward and has unfettered access to the breast. The child suckles at will, even if he is not getting any milk. The sucking reflex appears to be an

Natural Family Planning

According to Richard Lee, nursing in San women is "vigorous, frequent, given on demand, and spaced throughout the day and night." It has been known for quite a while that the stimulus of round-the-clock sucking suppresses ovulation. We make a distinction here between sucking and feeding. It is sufficient for there to be 24-hour, on-demand sucking to suppress conception. American mothers who follow this breastfeeding pattern experience a similar effect.[56] A decrease in the frequency of sucking/feeding results in the reappearance of menstruation and then ovulation.[57]

important aspect of what is called "contact comfort." Our close cousins, the chimpanzee and gorilla, exhibit the same behavior.

Carried on the hip in this side position, the child is looking at what the mother is seeing and has eye-level contact with other children. He has access to play with the ornaments and beads that are hung around the mother's neck. The total body contact time is much higher than with Western infants—75% of the time in the first few months, dropping to 40% at two years. Researchers note that boys get less contact time, dropping from 75% to 30% after one year.[58]

Almost as bad as weaning from mother's milk is the process of "weaning from the back"—when the mother ceases to carry a child once a new baby is born. From then on, the older child is not carried again. But children love to be carried, they delight in the physical contact with their mothers, and they hate the pressures imposed by toddling to keep up with the mother's foraging. Weaning from the back gives rise to similar kinds of behavior as breast weaning: temper tantrums, refusals to walk, demands to be carried, and refusal to be left in the village while the mother goes gathering.

Sibling Conflict

Squabbles between siblings have been a trial since the dawn of time. When the first child is born, he has the parents to himself. He has undisputed access to all his mother's resources. When the second child is born, he finds a rival already in place. This older sibling is bigger, smarter, and well-established. In the younger ones, being weaker genetically switches them to a subtle, indirect mode of operation. They tend to be better at provoking the older one into trouble and in playing one parent off against the other. The eldest child is bamboozled by this newcomer's magical ability to manipulate his parents against him. He is bigger, and the only weapon he knows about is violence. But violence, unlike needling, is readily visible to his parents. As he brings their reprimand down on his head, he feels the injustice keenly.

At another level, genes sitting in a child will try to improve his survival chances by restricting competition from newcomers. For a baby suckling at his mother's breast, the worst thing that can happen to his genes is if the mother gets pregnant too early. She will stop breastfeeding him, thus increasing his chances of dying. Hardwiring makes small babies ultra-sensitive to their mother becoming intimate with a man. If there is the slightest suspicion, the baby becomes demanding, tries to divert attention, cries, and bawls. The distraught mother drops any amorous intentions and seeks to find out what can be ailing the child. There is nothing wrong with him, but she is not to know that. This is one reason why young children want to climb into their parents' bed. Their chief, pre-programmed drive is to keep their parents apart. In other words, we are all descended from a succession of infants who were successful at slowing down the arrival of new, competing siblings.

Parent-Child Conflict

In a similar way, we can look at how mother genes and child genes have different agendas. At weaning, a child at the breast is leading a healthy, trouble-free, comforting existence. Quite reasonably, it could go on for a long while yet. The 3-year-old's genes are saying, "Survival is better assured by staying with breast-feeding." But the mother's genes are saying, "Wean the 3-year-old and start another baby." That is why weaning is always a battle. The San suffer from it just as much as Westerners. The important point to register is this: it is natural for there to be this conflict. The child is programmed for it: the mother must play her part properly and resist the child's demands. It is perhaps easier for a San woman, because she lives at a subsistence level and does not have the luxury of trying out trendy child-rearing theories.

Childhood

With the San, infants and children found themselves in an environment where they are rarely out of contact with adults and older children. They moved easily from one group of adults to another. They were all related in some way and the adults were fond of indulging the infants. Adults rarely reprimanded the children and they are only corrected when necessary to teach them to avoid danger. Infants are encouraged to sit up, and then stand up, as early as possible, and they develop motor coordination early. They are also advanced in cognitive development thanks to the high intensity of social contact and stimulating play opportunities.

Although a forager child circulates freely, he nevertheless has an acute sense of his place in the family tree. From an early age, he knows his mother and then identifies his father, brothers, sisters, and other relatives. He seems to have an instinct that immediately fixes the degree of genetic relatedness and therefore the degree of genetic investment that can be expected.

Children, once weaned from the woman's back, stay behind in the campsite with the older women and the men who were not hunting that day. The children were mostly left to play among themselves, but the grandmothers kept a watchful eye on them. Not many species have lifespans that cover three generations, so there must be an evolutionary reason why this should be—something about having grandparents around that promotes survival of their genes in their grandchildren. Researchers believe that grandparents, and in particular grandmothers, played a vital role in the survival of humanity.[59] Grandmothers are strongly programmed to nurture their grandchildren.

Both boys and girls would sometimes accompany the women on their foraging expeditions and thereby learn some foraging skills. However, they were not expected to forage on behalf of the family. From the age of about 11, boys were inducted into hunting with the men; girls never went on the hunt.[60]

There were not many children in the typical band, perhaps 20 or so from infancy to 14 years old.[61] Unlike in modern societies, where children of the same age are put together, each forager child found himself with only one or two others in a similar age group. Older children helped younger children and taught them what they knew, and younger children were dragged upwards in games by having to compete with older children.

Researcher Marjorie Shostak recorded the life histories of eight San women.[62] According to her account, older children were involved in sex play, including sexual intercourse. The adults regarded this as unexceptional, but scolded the children if they were not discreet. There is an innate prudery at all levels and no one likes to be observed. This may explain why daughters were married off before puberty—that is, before they get pregnant without a man to take responsibility. In this regard, it is interesting to consider the question of incest avoidance. Normally, children grow up with an aversion to having sexual relations with their close kin. This is a product of childhood "imprinting," the phenomenon we mentioned earlier in the section on taboo. Our brains are hardwired with an instruction that says: "If you have grown up with this person in your family, don't even think about being intimate with him." On the other hand, if a child is separated from his or her close kin at birth, there is no such imprinting.

An Indulgent Upbringing

With the San, a child is in intimate contact with the mother during the working day. Back at the camp, the child was never more than a few yards from its mother and other close relatives. At night, the child slept next to its parents around the family hearth. The same pattern is found in just about all forager societies. Is there any significance to all this close mother/child contact? Indeed, there is: the worst fate that can befall a small child is to be lost, overlooked, or abandoned. Children who allowed that to happen were less likely to survive into adulthood. On average, every child today is good at detecting being left alone and has a noisy panic attack about it. Looked at in this light, some modern ideas about leaving a child to cry himself to sleep in a nearby room seem misguided.

Children mostly stayed within the circle of the camp. The adults taught them about dangers, but, in reality, the risks of their life in the encampment were few. The adults kept a wary eye out for the children if they strayed out into the bush. On the whole, in their simple lives, there was little need for the adults to nag and scold the children. No worries about the children messing something up, being dirty, breaking valuable objects, or running into traffic. The general picture is of a carefree childhood with few responsibilities and the comfort of being surrounded by a benevolent community of relatives, leading to a well-adjusted existence.

When we look at both our ancient history and our understanding of genetic biology, we can identify some suggestive pointers for today. Ideally, it looks as though a woman should allow at least four years between births. She should allow breastfeeding/sucking for at least three years. She should provide plenty of intimate body contact and avoid giving the baby the impression that it is forgotten or abandoned; the child sleeps with her. The family would live in convenient daily contact with a large extended family of grandparents, aunts, and uncles. Grandmothers are on hand all the time and have a vital child-care role. The environment should allow an indulgent upbringing with little need for scolding.

These are apparently the desirable goals, but they are a long way from modern life. Perhaps only the first one—four-year birth spacing—would be simple to implement today. Nevertheless, once a mother understands these goals, she has a chance of steering her life in a helpful direction. She can avoid fighting harmful battles and focus on the necessary ones. Sibling rivalry is a genetically programmed feature of existence and parents have to battle it even-handedly as best they can. Parent-child conflict is normal in many areas: weaning is always a difficult time with tantrums and tears and the mother has to resist them in a sensible way. Weaning from the intimate body contact is also a difficult time: it is normal for the child to be depressed. Parents have to resist manipulation by the child's psychological warfare.

MYTHS AND RITUALS

In every culture, people lead intense spiritual lives expressed through dance, song, stories, rituals, and deep emotional attachment to the land. All peoples find their identity in tribal stories and myths. The primitive bands had no writing, so they passed down their cultural heritage by intensely disciplined repetition. The older members, who had memorized the entire folklore, would train the younger members to be word-perfect. This was how tribes preserved, with remarkable accuracy, events and stories going back thousands of years. Storytelling was a favorite pastime around the campfire. The children would listen in rapt attention as the tales unfolded, laughing in glee at the antics of some ancient trickster or gasping in dread at some tragedy. This time together, sharing the communal folklore, is at once a powerful release and a strong force knitting the members of the band together.

Many males were killed in battle, so there were not so many living well into old age, but one would be designated as the headman. He was the successful survivor of many life-and-death battles, the high-status "alpha-male," and he had many wives and children. The remaining elders were also venerated in some way, and they were the repository of know-how and tribal memory. Old men were indispensable sources of survival expertise and entertaining stories, the precious guardians of the tribal heritage. In contrast with today's society, old people were not only useful, they fulfilled an essential role in the well-being of the band.

People cluster in little groups during the day, often talking as they make artifacts or perform other tasks. At night, families talk late by their fires or visit other family fires with their children. Frequently, the men and women form their own groups. The subjects of discussion are quite distinct. "The men's imagination turns to hunting. They converse musingly, as though enjoying a sort of daydream together, about past hunts, telling over and over again where game was found and who killed it. They wonder where the game is at present, and say what fat bucks they hope to kill. They also plan their next hunts with practicality."[63] The women talk about who did or did not share food with them as well as their anxieties about not having food. They also complain about their arduous foraging day and the long trudge home. They talk at length about their lovers, husbands, sexual experiences, or the time they went into the bush to give birth. They would not dream of discussing such matters when a man is in earshot, because men had "their talk" and women had theirs.[64]

All primal peoples, whether we look at the San, Australian Aborigines, or Hadza, are deeply attached to their land and feel deeply connected to the nature that surrounds them. In tests made on people from all over the world, they consistently picked out a picture of blue sky, rolling parkland, and the occasional animal as being the most pleasing.[65] Other studies show that American children are less likely to suffer distress if they live in natural surroundings of greenery rather than in concrete buildings and asphalt-lined parking lots.[66] The closer we are to natural surroundings, the more comfortable we feel.

The San dance on many occasions. Both men and women dance, often all night long, working themselves up into a delirium. This kind of behavior is a human universal value and it does not require much imagination to see Western parallels with the atmosphere in nightclubs and discos. People everywhere like doing it and clearly there is some kind of healthy mental relief to be found from the experience. About once a week, the San adult males indulge in a sacred "fire dance" that goes on from dusk until dawn.[67] All the members of the band are present and the women sit in a tight circle singing and clapping and helping to raise the state of dancing frenzy. The men dance in a circle around the women until they go into a trance-like state, where they have mystical, hallucinatory experiences. In this state, and foaming at the mouth, they literally play with fire, skipping through the embers or even scooping up them up. The men describe their experience as a process of death and rebirth. "You give up what you are, give up your identity, enter the unknown, willingly going into fundamental mysteries and so enter the state of transcendence."[68] The American professor of comparative mythology, Joseph Campbell, describes this as the classic tale of the hero's journey into the unknown. The boy becomes a man and the man becomes a hero. After the dance, the Bushman is reborn as an ordinary, fully functioning man. These are deep themes, found all over the world and in all societies.

Rites of Passage

The need to turn boys into men is found in all societies. At some point, the boy, who has been attached to his mother, has to be removed from the world of women and incorporated into the world of men. It happens when the men believe that the boy has reached a suitable level of maturity (not necessarily puberty), probably around 10 to 12 years old. The process takes place over several months as the boy is instructed in behavior appropriate to the status of an adult male. It covers matters such as dress, speech, deportment, and morality.

Up to now, the hunt has been a mysterious activity of the mature, initiated males. They disappeared into the bush for hours or days on end and, on their return, related proud tales of valor, ingenuity, and derring-do. Often, they came back with the meat-prize, something which raised their status in the eyes of those who depended on them. It is a big moment in the life of a boy when he is allowed on his first hunt. This immediately separates him from his sisters and mother—this is something that the womenfolk will never experience.

In a similar way, many spiritual matters have been surrounded in mystery. "It is forbidden to talk of these things except by men who have been initiated in the mysteries of the dance," reported a Bushman to Laurens van der Post.[69] Now religious secrets are revealed. As part of this process, the initiate is required to commune for the first time with the "supernatural," which he does in trances induced by frenzied dancing, fasting, or the use of mind-altering plants. Often, body parts are modified as part of the ritual: penises are circumcised, noses are pierced, teeth are filed, or faces are tattooed. Without these modifications, the male is not a fully-fledged adult. Finally, the boy has to undergo an ordeal. The manner of the ordeal varies enormously from society to society, but they all have one thing in common: the boy has to show bravery worthy of a man. When he has finished, he knows in his soul that he is now a man.

In Western culture, there was, up until recent times, machinery that reflected similar processes, albeit in a much weaker form and with patchier coverage. Traditionally, these were provided by military academies, boarding schools, and various quasi-military cadet organizations. Civilian examples include the Boys' Brigade and the Boy Scouts. They all had their rituals, traditions, and ordeals. Now, the Boy Scouts have had to eliminate rough, body-contact games and, after a Supreme Court ruling, military academies are obliged to admit women. In many areas, initiation ceremonies have been driven underground and often take dysfunctional forms. Thus, clandestine university fraternity "hazings" and military initiation ordeals occasionally give rise to scandal, accusations of bullying, and even death of the initiate.

In many ways, we have dismantled male initiation rituals. We are raising a population of boy-men, in touch with their feminine side but hesitant in their masculinity. It should not be surprising, then, if some young men prefer life in a street gang or criminal activity. There, they find the excitement, danger, challenges, and combat that their souls crave. Of course, many men are able to divert their primitive instincts into ones that are more socially acceptable. For example, low-status males might find an outlet in competitive sports by becoming a star player at basketball or football. Schools used to understand this very well and made sure that every boy developed himself in competitive games; this is not necessarily the case anymore. Other men find satisfaction in intellectual pursuits, such as a fulfilling career as a doctor, journalist, or architect; these are the lucky ones. Most men still end up as bank clerks, assembly-line workers, and shop assistants. Males experience a midlife crisis when it dawns on them that they will never make it to the top—their fate is to join the ranks of the also-rans.

In our Pleistocene past, men were daily presented with opportunities to be heroic. This heroism was driven by the rewards: the admiration of the women-folk and the opportunity to win a new woman. It is a theme present throughout all folklore right up to the present day. Now, if a young man goes up to his sweetheart and says, "I want to prove myself to you, give me something dangerous to do," she is most likely to say "Don't be silly, you might get yourself killed." Most men today will live their lives never having been heroic. It is remarkable how many men now in their eighties, having led uneventful adult careers, revert to reminiscences of their youthful exploits in boot camp. It was the episode that defined their identity, just like an initiation rite, which in a way it was.

Heroism, of course, is a high-risk activity and the hero could lose his life. How did our forebears cope with the early deaths of young men? Part of the answer lies in the initiation rite. At this time, the mother experiences the brutal wrenching of her child away from her—she loses her "little boy" to the world of men and feels a sense of loss and bereavement. Today, we fight death at every turn and refuse to "go gentle into that good night."

LESSONS FOR TODAY

We have gradually built up a picture of what life must have been like for our Pleistocene forebears. The basic survival unit was the band of about 50 people, a grouping of people who were all related to each other by blood or marriage. They all socialized and supported each other and the children freely mingled among them.

Within this group, there were sub-groups, notably the family, consisting of mother and children plus father. A significant feature of the family grouping is that it is much more loosely knit than our so-called nuclear families of today. The ancient fundamental or nuclear family unit was the mother and child. This has been a special relationship down through the ages in all cultures. Fathers float-ed around in the inner circle, but were not part of the nucleus. It is to the cha-grin of many husbands when they find that, as soon as a child is born, they are no longer the center of their wife's attention, which is now focused on the baby.

As soon as the child was weaned from his mother's back, he was brought up in large part by the grandmother and other relations. The father played only a small role. In her daily life, the mother had long conversations with other mothers while foraging and with all women when back at the camp. The father was chiefly solitary while on the hunt and indulged in "man-talk" with the other men back at the camp. The husband interacted with his wife for short periods of the day, mainly to discuss factual matters and arrange the food sharing, most of which had been contributed by her.

In other words, the women mostly found their companionship with other women. The men found their companionship in their solitary communion with nature on the hunt and with the other men back at the camp. Even so, we must visualize these separate gatherings going on within the close confines of the encampment. The groups were only a few feet apart and, even if they had separate conversations, they would feel close to one another. The children would wander freely from one to the other.

This picture contrasts sharply with how Western society has evolved, in just the last 50 years. Not only today's mother but also the father are expected to be round-the-clock parenting machines. In fact, they are victims of the "Blank Slate" philosophy, bamboozled into believing that their children are amorphous lumps of putty who would stay that way unless they spend every moment of the day shaping them with constant entertainment, instruction, and "quality time." Parents are made to feel guilty for every misfortune and inadequacy that befalls their children. However, a host of studies, including those on identical twins brought up in different environments, show that they grow up with the same personalities. A parent can ensure that a child learns the piano where another does not, but as people they grow up just the same.[70] Mostly, the child's genes orchestrate how he or she turns out, even down to political affiliation and degree of religiosity.[71] In the words of cognitive scientist Steven Pinker, "All those differences among parents and homes have no predictable long-term effects on the personalities of their children. Not to put a fine point on it, but much of the advice from parenting experts is so much flapdoodle."[72]

In a similar way, there is an expectation among middle-class Western parents that they should be companions for each other. In one sense, they are: they operate as a team to ensure the survival and well-being of the genes lying in their offspring. However, in almost every other way, metaphorically speaking, men and women are from different planets. John Gray, in his book *Men Are From Mars, Women Are From Venus*, confronted head-on the doctrine that men and women should have identical drives and personalities.[73] As we have seen, they have different desires, objectives, ways of talking (and of not talking), ways of working, parenting, interests, innate talents, and physical attributes.

The relationship between husband and wife in middle-class Western society is one of the most vexed. It plainly is not working and has to be constantly maintained and repaired by a massive industry of marriage guidance coun-selors, self-help books, and talk show therapists. Many of them identify the symptoms quite accurately. However, no one outside evolutionary psychology draws the obvious conclusion: that the way we structure family life today is excruciatingly dysfunctional. It is as though we put a cat and a dog—both excel-lent creatures in their own right—into a sack and expect them to get along.

Men and women need to structure their joint lives differently. Today, we expect a man and a woman to coexist in intense proximity in a little box. How-ever, as we have seen, although a husband and wife might have concern and affection for each other, they do not make natural round-the-clock buddies. And if the reader feels we have focused more on the male predicament than the female one, this flows naturally from the state of affairs today. The Western world has become feminized to such an extent that the male qualities mentioned earlier—risk-taking, bravery, strength, aggressivity, heroism, female protection, ingenuity, hunting skills—have no place or role.

In forager society, each individual had a much higher degree of "social con-nectedness," a phrase sociologists use to describe the number and quality of links a person has with other members of the wider family. Husbands and wives had less intensity of contact with each other but a much richer and developed suite of contacts with everyone else in the band. This looser arrangement is the "natural" state.

In this chapter, we have explored the way our ancient ancestors lived their lives for eons. We have seen how many factors, such as the power of our genes, quite naturally lead to conflict in many situations and to harmony in others. This overview has brought out the major themes controlling our feelings, which in turn control the way we behave. In a great many ways, they operate at cross-purposes to the way our modern society demands. Since the farming revolution, humans, without realizing it, have been forced to pioneer new manners of liv-ing. In the process, many natural checks and balances have been removed and artificial ones have been instituted.

We have mostly avoided making formal recommendations and instead we lay out the issues for you to think about. Our society is structured with such rigidities that in many respects it is hard to change your own life within it. How-ever, examine the issues and question how they relate to your own circum-stances. You may find that you can make adjustments, subtle or otherwise, that help you get in touch with the naturally adapted heritage that makes you most comfortable.

Our evolutionary psychology illustrates how our current lives are out of sorts with our savanna-bred natures. This discord is adversely affecting our health just as our nutritional habits are. We must remember, too, that there is no going back. We have become so numerous that our prosperity and survival depend on structuring society in new, complex, and unproven ways.

9. Disease and the Bond Effect

We are fortunate that, in modern industrialized societies, a great many health scourges of the past are now a distant memory. Public health engineering, by bringing clean water and safely disposing of sewage and garbage, eradicated many diseases like cholera, typhoid, and bubonic plague. Medical science with its hygiene, antiseptics, drugs, and vaccinations brought deadly infectious diseases like smallpox, polio, tuberculosis, syphilis, and diphtheria under control. Nutritional science discovered how to eliminate deficiency diseases like scurvy, rickets, and pellagra. Surgeons learned how to cut out appendixes, amputate gangrenous limbs, and reset broken bones without killing us.

We have dealt with just about all the afflictions that nature can throw at us, so what is left? The answer is the reason for this book: self-inflicted ones. These are the diseases that were virtually unknown in prehistoric times: cancer, heart disease, diabetes, osteoporosis, arthritis, senile dementia, and many more. Most, if not all, of these "diseases of civilization" are quite avoidable. Many that have become entrenched can be abated or even cured. In all of them, our eating patterns are the major factor, although often other lifestyle factors play a role.

In our travels through this book, we have encountered many instances of how our choice of "body fuel" makes the machine run well or run badly. We looked at the type of feeding pattern that operated during the formative time of the human race in east Africa. We called it the "Savanna Model" and saw how the San still lived like that in recent history. They enjoyed enviable health and well-being, in spite of their rudimentary lifestyle in which there is an absence of both medical support and of many food groups that we think of as normal. We witnessed the radical change in dietary habits when humans first took up farming and saw how mass-marketing techniques were used to change and manipulate our feeding habits. We hinted at the kinds of diseases that humans began to suffer as a result.

In Chapter 3, we looked at the various food groups and spelled out some of the impacts on our health. Then, we reviewed the diets of various populations around the world and examined our biochemistry, digestive systems, and modern diet from a scientific point of view. We reached some conclusions about how dietary errors are making us sick. We drew up the "Owner's Manual" for the ideal food supply and eating pattern. Chapter 8 painted a picture of how our social environment diverges from our savanna-bred natures. This discord stresses us in many ways, another factor leading to ill-health.

Now, we draw all these threads together and present the material from the other side: that of specific diseases and the factors that make us vulnerable to them. Not surprisingly, there are many common factors. This reinforces the notion that adopting a lifestyle that mirrors our anciently programmed minds and bodies is the sensible way to go.

The human species is remarkable for how little its members vary genetically from each other, no matter where they live around the globe.[1] Chimpanzee populations show ten times the genetic variation that humans do. In other words, we are all still built to the same body plan and the same basic message is good for all of us. Nevertheless, there is some variation in our genetic makeup. We all have slight differences in susceptibility to disease, and our bodies have differing abilities to circumvent deficiencies in the diet. That is why, even though eating and living the same way, different people will break out in different illnesses.

This chapter is devoted to setting out our current knowledge of what aspects of our lives are helpful and what aspects are harmful for specific illnesses and what we should do about it. With regard to food, we know that there are literally tens of thousands of active compounds in the foods we eat, particularly non-starchy plant food. We can't define exactly how all these compounds work, but we know that they need to work together as a team.

We need to rid ourselves of the "magic bullet" mentality, the notion that there is a straight line from cause to effect, that for each disease there is one simple fix. On the contrary, most of our modern diseases are due to a complex interaction of many factors that are going wrong at the same time. We cannot micromanage or second-guess many of these processes. It is not good enough to cherry-pick from the menu of the Savanna Model. Ultimately, we have to nourish the body the way it was designed—with the complete package.

Finally, it is a fallacy to think that if you are sick with a modern degenerative disease, it is because it is "in your genes." Cancer, diabetes, osteoporosis, and other such diseases have been increasing alarmingly just in the last 50 years. But the genetic makeup of the population has not changed one bit in that time. The only thing that has changed is lifestyle! Some people will be genetically more vulnerable than others to certain diseases, but the vulnerability is only exposed—and expressed—when a discordant lifestyle pushes the body into failure. An extension of this fallacy is saying that a disease "runs in the family." What runs in families, apart from genes? Bad habits!

Our fate is not written in our genes—it is in our own hands. We just have to take responsibility and accept the idea of changing our habits. Note that putting your lifestyle right is not necessarily a substitute for medical treatment once you have got a disorder. However, by doing so, you will ensure that the medical treatment has the best chance of success.

CANCER

What causes cancer? Smoking? Sunlight? Radiation? Pesticides? Barbecued meat? Microwaves? These are some of the answers likely to be given by the average citizen, yet he or she would be wrong. All these have strong links to cancer, but they cannot be the root cause. Much of the population is exposed to these carcinogens, yet only a small minority actually suffers dangerous tumors as a consequence.[2]

You are probably aware that our bodies are made of trillions of cells. As a rule of thumb, a normal adult is considered to be made up of something like 30 trillion cells. They are the basic building units of living bodies. Some creatures, like bacteria, consist of just one cell. Cells are where a myriad of chemical reactions take place, where energy is generated, and, above all, where our genes are located. Just about every cell has a full copy of our genetic blueprint, the DNA.

Most cells either are damaged or wear out as time goes by. When this happens, they are programmed to die. Their life span depends on where they are in the body. It can be as little as a few days—the cells lining the colon are such a case. Red blood cells have a life span of four months; the tendon cells can live for as long as several years. To replace cells that die, living cells divide themselves into identical copies under instruction from nearby cells. That means carefully making a duplicate of every single piece of machinery in the cell, including the DNA and each strand of DNA is composed of over 10 million molecules. Ideally, all this copying takes place without a mistake.

Not surprisingly, something goes wrong from time to time: a cell does not self-destruct when it is supposed to and becomes immortal; a cell keeps dividing itself uncontrollably; or things go wrong with the copying process and rogue DNA is created. Sometimes these things happen all at once, and then we have the makings of a cancer cell. Such cells mean trouble, but there is worse to come. A small percentage of such cells have the diabolic ability to detach themselves from where they are, float around the body, and put down roots elsewhere. In this way, they spread seeds of cancer into every part of the body.

The 30 trillion cells must cooperate with each other to keep a human being healthy over the course of a lifetime. Because of the huge numbers involved, there are bound to be a few cells going cancerous every day; we are even born with precancerous cells. Why is it, then, that we don't all die of cancer at an early age? The chief answer is that the evolutionary mechanism has evolved a battery of defenses that fight cancer cells at every turn. These defenses are collectively known as the immune system.

The Immune System—An Overview

The immune system comprises many components working together. White blood cells known as phagocytes gobble up and kill offending cells by digesting them. T-cells and B-cells are known as "killer cells," which reside in the lymphatic system and bloodstream. They lock on to enemy cells and kill them by making them commit suicide. For all this to work properly, the immune system has to recognize which cells are legitimate and which ones are enemy. Alarms and signals must pass correctly between different elements of the immune system. The lymphatic system and bloodstream must pump these immune system cells quickly to the place where they are needed.

The immune system is an incredibly complex arrangement of parts. It can recognize and remember millions of different enemies, and it can produce secretions and cells to wipe out every one of them. The secret to its success is an elaborate and dynamic communications network. Millions of cells gather like clouds of bees swarming around a honey pot and pass information back and forth.[3] They must work together as a team for it to be 100% efficient.

Here is the essential thought to remember: the way we live our lives today depresses the efficiency of the immune system. In addition, lifestyle errors often cause it to go berserk—it attacks friendly cells and ignores enemy ones. Finally, by "living dirty," we often overload the immune system with too many tasks. We will find many instances of how our weakened, raggle-taggle, overworked immune systems allow disease to take hold. And sometimes our deranged immune systems actually cause disease.

The root cause of cancer is not, then, the various provocative factors (tobacco, radiation, pesticides, etc.), but rather a failure of the immune system. It is this lowering of the defenses that allows cancer to flourish and take hold. When that happens, conventional medicine takes over.

In spite of the hundreds of billions of dollars thrown into the "war on cancer" since the 1970s, progress has been slow. The chief tools are still the same: cut it out, poison it with chemotherapy, or nuke it with radiation. Certainly the techniques have become more targeted and sophisticated and success rates have climbed. There is more focus on detecting cancers early, so that these techniques have a better chance of winning out. Unfortunately, the outlook is often grim for cancers that have spread to other areas of the body (metastasized). In the United States, by the time they are discovered, 72% of lung cancers, 57% of colorectal cancers, and 34% of breast cancers have metastasized.[4]

Until recently, conventional medicine has not paid a lot of attention to repairing the defenses, let alone mobilizing the body's remarkable powers of self-repair. Often, cancer patients receive no nutritional or lifestyle advice. Such patients should ask themselves the question: "If I got cancer doing what I was doing before, what should I do differently now?" We would all agree that it would be best if people lived their lives so that their defenses against cancer are invasion-proof. If cancer has taken hold, it is even more important to repair the defenses and keep them that way.

There are three main weaknesses that can arise with the immune system. Two of them, depressed immune system and overloaded immune system, are particularly responsible for allowing cancers to flourish. The way we live often depresses and overloads our immune systems. By correcting these departures from the Savanna Model, we will give ourselves the best chance to avoid cancer and to recover from it.

Cancer Avoidance and Recovery

Strategy 1 Eat a Strictly Low-Glycemic Diet

The way we eat today drives blood sugar and insulin to abnormal, unhealthy levels. This is a common phenomenon: it is estimated that 90% of Americans and 75% of Europeans suffer from it, even though they do not feel it. However, those high insulin levels depress the immune system and allow cancerous growths to flourish. This is the first way in which the Western, high-glycemic diet is a culprit in the cancer epidemic.

The second consequence of a high-glycemic diet is more direct. Let me illustrate it with this example. When doctors want to highlight a cancer on an x-ray, they inject you with glucose. The cancerous cells gorge themselves on the sugar and they light up like a Christmas tree on the x-ray negatives. Cancers need food to survive—and the best food is a rich supply of blood sugar. In the West, we unwittingly oblige by gorging ourselves, and all those pre-cancerous cells in us, on a high-starch, high-sugar diet. By following the Savanna Model feeding pattern, the diet is automatically low glycemic, one that naturally starves cancers of nutrients and avoids undermining the immune system.

Strategy 2 Maintain a Low Percentage of Body Fat

We saw in Chapter 1 that cancer is absent from the San Bushman. Moreover, on the height-weight criterion, they have a low body-mass index (BMI), which averages around 19. This is considered to be at the low end of the "healthy" range in the West. In contrast, everything we know about being overweight tells us that it increases dramatically the risk of cancer. In fact, being slightly thinner than "normal" (like the San) is even better. Body mass index is a rather crude rule of thumb, which takes no account of stocky or slender build or degree of muscularity. The really important criterion is the percentage of body fat. The San, with their low BMI of 19, have a body fat percentage of around 10%. Westerners do not need to get that low, but they should aim for a maximum of 15% for men and 20% for women. It is also important to keep up lean muscle mass.

Strategy 3   Eat a Diet Rich in Non-Starchy Plant Food

Most people's bodies are starved for micronutrients. Non-starchy plant food is where all those tens of thousands of essential immune system–nourishing molecules come from. Thousands of studies confirm the beneficial effect that consumption of various fruits, salads, and vegetables has on cancer prevention and cure. Even the residues from plant food that arrive in the colon have their part to play: the "good" bacteria grow on them and feed the immune system with compounds called short-chain fatty acids (SCFAs), such as butyrate and propionic acid. These are absorbed through the colon into the bloodstream, where they act to depress cancer cell proliferation. There is a bonus—these SCFAs are also potent "bad" bacteria killers, cleaning up the colon from infection.

Strategy 4   Eat a Low-Fat Diet with Essential Fatty Acids in Balance

The Japanese have the lowest incidence of cancer in the industrialized world. This is due in part to their traditional, very low-fat diet—less than 10% of calories. A low-fat diet is cancer fighting. Furthermore, thanks to the absence of dairy products and animal meat in their traditional diet, their intake of "bad" saturated fats is minimal. Many studies have shown that saturated fats, particularly hydrogenated and trans-fats, are powerful immune depressors, allowing cancers to flourish. Finally, the traditional consumption of oily fish provides them with the "good" omega-3 oils. We are unwittingly depressing our immune system with a diet overloaded with omega-6 oils. Drive these out of your diet and favor the omega-3 oils at every opportunity. But don't go too far. The ideal is a 1-to-1 balance, but you don't have to micromanage it—just follow the Savanna Model and the ratio works out just fine.

Strategy 5   Good Colon Health

In Chapter 5, we emphasized how the colon, together with its contents of flora, should be functioning as a vital organ, contributing to the body's healthy operation. The way we eat today does the opposite: it leaves us with rotten colon health. The residues of the food we have eaten are the wrong kind: they nourish "bad" bacteria, yeasts, and funguses. Some kinds of foods destroy the intestinal villi, the incredibly fine hairs that absorb vital nutrients into the bloodstream. Some irritate the stem cells in the colon lining to the point where they become cancerous. Poor combinations of foods (for example, hamburger and bun) deliver poorly digested particles to the colon, where more bad flora feed on them. The immune system is designed to receive nourishment from a well-functioning colon that produces the vital compounds it needs to combat cancer. When they are missing, its efficiency is undermined.

The coup de grace is given by bad bacteria and the antinutrients found in cereals, pulses, and dairy that make the colon "leaky." Bad bacteria, yeasts, funguses, and even tiny food particles flood into the bloodstream. This is a major challenge to the immune system, which has enough to do fighting off infections and dealing with cancerous cells. When it is overwhelmed, it releases its grip on cancer cells, allowing them to slip through its defenses.

Strategy 6 Physical Activity

Physical activity plays an essential role in maintaining many kinds of body functions. In our ancestral past, a certain level of exercise was, by force of circumstances, occurring day in and day out. The human organism came to depend on it. One of these activities is to pump the circulation of the lymphatic system. Without physical activity, lymph does not circulate, it stagnates. That is bad because the lymphatic system plays an essential role in delivering the immune system's heavy artillery to the battle front (and carrying away the debris). This is one important, often neglected, aspect of physical activity. Exercise every day, just as happened quite naturally in the daily lives of our ancient ancestors.

Strategy 7 Get Enough Sunshine

In the human homeland, our ancestors were naked and exposed all day to the tropical sun. The San still live that way. Of course, their skin tone (copper color) is particularly adapted to that way of living. Skin color is one of the most obvious ways in which humans vary around the world. As humans spread to less sunny areas, their skin color became lighter, even white. It was necessary to absorb sunlight more readily, particularly as a large percentage of the body had to be covered with clothes. Avoiding sunlight is another unsuspected way we undermine our immune system.

We have overcompensated for fears of skin cancer by staying indoors too much! In a recent study, women who lived in the sunniest parts of the United States had three times less risk of breast cancer compared to those who lived in gloomy, overcast regions.[5] In another study, men who had the most exposure to sunlight had the least risk of developing aggressive prostate cancer later in life.[6] Other research shows that adults with good levels of vitamin D have half the risk of colon cancer.[7] Recent studies reinforce the message: sunshine helps melanoma sufferers recover and it prevents people getting lymphatic cancer.[8] Dr. William Grant estimates the yearly toll at 100,000 cases and 40,000 deaths from lack-of-sunshine cancers.[9] This is four times the mortality from skin cancer.

One big reason is that people living in gloomy parts of the world are starved of the vital immune system food, vitamin D, sometimes called the sunshine vitamin. People living in sunny areas were producing much higher levels of vitamin D under the influence of sunlight. We don't need much vitamin D—just 10 to 20 micrograms per day. It is toxic in large quantities. The body sorts this out just fine if the chief source is sunshine. The trick is to get sunlight regularly but avoid burning. A second reason is that sunlight regulates production of hormones such as melatonin and cortisol. When they are not being secreted in the right patterns, the immune system is depressed.

Strategy 8   Reduce Chronic Stress

The folkloric idea that major life stressors, such as divorce, death of a child, or loss of a job, can trigger cancer has yet to be proved. However, an unremitting level of background stress does depress the immune system, making us vulnerable not only to cancer but a wide range of diseases.[10]

Put another way, we have a stress response designed for the kinds of problems that occurred in savanna life. Most of the time our ancestors were living in harmony with their surroundings, so the stress response was only triggered in short bursts at irregular intervals. Our lives now are a continuous source of mental pressure. Stanford neuroscientist Robert Sapolsky observes, "Stress-related disease emerges, predominantly, out of the fact that we so often activate a physiological system that has evolved for responding to acute physical emergencies, but we turn it on for months on end, worrying about mortgages, relationships, and promotions."[11] It is certainly a challenge to restructure our lives so as to limit this level of background or "chronic" stress, but do it we must.

Breast Cancer

Everything said about cancer in general applies to breast cancer in particular. Nevertheless, there are some special considerations. "We are what we eat" might be a cliché, but it is particularly apt for women's breasts. A woman who eats a lot of saturated fats and trans-fatty acids (hydrogenated fats) has more of those bad fats stored in her breasts. Such women are at a higher risk of developing breast cancer.[12] Those who have good levels of the omega-3 oils, whether fish oils or alpha-linolenic acid (ALA), have a lower risk.[13]

Breast cancers mostly develop from milk-producing cells in the breasts that are stimulated to divide by estrogen. This stimulation occurs through a molecule on their surface called an "estrogen receptor." The purpose is to multiply milk cells every month in preparation for a possible pregnancy. However, the more estrogen receptors there are, the more likely something will go wrong in a cell and it will multiply out of control. What agent might do this? A major one is the powerful hormone insulin. Abnormally high insulin levels increase the number of estrogen receptors in the breast by a factor of 12.[14] With 12 times the number of receptors, there are 12 times as many chances that one of the milk-producing cells will become cancerous. This is another way in which the high-glycemic Western diet particularly encourages breast cancer.

A second factor is the lifetime exposure of a woman's breasts to estrogen. Today, girls are arriving at puberty much earlier than nature intended. Their breasts are exposed to estrogen for a longer period, so they are more likely to develop breast cancer later in life. A girl who starts menstruating at age 10 has three times the risk of breast cancer compared to starting at 15.[15] On the other hand, menopause around 50 is quite normal. Nevertheless, the same mechanism is at work: menopause at 55 doubles the risk of cancer compared to menopause at 45 and triples it compared to menopause at 35.

Why is it that girls' periods start earlier these days? Obesity, a high-fat diet, a high-glycemic diet, and a diet rich in dairy and soy products are all factors driving their bodies in this unhealthy direction. Soy products can also promote breast cancer directly.[16]

In another twist, women who have children, who have children early and/or have many children, and who breastfeed all have a reduced risk of breast cancer.[17] There are many complex hormonal operations that science has yet to unravel and understand, but it all comes back to estrogen, progesterone, and other sex hormones. In our ancestral past, women were breastfeeding almost continuously for some 30 years while they were fertile. We might suppose that the body depends on this format to function properly. It is tough to emulate this pattern in today's world. Nevertheless, it is one more strong argument for breastfeeding and doing it for as long as possible.

Finally, breast cancer is practically unknown outside the West. You don't even have to clamber over the Himalayas or the Andes to find peoples who live free of breast cancer. Take a comfortable plane to Tokyo, Singapore, or Hong Kong and you will immediately be among peoples who live longer than Westerners do and whose women do not suffer from breast cancer. Their secret? Traditionally, they have very low-fat, low-glycemic diets. That might not last for much longer: the Japanese diet is becoming Westernized, and the rates of breast cancer are rising.

Lung Cancer

Lung cancer is entirely due to smoking, right? Wrong—many people who have never smoked get lung cancer, and many smokers never get it. The Japanese are one of the heaviest smoking populations in the world—and yet one of the longest lived. Japanese longevity is not due to smoking but in spite of it. But they get away with smoking because their diet, while not perfect, is a lot better than the one that is common in the West. In other words, the Japanese diet, turns out to be closer to the ideal diet for the human species than what is eaten elsewhere. Their focus on fish (which contains omega-3 oils) instead of meat is beneficial.[18] In general, researchers find that the micronutrient connection is critical.[19] People who have a high consumption of non-starchy plant food are much less likely to get lung cancer, whether or not they are smokers.

Colon Cancer

With approximately 135,000 new cases reported each year, colon cancer is the third most commonly diagnosed cancer in the United States, and it is one of the leading causes of cancer-related deaths. Studies have shown that a variety of diet and behavioral modifications reduce colon cancer risk in the general population.

It is hardly surprising that what you put into your mouth can have dramatic effects on what happens at the far end of the digestive tract. You don't even have to eat like a primitive tribesman to avoid colon cancer. It is virtually unknown among many societies such as the Japanese and Chinese. Some of the causes are really surprising—who would have thought that high insulin levels might be a factor? But they are.[20] So, too, are high-fat diets, the consumption of saturated fats and trans-fats, and diets that are dominant in omega-6 oils.[21]

Of course, the remarks about colon health (Strategy 5) have a direct bearing on colon cancer. Not only does poor colon health contribute to cancers developing in other parts of the body, it contributes directly to cancer developing in the colon itself.

Prostate Cancer

Asian men have much lower rates of prostate cancer than Western men.[22] The same factors that are good for suppressing cancer in general, work well on the prostate too. The Asian diet, low in animal fat and dairy, high in omega-3 oils, and rich in non-starchy plant food is good.[23] In contrast, a high intake of omega-6 oils encourages prostate cancer.[24]

Abnormal testosterone production is a major risk factor for prostate cancer. Some compounds, such as lignans, lock up testosterone and stop it from creating damage. Lignans are a kind of plant fiber. The highest concentrations of lignans are found in flaxseed, followed by squash, broccoli, carrots, and asparagus. Studies on flaxseed, which also contain high levels of omega-3 oils and fiber, show that they are indeed great cancer fighters.[25]

Sunshine is also protective. Dr. Esther John found that men who had received the most sunshine during a lifetime were 50% less likely to develop prostate cancer than those who received the least.[26] Ejaculation is good, according to research by Dr. Graham Giles. The more often men ejaculate, between the ages of 20 and 50, the less likely they are to develop prostate cancer; the greatest protective effect is for a man in his twenties.[27] Dr. Giles speculates that frequent ejaculation keeps carcinogens from accumulating in the prostate gland.

CARDIOVASCULAR DISEASE

Heart disease, atherosclerosis, thrombosis, strokes, and high blood pressure—this cluster of diseases has only become common in recent times, and chiefly in Western, industrial societies.[28] They were unknown among primitive tribes, such as the Australian Aborigines, the Tarahumara hill tribe of Mexico, the Eskimos, and the San Bushman.[29] Studies on tribes such as the Vilcabamba of the Andes and the Tarahumara of Mexico show that they have low blood pressure and an extremely low incidence of cardiovascular disease. Rarely does their blood pressure exceed 130/75, even among centenarians, and they have 13 times the rate of centenarians as America.[30] As recently as the 1930s, heart disease was rare in America.[31] Even today, Okinawans and Cretans do not suffer these diseases. As far as we can tell, they were unknown amongst our Pleistocene forebears.

What is at the root of these illnesses? Heart disease is any disorder that affects the heart's ability to function normally. The most common cause of heart disease is narrowing or blockage of the coronary arteries, which supply blood to the heart itself. This happens slowly over time. Arteries start to block when they are inflamed. This process, known as atherosclerosis ("hardening of the arteries") can happen anywhere in the body, including the brain. Special white blood cells called macrophages respond to this inflammation by rushing in to help "clean up" the damage. However, in doing so they also damage the artery walls, which in turn become ideal sites for fatty plaque to accumulate. Repetition of this cycle narrows arteries and raises the potential for clots, heart attack, and stroke.

Sometimes, under abnormal conditions, blood coagulates and forms a clot in a blood vessel. This is not supposed to happen, but when it does it is called a thrombosis. The consequences are serious: the clot blocks the blood supply to the affected part and can cause it to die. When a thrombosis occurs in the brain, it is called a stroke; in the lung, it is a pulmonary embolism; in an artery supplying the heart, it is a heart attack.

Aspirin and Heart Disease

Various studies have demonstrated that aspirin quenches many of the "bad" prostaglandins. This remarkable result led doctors to recommend that cardiac patients should take an aspirin a day as a preventative measure. And it works: heart attacks can be reduced by up to 40% in vulnerable patients. So, doctors started recommending that even perfectly healthy people should regularly take aspirin "just in case."

However, there is no such thing as a free lunch. Aspirin works by knocking out all prostaglandins, both good and bad. Blood may then clot poorly (giving rise to internal bleeding) and stomach acidity is disrupted (leading to ulcers). Over the longer term, the immune system is depressed and sensitivity to allergies is increased. In fact, aspirin, while fulfilling a great role for emergency relief, does not deal with the fundamental problems. The good news is, we have the ideal drug right in front of us: our food. Get that right and the fundamental problems disappear.

High blood pressure can occur for several reasons. When arteries become blocked, the heart has to pump harder. For example, kidneys, to filter blood properly, need to have a decent pressure across the filters. Loss of pressure can occur if the arteries in the kidney are partly blocked by atherosclerosis; it then sends signals to the heart to pump harder. In another example, the body can secrete hormones that cause blood vessels to constrict, which causes the heart to pump harder to maintain flow. Similar hormones may cause the blood to be thicker than normal and again the heart has to pump harder. The result is that the heart has to step up the pressure to force the blood to flow where it is needed—hence, high blood pressure.

What causes blood to thicken and clot abnormally, blood vessels to constrict, and arteries to become inflamed? There are several factors, almost all of them dietary. Overconsumption of omega-6 oils such as sunflower oil, peanut oil, and corn oil produce "bad" prostaglandins that increase blood clotting, blood pressure, and inflammation, clogging arteries with plaque. These hormones also encourage the liver to overproduce cholesterol and stimulate the pancreas to overproduce insulin. Right here we have one reason why heart disease only became common since the 1930s: these vegetable oils only became abundant after World War II. In contrast, the omega-3 oils produce "good" prostaglandins that do the opposite: decrease blood pressure, decrease coagulation, decrease inflammation, and reduce plaque.[32]

A second powerful effect is provided by the hormone insulin, which is produced in abnormal quantities by a high-glycemic diet. Insulin acts in ways that provoke the overproduction of similar blood clotting and blood pressure factors.[33] Insulin itself inflames the artery walls directly. In other words, foods that are glycemic and/or insulinemic—and combinations of such foods—are part of the problem. This means that the principle culprits are starches like grains and potatoes, sugars, and insulinemic foods like yogurt and potato.

Some saturated fats also inflame arteries. The chief perpetrators are myristic acid and palmitic acid, which are the kinds of fats found in dairy products, tropical oils (like palm oil), and red meats (beef, pork and lamb). That is why all nutritional professionals say we should avoid them. But there are worse: the artificial saturated fats called hydrogenated and trans-fats are even more harmful to the arteries. The American Institute of Medicine states that the only safe level of trans-fat is zero.[34] Trans-fats and hydrogenated fats are found in vegetable shortening, margarine, potato chips, crackers, doughnuts, cookies, fried foods, cakes, pies, and pizzas.

A high-salt diet is not helpful. Salt, just by being in the bloodstream in abnormal amounts, damages arteries.[35] For a high percentage of the population, salt also raises blood pressure. It is significant that strokes are the biggest killer in Japan. Japanese smoking and high salt intake (from soy sauce) have something to do with it. In contrast, high blood pressure yields well to a high plant-food diet.[36]

The story on artery damage is not yet finished: where proteins come from is also significant. Animal protein is potentially atherogenic (artery damaging) and milk proteins, notably the casein in cheese, particularly so.[37] How can this be? After all, we are naturally adapted to consuming animal proteins, albeit in modest proportions. The answer lies with a waste product from animal protein digestion called homocysteine. Homocysteine, if it is not swept up quickly by the body, does a lot of damage to arteries. The naturally adapted "sweepers" are micronutrients readily found in non-starchy plant food. Fruits, salads, and vegetables are the natural—and essential—companions to the consumption of animal matter.[38]

Proteins, Amino Acids, and Homocysteine

Proteins are composed of a cocktail of compounds called amino acids. The composition of the cocktail varies with the foodstuff. Eight of these amino acids are essential: the body must obtain them from food. One of these essential amino acids is called methionine. When methionine is digested, it produces a toxic waste product called homocysteine. Proteins of animal origin tend to contain much more methionine than proteins of plant origin. Compared to plant proteins, animal proteins, therefore, produce a higher toxic load of homocysteine.

Research also shows that blood pressure, on average, increases the further one lives from the equator. The evidence suggests that it is the lack of sunshine that causes the problem. More precisely, it is the absence of the sunshine vitamin, vitamin D.[39] Get enough sunshine, you make enough vitamin D and reduce your blood pressure.

How reversible are these diseases? That depends. The main objective has to be to stop the rot. The risk of strokes and thrombosis can be quickly reduced by changing dietary habits. Thromboxane, the prostaglandin chiefly responsible for abnormal blood clotting, is reduced almost overnight by cutting bad fats. High blood pressure is brought down to a greater or lesser degree over a few months. It is even possible to reverse atherosclerosis both by eating plenty of plant food and by losing any excess weight.[40]

The Role of Cholesterol

Cholesterol levels of hunter-gatherers are low. Stuart Truswell and John Hansen found that the San Bushmen have one of the lowest cholesterol levels in the world.[42] Total cholesterol levels for all age groups (including old people) are around 120 mg/dl. Other researchers found that African Pygmies (110 mg/dl),

Australian Aborigines (140 mg/dl), and Tanzanian Hadza (110 mg/dl) all have total cholesterol levels in the same ballpark.[43]

Cholesterol comes in several varieties. Two of them, low-density lipoproteins (LDL) and very low-density lipoproteins (VLDL) are dubbed "bad" cholesterol and high-density lipoproteins (HDL) are dubbed "good" cholesterol. Bad cholesterol has been portrayed as the Darth Vader to our arteries and our heart, but what does it do? It fell under suspicion because inflammatory particles of oxidized cholesterol build up in the arteries to create the dreaded plaque. However, the real question should be: "Why is the body causing cholesterol to oxidize, and why is it allowing it to settle in arteries?"

Our internal plumbing is not like boiler pipes that passively fur up. Rather, our arteries are made of living tissue that inflames, scars, produces hormones, and sends signals to other parts of the body. Why do the cells that line our arteries decide to capture cholesterol molecules, allow them to oxidize, and allow them to build into plaque?

The answer seems to be that immune system cells, the macrophages, which have been summoned to repair artery damage, latch on to the cholesterol particles and try to pull them through the artery wall where they get stuck. With the passage of time, the cholesterol particles oxidize and create inflammation, and so the inflammation and the cycle starts all over again. So, the problem is not the cholesterol as such, it is the problem of previous damage to the artery wall. Even so, all need not be lost if the cholesterol does not oxidize. This is the case for those who consume sufficient quantities of oxidation fighters, antioxidants, which are found almost entirely in non-starchy vegetation.

Erectile Dysfunction (Impotence)

As Shakespeare's drunken porter in Macbeth said about strong drink: "It provokes, and it unprovokes; it provokes the desire but it takes away the performance." We might suppose that the porter recovered his powers when he sobered up. However, for many men, sexual performance is a constant source of difficulty.

There are several reasons why this might be, but one biological reason is fundamental. If the artery in the penis has blockages, it cannot rise to the occasion. The blockages, of course, are of the same nature as blockages in arteries elsewhere in the body: in the heart, lungs, and brain. The phrase applied to this condition, "hardening of the arteries," seems like a bad joke in this context. In other words, erectile dysfunction is very often a symptom of cardiovascular disease. The linkage is so strong that researchers say that erectile dysfunction is the earliest predictor of looming cardiovascular trouble.[41] For erectile dysfunction, then, the wisest and most urgent course is to follow the guidelines for cardiovascular disease.

The conventional view is that heart disease would be reduced if people had lower levels of cholesterol circulating in the blood. In a crude way, this is true: with less of the stuff to be trapped and oxidized, the slower the buildup of inflamed plaque. But lowering cholesterol by itself does not deal with the fundamental problem: inflammation. In fact, the links between cholesterol levels and heart disease are rather weak, but they are much stronger with homocysteine. This is not surprising, since homocysteine is a strong provoker of inflammation.

Nevertheless, we might ask ourselves why modern Western populations have such high levels of cholesterol. The basic answer is that our bodies make it in abnormal amounts as a reaction to dietary errors. The chief one is the abnormally high level of insulin, which provokes the liver into making abnormal amounts of cholesterol—yet another wickedness perpetrated by a high-glycemic, high-insulinemic diet.

In contrast, bad cholesterol is reduced by a diet rich in soluble fiber.[44] This is something that most Westerners do not have, yet which our bodies expect to receive. Other studies show that exercise reduces cholesterol levels. And stress, by provoking hormones like cortisol and adrenaline, has the side effect of raising cholesterol levels. In complex biological organisms, everything is interconnected in ways that we cannot imagine.

Contrary to the prevalent myth, consuming high-cholesterol foods like eggs has little effect on cholesterol levels, if the diet conforms to the Savanna Model.[45] As Paleolithic expert Boyd Eaton observes, the San Bushmen consumed just as much cholesterol as the average American, yet they maintained very low levels of cholesterol in the blood.[46] The message is the same: give the body the right tools and signals, and it sorts out these matters just fine.

So, high cholesterol levels are simply a pointer to possible cardiovascular disease. Reducing them with medication, in spite of the promotional hype, has little effect on your chances of dying of a heart attack.[47] Worse, medications increase your chances of getting depression, suicidal tendencies, cancer, and stroke. Pfizer, the maker of Lipitor, the most common cholesterol drug, states: "The patient should be put on a cholesterol-lowering diet before receiving Lipitor."[48] These medications work by blocking the liver from making cholesterol. So, what they are really doing is papering over the cracks caused by dysfunctional, insulin-producing diets.

Twelve Ways to Combat Cardiovascular Disease

1. Adopt a low-glycemic diet.
2. Consume a diet rich in non-starchy plant foods.
3. Consume animal protein only modestly.
4. Avoid dairy products.
5. Consume a diet low in animal fat and palm oil.

6. Adopt a diet that eliminates hydrogenated and trans-fats.

7. Consume a diet that severely limits omega-6 oils.

8. Consume a diet rich in omega-3 oils.

9. Stop smoking.

10. Reduce salt intake to a minimum.

11. Practice at least the minimum amount of physical activity.

12. Change the way you lead your life to make it less stressful.

We have seen that cardiovascular disease is a phenomenon that has hit us just in living memory. The causes are easily identifiable and easily put right. Take control of your life in the way nature intended and put behind you concerns of ever developing heart disease. If you already have it, you can bring it under control—it is reversible! Regarding the "noble savage," who has perfect cardiovascular signs, how does he live? A lifestyle conforming to the Savanna Model in terms of diet, social environment, and physical activity. He eats plenty of non-starchy plant food and little bad protein, no bad fat, no bad carbohydrates, no sugars or grains, no potatoes, and no dairy products.

DIGESTIVE PROBLEMS

Indigestion

There used to be a TV commercial in which a New York cab driver suddenly hunches over and clutches his stomach in pain. "Aw, gee!" he gasps, "It must have been that pastrami sandwich." So, what does he do? He reaches over to the glove compartment where he keeps a bottle of pills. This little sketch neatly encapsulates many things that are wrong with us today. Indigestion is a huge problem in the West, particularly America. Indigestion remedies are the biggest selling class of over-the-counter medications. As illustrated in the commercial, people have become so accustomed to indigestion that they keep bottles of pills available for every occasion. However, like the cab driver, no one stops to think about what they must be doing wrong. It didn't even occur to the cab driver to stop eating pastrami sandwiches!

One of the major causes of indigestion is bad food combining. The cab driver, with his pastrami sandwich, had just eaten a bad food combination, protein with starch. Other bad combinations are dairy all by itself or with anything else, and fruit with anything. In the Savanna Model, bad food combining cannot really happen, because we are not consuming the food groups that give us problems: starches, dairy, and sugary fruit. Most people find they get immediate relief when they cease bad food combining. Other causes of indigestion are more obvious ones: eating too much, eating too late at night, eating on the run, alcohol abuse, and stress.

Constipation and Diverticulosis

Over-the-counter constipation remedies follow closely after indigestion tablets in popularity, yet constipation is not a normal thing to be happening. Primitive societies consume up to 100 grams (g) of fiber a day from vegetation and fruits. Their intestines were healthy and they never suffered from intestinal diseases. The average American consumes only 11 g of fiber per day. Don't be sidetracked into eating bran products. Bran is abrasive and not at all what the intestinal tract is designed for. On the contrary, our Pleistocene past designed it for the "soft" soluble fibers like pectin and guar that are found in non-starchy plant food.

Again, the solution is extraordinarily simple. Follow the Savanna Model and consume high volumes of non-starchy plant food, up to 15 servings a day. This is not only best way to get regularity back to normal, but it is also best for colon health. No one will develop diverticulosis doing that either. If you already have it, this is the best remedy to get it under control and into remission.

A cautionary note: most people's digestive tracts have been hardened into working only when whipped into action by harsh, insoluble fibers, so shift the emphasis to the soft fibers over a period of several weeks. Give the intestinal muscles time to respond to the subtler signals and time to find their natural tone again.

Inflammatory Bowel Diseases
(Irritable Bowel, Crohn's Disease, Colitis, Celiac Disease)

Medical science struggles with "syndromes" like inflammatory bowel disease because it is missing an essential piece of the puzzle, a proper knowledge of nutrition. That is where other branches of science (like ours) come in. We know how the modern diet puts immense stress on the digestive tract and why the large bowel (colon) often gives way.

Antinutrient Connection. The main error is the consumption of grains, dairy products, and pulses. The human digestive tract cannot handle their content of allergens (such as gluten and lactose) and plant poisons (such as lectins). They inflame the gut, strip the delicate lining raw, and encourage bad bacteria, their toxins, and funguses.

Bad Food Combining Connection. Bad combinations of foods add to the misery. Starch and protein combinations are particularly harmful: not only do they feed inflammatory bacteria, the insulin reaction provokes wrenching gut spasms (digestive neuromuscular disease). The modern diet is also loaded with sulfides, often used as a preservative. Sulfides encourage overgrowth of "bad" sulfate-eating bacteria in the colon, which in turn provoke inflammatory bowel diseases. Not surprisingly, hot spices irritate the colon, so you should avoid chili, paprika, and cayenne pepper.

Allergen Connection. Celiac disease is a clear case of an allergic reaction to gluten. Humans should not be putting gluten into their bodies because, whether or not they notice any reaction, damage is being done anyway. The remedy is straightforward: eliminate grains and all their derivatives, just as in the Savanna Model.

Sunshine Connection. The incidence of inflammatory bowel is rare near the equator, where ultraviolet light from the sun is intense and people produce abundant vitamin D. Dr. Margherita Cantorna of Pennsylvania State University tested the effect of vitamin D on inflammatory bowel disease and found that symptoms diminish or disappear with an adequate supply of vitamin D.[49]

Plant Food Connection. A diet rich in the soluble fiber found in plant food is soothing and beneficial for inflammatory bowel. This is the kind of material that nature designed our colons to work on.

Gastroesophageal Reflux Disease (Heartburn, Acid Reflux)

Heartburn occurs when stomach acid flows back into the esophagus and, quite literally, burns it. Heartburn affects a quarter of the population, representing a terrible burden of suffering, particularly because eliminating the cause is so easy. When put on the Savanna Model, I have seen some heartburn sufferers experience relief overnight. When gastroenterologists have tried it in their own practice, they too have found excellent results.[50] The chief decisive factors are good food combining and the absence of dairy products.

Researchers have identified other risk factors for heartburn, such as the consumption of hot spices like chili, cayenne, and paprika. Another study found higher risks of heartburn in obese people. The same study found that those who drank one or more carbonated soft drinks a day increased their risk of developing heartburn at night by almost a third, compared to patients who stayed away from them.[51]

IMMUNE SYSTEM DYSFUNCTION

Sometimes the immune system goes berserk and actually causes disease. This happens when the immune system launches an attack when it should not. There are two types of target for such "rogue" attacks: foreign particles originating from outside the body and internal body tissues.

The immune system has a subtle job to do in deciding quickly whether or not to attack a foreign particle. A healthy immune system is extraordinarily good at this and rarely makes a mistake. However, a poorly tuned immune system often fails to recognize which particles are friendly (like many food proteins) and which are "enemy" (like viruses and bacteria). When it makes a mistake like this, the response is called an allergy and the foreign material is referred to as an allergen. Instead of ignoring the harmless foreign particles, the immune system unleashes its counterattack of inflammation, swelling, and mucus secretion. We perceive this inappropriate response as various ailments such as allergies and asthma (or "allergen diseases").

Rogue attacks on the body's own tissues occur when the immune system fails to recognize its own body cells as "self" and launches an attack on various parts of the body. Killer T-cells, when they forget who hired them, attack innocent cells with friendly fire. We perceive the destruction as various ailments such as arthritis and multiple sclerosis (or "autoimmune diseases").

Allergen Diseases

What causes an allergen disease? Pollen? Cat dander? Shellfish? Peanuts? These are some of the answers likely to be given by the average person, yet he or she would be wrong. All of these substances certainly have strong links to allergic reaction. Indeed, allergy counselors would add milk, soy, and wheat to the list.[52] However these cannot be root causes. If so, everyone would suffer from allergen disease. The root problem is not the triggers (pollen, peanuts, etc.), but a failure of the body's defenses, the immune system.

Of course, you need to pay attention to the triggers, but you should not be sidetracked into thinking they are all-important. The chief priority is to restore sanity to the deranged immune system. Allergen disease is a disease of modern industrial societies for similar reasons that cancer has become much more common.

Usually, the sufferer is sensitive to quite a few allergens and the allergy only breaks out when several of them have accumulated. Then, it is the last one that gets the blame. Even worse, often the reaction can be delayed up to 24 hours after exposure. The average sufferer has no way of making the link between the trigger and the onset of the allergic reaction. That is why it is difficult to isolate the culprit: there are many of them and the exposure from day to day will be in a different order. Many of these complications are removed when we eat in conformity with the Savanna Model. As soon as we stop eating grains, dairy, and legumes, we remove a massive burden of allergy triggers.

Many of our dietary errors aggravate allergy symptoms such as inflammation, swelling, and mucus production. The first error is an overconsumption of omega-6 oils, which produce "bad" prostaglandins that instruct cells to inflame, swell, and secrete mucus. They also increase histamine production. In contrast, omega-3 oils produce "good" prostaglandins that suppress histamine, inflammation, and swelling. That is another reason why it is vital in fighting allergen diseases to have the essential fatty acid ratio in balance. The second error is abnormally high insulin levels, which also generate abnormal levels of histamine and other allergic reaction chemicals. That is why it is important to consume a low-glycemic diet.

A major reason why allergens have their effect is that their molecules closely resemble a genuine enemy molecule, such as a virus. A sweetly tuned immune system has no difficulty distinguishing them, but a crazed immune system just lashes out indiscriminately. It sets in motion an unstoppable chain reaction and sometimes sets up the sufferer for a lifetime of allergic reactions.

Histamine and Allergic Reactions

Histamine is a substance that is released from the body's tissues during conditions of stress, inflammation, and allergy. It provokes the familiar allergic reaction of runny nose, watery eyes, and tissue swelling. Many allergy sufferers are familiar with "anti-histamine" medications designed to neutralize the histamines produced by the immune system.

This is how it happens: the immune system labels bad guys with a criminal record. That way, if it comes across them again, it knows straight away to give them a hard time. It does this all the time with virus infections and other foreign invaders. For example, when you have a disease like measles, the body remembers it for a very long time and you are unlikely to suffer it again. This works fine as long as the "criminal" label is correctly applied. But this is not always the case: the confused immune system sometimes labels harmless molecules as "criminal." When that happens, the immune system launches an attack that is even more rapid and violent when it meets that falsely labeled "criminal" on subsequent occasions. This condition is known as hypersensitivity and is why allergies can take a long time to shake off. We have to give the immune system time to "forget" the falsely applied "criminal" label, which can take many months or even years.

Allergies

Allergy symptoms range from the mild response of sneezing and a runny nose to the sometimes life-threatening reaction called anaphylactic shock. During an anaphylactic reaction, the airways in the lungs constrict intensely, making it impossible to breathe, and the blood pressure falls precipitously.

Allergen Connection. A deranged immune system is capable of taking exception to foreign particles from almost any source. However, the biggest sources of allergens are the following:

Grains. All grains (wheat, rye, barley, corn, rice, oats, etc.) are allergenic.

Milk and Dairy Products. A number of constituents of milk are highly allergenic: lactose, casein, and lactalbumin are the main examples. All milks and their products are concerned—milk itself, yogurt, and cheese. And it doesn't matters if they are low fat. Dairy products from other creatures (such as sheep and goats) are just as bad.

Legumes. Lentils and beans contain many allergenic substances. Soy, however, is the biggest problem. It has the most powerful allergens, and soy in various forms is an all-pervading, ingredient in a huge range of processed foods. A Swedish study found that in four out of five fatal reactions to food the deaths were due to soy.[53] The amount of soy needed to kill was small: between 0.25–2.0 teaspoons.

Essential Fatty Acid Connection. Many studies have demonstrated that a high intake of omega-6 oils is harmful. The ideal is to have a rich omega-3 intake in balance with omega-6.[54]

Colon Health Connection. Hot spices encourage allergic reactions. Hot spices such as paprika, cayenne pepper, and chili pepper interact with the lining of the digestive tract and allow allergens to invade the body.[55]

Stress Connection. There are many non-dietary triggers of allergies and one of the most common is stress. Stress hormones deregulate powerful immune system chemicals called cytokines, causing them to unleash allergic reactions.[330]

If you are bringing up young children, you have a chance to ensure they start life with a properly developed immune system. In order to mature properly, a child's immune system needs to be constantly challenged by naturally occurring foreign particles. That way, the immune system is properly programmed with the right responses. One study found that children growing up in a large family, sharing bedrooms with siblings, and having a dog reduces the risk of developing allergies in adulthood.[56]

Asthma

Asthma is an inflammatory process with abnormal spasm of the bronchial tubes, mucus production, fluid in the lungs, and inflammatory cell migration. The prevalence of asthma has increased dramatically in recent years.[57] What has changed so much to cause this?

Essential Fatty Acid Connection. Spasms, mucus, fluid, and inflammation are all conditions driven by powerful "bad" prostaglandins. Once again, the culprit is overconsumption of omega-6 oils.[58] The increase in asthma in the last half century is directly linked to the increased consumption of corn oil, sunflower oil, peanut oil, and other omega-6 vegetable oils.

Colon Health Connection. A leaky colon increases the risk of asthma.[59]

Allergen Connection. The consumption of dairy products increases the risk of getting asthma.[60]

Non-Starchy Plant Food Connection. Studies show that lung performance is better in those who eat fresh fruit at least once a day,[61] those who eat at least five apples a week,[62] and those who have a high intake of fruit and vegetables.[63] In other words, poor lung function, including asthma, is in large part due to a deficiency of plant food micronutrients.

Sunshine Connection. Dr. Peter Black of Auckland University, in New Zealand, found that the sunshine vitamin, vitamin D, improved lung function, even in ex-smokers.[65]

Migraine

Migraine is a mechanism in the brain that becomes activated in response to various trigger factors, such as routine stress, hormonal fluctuations, sleep disturbances, certain foods, or even changes in weather conditions. The migraine mechanism involves many parts of the brain, various neurotransmitters, and, ultimately, the activation of nerves and swelling and inflammation of blood vessels around the head. The greater the degree of blood vessel swelling and inflammation, the worse the headache.

Allergy Connection. A number of allergens may play a role in migraines:

Grains. Gluten has a particularly strong connection. Sufferers of full-blown gluten allergy (celiac disease) are also much more likely to suffer migraines.[66]

Dairy. Dairy, in particular dairy protein.[67]

Pain-killers. Sometimes the medication that one takes to relieve pain actually makes it worse, a phenomenon called "rebound." The only solution is to grit your teeth and cut out your usual pain relievers.

Histamine. This powerful chemical is contained in many fish, many cheeses, and some vegetables.[68]

Non-Starchy Plant Food Connection. A low plant food diet, deficient in micronutrients, notably magnesium[69] and riboflavin (vitamin B_2),[70] sharply increases the likelihood of developing a migraine.

Blood Sugar Control Connection. High abnormal insulin levels have the effect of manufacturing abnormal levels of histamine. Diabetics are much more vulnerable to migraine.[71] The low glycemic diet is how nature intended.

Autoimmune Diseases

In autoimmune diseases, the immune system turns against the body's own organs and tissues. Many of the same processes are at work as for allergen diseases.

Rheumatoid Arthritis

Rheumatoid arthritis is more common in women than in men and usually strikes between the ages of 20 and 40. It is due to an abnormal immune reaction in which the immune system attacks and destroys the lining of the joints. The consequences are pain, inflammation, swelling, and eventually deformity of the joints and disability. Not content with producing these unpleasant symptoms, the immune system then launches a second wave of attack. Its killer T-cells swarm to the area where it has previously created inflammation. In the process, the T-cells produce a substance called OPGL, which cannibalizes and attacks cartilage tissue.[72] Studies over the years point to three main factors causing rheumatoid arthritis.

Fatty Acid Connection. The production of inflammatory chemicals caused by the overconsumption of omega-6 oils is one factor. Omega-6 oils are transformed into chemical messengers that instruct cells to inflame, swell, and secrete mucus. This is the perfect recipe for encouraging rheumatoid arthritis. In contrast, omega-3 oil consumption calms inflammation and swelling. Cutting down on omega-6 oils and boosting omega-3 oil intake is helpful.[73] A second culprit is saturated fat in all of its forms: animal origin, plant origin, and man-made (margarine, trans-fatty acids, and hydrogenated fats). Saturated fats block and interrupt the work of helpful chemical messengers from omega-3 oils, encouraging inflammation.[74] It is essential to eliminate saturated fat.

Non-starchy Plant Food Connection. The body needs antioxidants to quench the aggressive action of free radicals on joint tissue. Studies have found that people with rheumatoid arthritis are much more likely to have lower blood levels of antioxidants such as vitamin A, vitamin E, and beta-carotene in the years before the disorder is diagnosed.[75] There is only one source of the cocktail of antioxidants that works: non-starchy plant food.[76]

Allergen Connection. Arthritis is often triggered by an allergic reaction. Some of the most common suspected allergens are grains, especially gluten,[77] and milk and dairy.[78]

Osteoarthritis

Osteoarthritis (degenerative joint disease) is a disorder of the joints in which the cartilage disintegrates and bone rubs on bone. It is the most common joint disease, affecting more than 80% of those who reach the age of 70. Osteoarthritis is, in part, due to poor bone and cartilage building. As soon as humans took up farming grains, they started to suffer osteoarthritis.[79] Two factors were at work. First, the presence of wheat antinutrients irritated joint lubrication. Second, the drudgery of grinding the wheat, day in and day out, between two large slabs of stone put an unnatural strain on joints that were not designed for it.

Grain Connection. Grain antinutrients, notably lectins, depress cartilage building.

Mechanical Load Connection. Unusual mechanical wear-and-tear on the joints can lead to osteoarthritis. Today, osteoarthritis is most common in the load-bearing joints of the body, the hips and knees. Hip and knee replacement surgery is growing astronomically. Just in the 13 years from 1990 to 2002, hip replacements increased by 50% and knee replacements by 200%.[80] The main problem? Overweight and obese bodies. Nature never designed the hips and knees to support that kind of weight. This is one factor which is easy to understand and remedy.

Essential Fatty Acid Connection. Omega-6 oils depress the hormones that build bone and cartilage, while omega-3 oils encourage bone and cartilage building.[81] Once again, we need to cut down sharply on omega-6 oil intake and boost omega-3 oil intake to the point where the two are in balance.

Multiple Sclerosis

Multiple sclerosis (MS) is an autoimmune-induced inflammation that destroys the fatty insulation (myelin sheath) surrounding the nerves. Surprisingly, there are strong links between MS and lifestyle.

Allergen Connection. Wheat gluten is the strongest allergen that we know of. It tricks the immune system's killer T-cells into attacking myelin molecules because of their similarity to virus proteins.[82] There are many reports of complete remission of MS on gluten-free diets.[83] Milk is the second most powerful allergen and studies show that it also causes the immune system to attack myelin.[84]

Colon Health Connection. A leaky colon allows vast quantities of milk and gluten allergens to invade the bloodstream and create their mischief throughout the body. In a double whammy, the colon is made leaky, in part, by the allergens themselves.[85]

Fatty Acid Connection. For a long time, scientists have suspected that omega-3 essential fatty acids play a vital role in the maintenance of the myelin sheath.[86] The suspicion hardened when studies on Greenland Eskimos (who have a high omega-3 diet) found that they had a complete absence of multiple sclerosis.[87] Surprisingly, no one has done a high-quality clinical trial to answer the question once and for all.[88] Nevertheless, many studies are suggestive of the importance of having a good omega-3 oil intake and avoiding overloading on omega-6 oils.[89] In other words, get the essential fatty acids in balance.

Sunshine Connection. Multiple sclerosis is less common in sunny climates than in gloomy ones. Kassandra L. Munger, of the Harvard School of Public Health, found that the sunshine vitamin (vitamin D) has a protective effect against MS. In two ongoing studies of 187,500 U.S. nurses, women getting at least 400 IU of vitamin D per day showed only a 60% risk of developing MS compared with women getting less of the vitamin.[90] In confirmation, researchers at Pennsylvania State University found that vitamin D puts a restraining order on the killer T-cells.[91]

Ways to Alleviate Immune System Dysfunction

Allergic and autoimmune disorders are primarily a failure of the immune system. Repairing immune function will fix the root of the problem. We looked at the factors that make the immune system have a nervous breakdown. The remedial measures are simply stated: adopt a lifestyle that is close to the way nature intended, the Savanna Model.

1. Eat a strictly low-glycemic diet: eliminate starches and sugars.

2. Have a low-insulinemic diet: eliminate starches, sugars, and certain proteins like yogurt.

3. Eat a diet rich in non-starchy plant food: load up on salads, fruits, and vegetables.

4. Have a conforming fatty acid profile: eliminate saturated fats, sharply reduce or eliminate omega-6 oils, and load up on omega-3 oils.

5. Consume a high amount of plant food micronutrients: load up on salads, fruits, and vegetables.

6. Have a low plant poison intake: avoid grains, legumes, and potato.

7. Have a low antigen (allergen) intake: avoid grains, legumes, and dairy.

8. Be hungry some of the time and have a low percentage of body fat.

9. Maintain good colon health.

10. Get the right amount of physical activity.

11. Get sufficient exposure to sunshine.

Two other points from the Owner's Manual are relevant: acid / alkali ratio in balance and a low salt to high potassium ratio. In terms of immune function, we do not know if getting those right will make a difference, because no one has done the studies. But in our view, it is only wise to get your lifestyle in tune with the Savanna Model and give yourself the best chance to straighten out the rogue immune system.

BRAIN HEALTH

The brain is an organ of the body just like the heart or liver. It was built from food, is repaired with food, and its fuel is food. The way we nourish the brain deeply affects its health—yet, amazingly, few people think of it like that. Most people readily consume alcohol or coffee to alter their mood, accepting, without acknowledging it, that what we put in our mouths changes something in the brain.

For most of the 20th century, the psychiatric teachings of Sigmund Freud and Carl Jung dominated problems of mental malfunctioning. They found that mental problems had grown quickly during the years that they were formulating their ideas. For example, the incidence of schizophrenia increased dramatically during the Industrial Revolution. Researchers are now realizing that our mental state is affected not only by psychological stress but also by nutritional and other lifestyle errors. This insight has opened up an extraordinary revolution in the treatment of mental illness.

The scale of the challenge is enormous. Disorders affecting mental health are very common and affect all societies and all ages. These conditions include depressive disorders, Alzheimer's disease, attention deficit / hyperactivity disorder, schizophrenia, and Parkinson's disease. Mental health problems affect more than 25% of all people at some point in their lives. At any one time, about 10% of the adult population is suffering from a mental or behavioral disorder. The World Health Organization (WHO) estimates that mental or behavioral problems affect one family in four.[92]

Presently, depression is the leading cause of disability worldwide. At current rates, WHO predicts that depression will become the second highest cause of the global disease burden within the next 15 years.[93] Five other mental health conditions figure in the top 20 causes of disability in the world. The San Bushmen did not suffer mental disease in this way, nor did any other forager tribes that we know of. So, what is going wrong? Let us look first at how the brain works.

The brain is partially constructed from billions of nerve cells (neurons). When the brain is "working," these neurons communicate with each other in highly complex ways, just like a parallel-processing supercomputer. This communication takes the form of electrical or chemical signals shuttling between the billions of neurons. There are over 100 types of chemical signaler or neurotransmitter. Some of them have become household names, such as serotonin and dopamine; other examples are norepinephrine and acetylcholine. The brain makes most of these chemicals from the food we eat. If we don't eat the right foods, the brain cannot function properly.

The brain is mostly composed of various types of fat and water. About 60% of the brain's "dry weight" is fat, mostly composed of highly unsaturated fatty acids.[94] Neurons, and especially their outer skin (membrane), are composed mostly of special polyunsaturated fats. The neuron's membrane plays a vital role in absorbing nutrients and it is also very supple, allowing rapid changes in the membrane's shape. These qualities (suppleness and nutrient absorption) are vital to the successful communication between the billions of cells in the brain. If the neuron membrane is not supplied with these special fats, it will not work.

What are these special, highly unsaturated fatty acids? None other than the essential fatty acids, omega-3 and omega-6. Furthermore, for good brain health, these fatty acids must be present in equal amounts, just like in the Savanna Model.[95] In particular, omega-3 is critical to the growth of brain cell membranes. That is where the all-important neurotransmitters bounce between cells communicating messages, including those related to feelings of well-being.

The brain makes neurotransmitters mostly from amino acids (proteins). A number of amino acids are considered "essential," meaning the body (and brain) must obtain them from the diet. If the diet is deficient, the brain lacks the neurotransmitters it needs. On the other hand, the brain does make a few neurotransmitters from essential fatty acids. In fact, the brain converts omega-3 and omega-6 fats into a wide range of compounds to regulate many vital brain functions. Copper and vitamin C play a role in the creation of neurotransmitters, and zinc and magnesium stimulate certain neurotransmitters.[96] Antioxidants play a role in protecting brain tissue from oxidation,[97] which occurs when free radicals batten onto and destroy the good molecules. Vitamins C and E come to the rescue and extinguish free radicals, and vitamin E also prevents oxidation of polyunsaturated fats.[98]

Micronutrient deficiency ought to have given us the hint long ago that diet had profound effects on mental state. Often, mental disturbances are the first sign of deficiency.[99] For example, irritability and a general malaise often precede scurvy, caused by vitamin C deficiency. However, remember that no nutrient works alone. Since they have to work together as a team, the tens of thousands of micronutrients essential to human health can only be obtained from plant food.

Many other substances actively undermine brain health. Plant poisons (antinutrients) in beans and grains, and allergens in dairy products, beans, and grains all affect mental health for the worse. Saturated fats obstruct essential fatty acids from being absorbed into the brain.[100]

The brain must receive a nourishing diet of essential fatty acids in the right ratio, proteins of the right kind, and a complex cocktail of micronutrients in order to remain healthy. Furthermore, we must not allow antinutrients and other compounds to disrupt its delicate circuitry. Let us look at how these factors, and other lifestyle factors, come together to generate a range of common brain disorders.

Alzheimer's Disease and Dementia

Dementia is any chronic deterioration of intellectual function that is severe enough to interfere with the activities of daily living. Alzheimer's disease is the most common form of dementia. It is a progressive, physical disease of the brain, in which plaque builds up and causes inflammation of the neurons.[101] Studies show that chemicals called cytokines create the plaques and then inflammation directly damages neurons. Symptoms include loss of memory, confusion, mood swings, and withdrawal.

Alzheimer's disease has become much more common in the past 50 years. Since our genes have not changed, it must be lifestyle factors that are causing the increase. Indeed, immigrants to industrialized countries become just as vulnerable once they take up a Western lifestyle.[102] Evidence linking Alzheimer's disease and diet, either from population studies or from studies on large groups of people over many years, shows that Alzheimer's disease is very much a result of modern lifestyle.

What Increases the Chances of Alzheimer's Disease?

Too Much Fat and the Wrong Fats and Oils. A high fat intake, including saturated and hydrogenated fats, is a risk factor for Alzheimer's disease.[103] Deficient omega-3 and omega-6 intake is another problem. Alzheimer's patients have lower levels in their blood when compared to healthy people of the same age. Furthermore, autopsies of Alzheimer brains show low omega levels compared to healthy brains.[104]

High-Glycemic Diet. High insulin levels stimulate a protein called tau, which tangles brain cells into Alzheimer knots.[105]High blood sugar levels shrivel the hippocampus, the region of the brain where short-term memory is stored. The higher the blood sugar levels, the more it fogs memory.[106] Long-term obesity by itself predicts an increased risk of Alzheimer's.[107] In addition, obesity is connected with damaging high insulin and high glucose levels.

High Consumption of Plant Toxins (Antinutrients). Soybean antinutrients in the form of tofu consumption can double the risk of Alzheimer's disease.[108]

Low Consumption of Plant Micronutrients. High levels of homocysteine increase brain inflammation and are a risk factor for Alzheimer's.[109] A high intake of plant food micronutrients is required to clear homocysteine from the blood.

Lowering Your Risk for Alzheimer's Disease

A life lived out of harmony with the Savanna Model sharply increases the risk of Alzheimer's disease. A common thread has to do with inflammation—the same problems mentioned in regard to cardiovascular disease, obesity, and diabetes. It is not a surprise, therefore, that many of the factors that prevent inflammation also help you avoid Alzheimer's disease.

The Right Fatty Acid Profile. Our ancient ancestors had high intakes of omega-3 fatty acids from sources that included fish and shellfish from lakes and rivers.[110] Both a high consumption of omega-3 oils, including fish and fish oils,[111] and the absence of saturated fats help lower your risk.[112]

Low Energy Intake. Fasting gives the body's cells a "workout" similar to how physical exercise limbers up muscle cells. Brain neurons are strengthened, leading to reduced rates of Alzheimer's, Parkinson's, and Huntington's diseases.[113] A low-calorie diet is also protective[114] and it is important to avoid a high-glycemic diet.

High Plant Micronutrient Intake. A high intake of plant nutrients is critical, because the micronutrients quench brain-destroying molecules like homocysteine and free radicals. Plant food micronutrients include folate, vitamin B_{12}, and antioxidant flavonoids such as resveratrol, quercetin, catechins, and anthocyanins.[115] Alzheimer's patients have lower antioxidant levels in their blood than healthy people;[116] they also have correspondingly higher levels of oxidized fats. Another study reported low levels of folate and vitamin B_{12} in the blood of patients diagnosed with Alzheimer's, and found elevated levels of homocysteine.[117] A vegetarian diet is less risky than a high-meat diet for Alzheimer's disease.[118]

Physical Exercise. Old people who walked two miles or more a day had only half the risk of Alzheimer's as those who walked only 0.25 miles per day.[119] Exercise reduces brain levels of amyloid, a sticky protein that clogs the brain in Alzheimer's patients. It also boosts levels of hormones necessary for nerve cell production and increases blood flow to the brain. Our ancestors walked and ran several miles a day. We know that our bodies depend on it, and the brain does too.

Brain Exercise. "Use it or lose it." Brain scans show that when people use their brains in unusual ways, more blood flows into different neural regions and new connections form. To exercise the brain, do a new type of puzzle, learn to play chess, take a foreign language class, or solve a vexing problem at work.

Can Alzheimer's be reversed? No one knows, but it can certainly be slowed down by adopting these helpful measures. There is even evidence that brain cells can regenerate.[120] The fundamental lesson is that we have to live our lives in such a way as to avoid driving our brains into Alzheimer's in the first place. Remember (while you can!) the maxim, "an ounce of prevention is better than a pound of cure."

Attention-Deficit/Hyperactivity Disorder (ADHD)

ADHD is a brain disorder marked by impulsivity, hyperactivity, and an inability to sustain attention. It is most common in children and often, but not always, fades away in adulthood. There is a strong overlap with autism and dyslexia. Around 5% of children today are considered to suffer from ADHD, which means that a classroom of 25 to 30 children will have at least one who has ADHD. The "disorder" was first described at the beginning of the 20th century, but it only became routinely diagnosed in the 1980s. Since then, the number of children considered to suffer this condition is increasing sharply. What can be causing this sudden increase in cases?

Some of the usual culprits are suspected. Plant antinutrients such as gluten have been found guilty. Youngsters with full-blown gluten allergy (celiac disease) are at greater risk of ADHD.[121] So, too, are those who consume a lot of sugar.[122] Additives have also been linked to ADHD.[123] A double-blind, placebo-controlled study in the United Kingdom found that additives put in sweets, biscuits, and carbonated drinks trigger behavioral changes in up to 25% of toddlers. A group of 1,873 three-year-olds were given juice containing artificial colorings and preservatives each day for a fortnight. (The additives in question were Tartrazine E102, Sunset Yellow E110, Carmoisine E122, Ponceau 4R E124, and Sodium Benzoate E211.) The scientists found that the artificial additives had a "substantial effect" on children's tempers, concentration, sleeplessness and irritating interruptions.[124]

At the Appleton Alternative High School, in Wisconsin, the kids used to be out of control until 1997. Then, fast-food burgers, fries, and burritos in the cafeteria gave way to fresh fruit, fresh salad, and meats "prepared with old-fashioned recipes." Good drinking water replaced carbonated beverages. "Grades are up, truancy is no longer a problem, arguments are rare, and teachers are able to spend their time teaching," pronounced Principal LuAnn Coenen.[125]

Other studies find that ADHD sufferers have low essential fatty acids,[126] particularly a poor omega-3 intake,[127] and an imbalance of omega-6 oils.[128] They have micronutrient deficiencies in minerals such as zinc, iron, and magnesium.[129]

There is also a fascinating insight concerning the mismatch with our natural inclinations. Children who spent the most time in "green" settings had reduced ADHD symptoms in a study by Frances Kuo on 400 children. In the study, activities were done inside, outside in areas without much greenery (such as parking lots), and in "greener" spots like parks, back gardens, and tree-lined streets. The kids showed fewer ADHD symptoms after spending time in nature. Rural or urban, coastal or inland, the findings held true for all regions of the country.[130]

ADHD is clearly a disorder of modern industrial societies. The science is clear on some points and quite incomplete on many others, but the message is clear: adapt your child's life as closely as possible to the Savanna Model. Make sure that he or she avoids grains and dairy, remove sugar from the diet (be particularly ruthless about sugary soft drinks), and avoid processed foods with its artificial additives. Ensure that your child gets essential fatty acids, particularly omega-3 rich seafood, eliminate saturated fat and trans-fats, and keep omega-6 intake under tight control. Make sure he eats plentiful salads, fruits, and vegetables with their valuable cargo of micronutrients. Finally, get him away from the TV, computer console, and video games and into natural, green (savanna-like) surroundings.

Depression

In the past century, the prevalence of severe depression has increased dramatically, as much as 20-fold since 1945.[131] Not only have the numbers risen, sufferers are getting younger, with more cases reported in adolescents and young adults.[132] These increases are not due to better diagnosis—rather, there has been a genuine rise in the numbers of individuals suffering from depression.[133] Explanations for the rise have included increased life stress and changing social networks. However, the weight of evidence points to changes in nutrition that have occurred simultaneously.

Essential Fatty Acid Connection. There is a massive body of evidence that links low omega-3 oil intakes to manic depression, suicide, and post-natal depression. The incidence of major depression is nearly 60 times greater in New Zealand than in Japan. The New Zealanders' average seafood consumption is 40 pounds per person per year; the Japanese average is nearly four times that much.

Post-natal depression is 50 times more common in countries with low levels of seafood consumption.[134] Eskimos, when they abandon their traditional, omega-3-rich fish diet for industrial foods, suffer more depression.[135] Another study on Finns, which compared high fish consumers with those who were not, had a similar result.[136]

What about tests under laboratory conditions? Researchers have not been slow to try omega-3 therapy in controlled trials. In one celebrated study, Harvard researchers gave two groups of hospitalized depressed patients diets that were high in omega-3 oils and omega-6 oils, respectively. The omega-3 group had such dramatic improvement that, after three months, the scientists stopped the experiment and allowed the omega-6 group to benefit from the therapy.[137] Many other studies have confirmed the importance of boosting omega-3 consumption and driving omega-6 down.[138]

Micronutrient Connection. Researchers have carried out many studies to find some "magic bullet" vitamin pill for depression. They did not find the magic bullet, but their labors did establish the vital role that micronutrients play in brain health. They found that people who had low micronutrient intakes were more likely to be depressed. The closest associations were with folate and vitamins B_1, B_2, C, and B_{12}.[139]

Blood Sugar Control Connection. A high-glycemic diet provokes a switchback of blood sugar, leading to abnormal lows of sugar in the blood. This state of hypoglycemia gives rise to the so-called "sugar blues."

Lifestyle Connection. Lack of sunshine affects mood. For example, the depressive condition known as SAD (seasonal affective disorder) is most common in areas with long winter nights, like Alaska, Finland, and Sweden.[140] Sunlight even helps the body clock stay synchronized. Exercise, particularly with depressed people, helps lift them out of their moodiness.[141] The way we live today drives more and more people into depression. Undoubtedly, the dysfunctional structure of society has a great deal to answer for. Reappraise your personal situation and see if you can restructure your life to relieve unnecessary subconscious (and conscious) distress.

There are still many areas where we can take control for ourselves. In particular, follow the Savanna Model in matters of nutrition and lifestyle. The most important factor is to get omega fatty acids in balance, especially by stoking up on omega-3 oils and eliminating omega-6 oils. Also, increase your consumption of plant food, which is rich in micronutrients. Finally, follow a low-glycemic diet. Remember our tropical ancestry: we are creatures who need sunlight. If you cannot obtain it naturally, use a sun-bed or a light box. Think about the greater degree of social connectedness of our forager band—people who have this in their modern lives are much less likely to suffer depression. Finally, the savanna life designed our bodies on the assumption that physical activity is a constant factor in our daily lives and this helps too.

Schizophrenia

The principal signs of schizophrenia are delusions, hallucinations, incoherent thought processes, deficient feelings, and a withdrawal from reality. The incidence of this disease rose sharply during the Industrial Revolution in the 19th century. We have no evidence that forager societies suffered the disease at all, although this is possible. Nevertheless, there is mounting evidence that a lifestyle mismatch with our naturally adapted origins is greatly responsible. Generally, people in poorer countries fare better. For example, remission rates in India after two years of treatment were 54%, while they were only 3% in United States.[142] According to the World Health Organization, "This undoubtedly means that environment plays a crucial role as an outcome determinant in schizophrenia."[143]

Essential Fatty Acid Connection. Many studies and trials show that when patients consume a normalized intake of essential fatty acids, their schizophrenia is improved. That is, consumption of omega-3 oils is increased and omega-6 oils are sharply reduced to bring them into balance.[144] One of the fish oils, EPA (eicosapentaenoic acid), seems to play a crucial role.[145] Normally, the body can make EPA from an omega-3 oil of vegetable origin, but it is possible that some schizophrenic bodies have difficulty doing so. Other studies suggest that a high consumption of animal fats (which block essential fatty acids from working properly) worsen symptoms.[146]

Sugar Connection. An analysis found links between sugar intake and schizophrenia. It found that "a higher national intake of refined sugar and dairy products predicted a worse two-year outcome of schizophrenia."[147]

Antinutrient and Allergen Connection. A number of studies suggest a link between schizophrenia and the consumption of grains.[148] Furthermore, the incidence of schizophrenia is 30 times greater in patients with celiac disease (gluten allergy).[149] The same analysis that found links with sugar intake also found connections with dairy intake.[150] Similarly, a milk-free diet yields much quicker remission.[151]

The World Health Organization thinks that environment plays a "crucial role" in the remission of schizophrenia, but there is a great deal more to be studied on just what factors make a difference. Certainly social factors, especially those arrangements of work, family, and society that conform to the Savanna Model, are helpful. In dietary terms, paying attention to the essential fatty acid profile is the most important. Keeping to the low-glycemic diet, which automatically keeps sugar at bay, is also a sensible thing to do. Food allergens, like those from grain and dairy, also play a role, but more research is needed. Of course, grains and dairy are best omitted from the diet anyway.

Parkinson's Disease

Parkinsonism was first described in 1817 by the British physician James Parkinson. He was the first to categorize a particular variety of palsy called "shaking palsy," a condition brought about by neuron degeneration in a brain region called the substantia nigra. When this happens, they stop producing the neurotransmitter dopamine. The adjacent region of the brain, responsible for masterminding movement, cannot function properly without dopamine. The result is a variety of symptoms of which uncontrollable tremors are the earliest and most visible. Although the conventional treatment uses drugs such as L-dopa, many studies show that there are strong lifestyle risk factors linked to Parkinson's disease.

Allergen Connection. A number of studies point to dairy consumption as a major risk factor.[152] The Honolulu Heart Program found that those who consumed more than 16 ounces of milk each day were 2.3 times more likely to develop Parkinson's disease than those who didn't drink any milk.[153]

Low Plant Food Connection. Low intakes of folate and other micronutrients allow homocysteine to cause damage in the brain. High homocysteine levels are a strong risk factor for developing Parkinson's.[154] Findings from the Honolulu Heart Program found that infrequent bowel movements lead to increased risk of Parkinson's. Those with fewer than one bowel movement per day had 2.7 times the risk of those with one bowel movement per day and four times the risk of those who had two bowel movements per day.[155] What do we make of this? Earlier, we highlighted the hundreds of subtle ways in which the bowel, and its contents, have a powerful influence on the body's health. Here we have another, quite unintuitive example. Who would have thought that a mucky bowel could affect dopamine levels in the brain?

Bad Fat Connection. Many studies conclude that diets high in animal fat are associated with a substantial increase in risk for Parkinson's disease.[156]

Parkinson's disease is a degenerative disease, and lifestyle certainly has something to do with it. All the evidence points to departures from the Savanna Model as being risk factors. So, be sure you have a voluminous non-starchy plant food intake and avoid dairy and saturated fat. You do not have to give up all pleasures, though—studies suggest that caffeine is all right, even beneficial.[157] Parkinson's is a progressive disease, so if you already have it, then you have no time to lose—go on the Savanna Model program straight away.

Autism

The term *autism* was first used by the psychiatrist Leo Kanner in the 1940s to describe children who appeared to be excessively withdrawn and self-preoccupied. The incidence of autism has risen from about 1 in 10,000 individuals in the 1970s to 1 in 200 now.[158] It is four times more common in boys. Media scares have condemned vaccinations and mercury poisoning, but the evidence for this connection is slight. On the other hand, many studies show strong connections with more everyday lifestyle factors. Dairy products, particularly the protein casein, are a high risk factor.[159] Grains, notably the allergen gluten, are another.[160] "Bad" bacteria in an unhealthy colon release toxins that favor autism.[161]

There is also evidence of a phenomenon that it is difficult to do anything about. Male fetuses receive strong doses of testosterone in the womb, which has the purpose of turning the fetus into a boy. Among other things, it wires the brain with male circuitry. Heavier doses of testosterone increase the risk of autism to the point where some researchers suggest that some autistic brains are simply "extreme" male brains.[162] Even if this is true for some autistic boys, it cannot be true for girls at all. So, an autistic child will always do better on the Bond Effect, in particular, by eliminating dairy and grains.

Achieving Brain Health

The brain is a living organ, throbbing with life, just like any other vital organ in the body. Moreover, it is a fantastically complex, three-dimensional network of microcircuits carrying out billions of operations per second. It is continuously processing information from the outside world and, using this data, calculating and directing our bodies to function in a challenging environment. Our instincts, reflexes, emotions, and moods are the puppet strings by which it directs us.

Already the brain is under enormous strain. Our homeland environment hardwired it for and installed the software for optimum functionality on the savannas of east Africa. We now live lives that are strongly at variance with this environment. The brain has to cope with the conflicts between hardwired reflexes and the restraining calculations necessary for today's world. One example is when the male aggression reflex has to be subordinated to the restraining influence of "civilized" behavior. It does not always succeed when we consider how phenomena like road rage can overtake the most mild-mannered driver. Freud began his career by analyzing hysterical bourgeois women. He put their hysteria down to the subconscious conflict between hardwired sexual feelings and the repression imposed by their "respectable" middle-class culture. Hysteria and road rage are just extreme examples of the conflicts that the brain is resolving many times a second. As Freud observed, the vast majority of these conflicts are taking place in our subconscious. Only occasionally does the fallout surface as a psychiatric problem.

That is what happens when the brain is functioning normally. It is already a bleak picture. But we add to the difficulty by throwing a screwdriver into the workings of the brain. In industrial societies, we feed the brain badly, deprive it of vital nutrients, encourage sickening inflammation, poison it with natural toxins, and irritate it with allergens. It is not surprising that some brains have a "brainstorm" and fail to function properly.

The lesson is that we must attempt to align our lifestyles again with the Savanna Model. We need the sunshine and the physical activity. We need to nourish the brain with the correct fatty acid profile and an abundance of micronutrients from plants. We need to avoid sabotaging brain health by consuming plant poisons, notably those in grains and legumes. We should avoid the allergens contained in grains, legumes, and dairy products. We must avoid inflaming the brain (and also giving ourselves wild mood swings) with a high-glycemic diet. In other words, follow the Owner's Manual for optimum brain health.

OBESITY AND DIABETES

Obesity and diabetes, as we will see, are really two sides of the same coin. Everything we know about our prehistoric ancestors is that they were lean and did not suffer from diabetes. Most of the time, they were slightly hungry and we can imagine why: getting food required work. They were constantly balancing the inconvenience of obtaining food with the satisfaction of consuming it. If they finished lunch hungry, they had a choice. Go off for an hour or two and find more food or have a siesta during the heat of the day. Thus, there was an automatic mechanism controlling the intake of food. You had to really want the food to go to the effort of getting it.

Unlike some creatures (gorillas, for example), humans were not living surrounded by their food. We do not have a well-developed "satiety reflex"—our bodies do not have strong signals telling us when to stop eating. For our ancestors, food bonanzas were rare, so we have a little voice inside us urging us to keep eating while the going is good.

Hunger Signals

Our bodies rely on a complex interplay of signals to regulate food consumption. Hormones and nerves are constantly relaying "eat" or "don't eat" messages to our brain and back again to various parts of our digestive system.[163] The details of this "chaotic" system are still not fully known and they are extraordinarily difficult, if not impossible, to analyze. However, one thing is clear: a wide variety of factors disturb the naturally adapted "eat" or "don't eat" instructions. To date, two dozen chemical agents have been identified that stimulate appetite, and a similar number that suppress appetite. These agents, many of them hormones, have names like ghrelin, PYY, agouti, and leptin. These complex signals get misrouted when we live in ways they do not recognize. For example, compared with other people, the obese remain hungry longer and don't feel full as quickly.[164] Lack of sleep generates signals that drive up hunger pangs.[165]

Pharmaceutical companies are trying to find drugs to change these signals, but with little prospect of success. The chaotic nature of the interactions means that they cannot be micromanaged. Of course, we advocate dealing with root causes and not trying to second-guess nature. Appetite signals go haywire because our whole lifestyle is out of whack. Get it back into line with the Savanna Model and appetite sensations will fall into line too.

Today, of course, in the affluent countries, we are surrounded by food. We can, with no effort, satisfy our desire to eat. As one wag observed: "When you hunt animals, you might succeed or you might not. But when you open the fridge door, you will succeed 100% of the time." Instead of the discipline being exerted on us by our environment, we have to exercise self-discipline. Prosperous times do have drawbacks! A second factor is the free-for-all in the supply of food. Supermarkets are modern-day Horns of Plenty, overflowing with substances, most of which are not proper human food at all. So, we have a double challenge: to exercise self-discipline in regulating both the quantity and the nature of what we eat.

Obesity

Carrying extra fat is not just a cosmetic issue. Everything we know about our biology is that it is unhealthy to have too much body fat—it is not how nature intended. Fat in your abdomen (a potbelly) is not just sitting there as dead weight—it produces all kinds of inflammatory chemicals called cytokines. By eliminating fat, you also get rid of a very dangerous inflammation-producing organ. Inflammation is linked to many chronic illnesses, including heart disease, syndrome X, dementia, depression, cancer, osteoporosis, and autoimmune diseases.[166]

In Chapter 1, we saw how San and Aborigine foragers had low body fat. So, why do our bodies make it so easy to put on weight? On the savanna, our bodies had to be good at storing excess food in times of abundance to see them through the times of scarcity. This storage mechanism has no upper limit: there was never a need to have one in the Pleistocene past, because scarcity was as common as abundance. Today, times are always abundant and our waistbands expand indefinitely to store the available food.

There are two major ways that food gets turned into fat. The body works to keep the level of blood sugar just right, neither too little nor too much. To do this, it uses the body's fat cells like a bank. Sugar is not actually stored as sugar, it is stored as fat. Fat is a concentrated, space-saving form of sugar. When there is too little blood sugar, the pancreas sends out the hormone glucagon to the fat-cell bank to draw out some sugar. When there is too much blood sugar, the pancreas sends out the hormone insulin to deposit surplus sugar in the bank. In a body that is living like nature intended, these banking transactions are going on all the time. Half the transactions are credits and half are debits. In the long run, our bank balance stays modestly in credit.

In the case of obesity, far more sugar is being deposited than is being drawn out. Where does this excess blood sugar come from? By far the biggest source is "bad" carbohydrates, chiefly grains, starchy vegetables, most sugars, some drinks, and some fruits. A secondary source of blood sugar is the liver: it converts some excess protein into sugar and puts it into the bloodstream. If there is too much sugar in the blood already, it gets deposited in the fat-cell bank.

The second major way in which we get fatter is more straightforward: the fat-cell bank also accepts deposits of fat directly. However, to do this, the bank requires special instructions or the deposit will not be accepted. These instructions are given, once again, by the hormone insulin—no insulin, no deposit. This explains why Eskimos, who eat a high-fat diet, are skinny under their voluminous furs. Their diet contains no carbohydrates whatsoever to trigger insulin release. Neither Eskimos nor San Bushmen make much insulin.

So, starch is stored as fat, sugar is stored as fat, protein is stored as fat, and fat is stored as fat. With all these alternatives, it is not surprising that the way we eat today is fattening. Insulin is the common factor in these activities. Nevertheless, in natural circumstances, neither protein nor good carbohydrates cause it to be secreted in large amounts.

Finally, let us look at one more factor working to make us fat. Although protein on its own does not provoke much insulin, when we eat protein together with bad carbohydrates, the effect is multiplied.[167] Insulin levels skyrocket, meaning that certain combinations of foodstuffs are exceptionally fattening. Popular foods combine bad carbohydrates, protein, and fat all the time. Examples are hamburger (bun and meat patty), hot dog (roll and sausage), french fries (potato and cooking oil), pizza (pastry and cheese), pasta (spaghetti and meat Bolognese), BLT sandwich (bacon and bread), deep-fried breaded chicken, and so on. We do not have to look far to see why Americans, and industrialized populations generally, are becoming obese.

Our diet, high in bad carbohydrates and fats, is making us fat. We put too much blood sugar and fat into storage and do not withdraw it often enough. We need to feel hungry on a regular basis, a signal that the "slimming down" hormone glucagon is operational and drawing down fat. We also need to consume fat frugally and bad carbohydrates not at all.

Seven Ways to Reduce Obesity

These steps for reducing obesity are all in accordance with the Savanna Model.

1. Consume a strictly low-glycemic diet (no starches or sugars).

2. Adopt a low-fat diet.

3. Consume protein-rich foods modestly.

4. Keep a check on alcohol intake and avoid "empty calories." Alcohol gets in the way of glucagon working properly, so that withdrawals are harder to make from the fat-cell bank. Also, alcohol loads the body with calories that serve no useful nutritional purpose. The body uses these up first, putting calories from other sources in the fat cells. Plus, many alcoholic beverages are glycemic. Beer, with its malt sugars, is a common example. Heavy beer drinkers are much more likely to develop a "beer belly" and suffer from the diseases of a high-glycemic diet.

5. Practice the recommended amount of physical activity every day. Physical activity performs an essential role in making our body function properly. This applies just as much to weight control. The more active we are physically, the

more likely we are to burn off a high intake of calories. Physical activity, at levels which conform to our naturally adapted pattern, makes wondrous improvements to blood sugar control and fat burning.[168] In particular, glucagon is encouraged to withdraw fat from the fat-cell bank. Physical activity also suppresses appetite, especially in obese people.[169]

6. Feel hungry several times a day.

7. Get proper sleep.

Diabetes

Diabetes is the condition in which the body either does not produce enough insulin or the fat cells do not react to insulin's signal. In other words, diabetes results when the blood sugar control mechanism goes haywire. There are three main types of diabetes: type 1, type 2, and gestational diabetes. Here, we feature type 2 diabetes, which is by far the most common (90% of all cases) and it is also a purely lifestyle disease.

Type 2 diabetes can occur for either or both of the reasons cited above: not enough insulin is made by the pancreas or the fat cells do not listen to insulin's instructions. The latter scenario is called "insulin resistance." In insulin resistance, the pancreas (under instructions from the brain) senses the danger and churns out yet higher amounts of insulin. The fat cells sense this flood of insulin and become yet more resistant, a vicious cycle of high glucose levels and often high insulin levels. The result is that dangerously high levels of sugar remain in the bloodstream. Over time, this leads to gangrene, limb amputations, blindness, kidney failure, and nerve death. High insulin levels increase the risk of stroke, clots, heart disease, cancer, and other serious ailments.

Diabetes wreaks havoc on the body. Half of all amputations of hands and feet in the United States are due to diabetes. Similarly, it is a leading cause of

Insulin Medication

An outstanding event of early 20th century medicine was the discovery of insulin by the Canadians Sir Frederick Banting, Charles H. Best, and J.J.R. Macleod in 1921. Almost overnight, the fate of diabetics changed from a sentence of almost certain death to a prospect of a long and healthy life. For many decades, it was thought that insulin was a miracle cure. However, the medical establishment has come to realize that there is a dark side to insulin injections. As a powerful hormone, insulin acts on all sorts of other body functions that give rise to the higher risk of cardiovascular and many other diseases. Perhaps half the number of diabetics do not actually need insulin injections at all. In spite of that, their risks are hardly lower. They still have insulin levels out of control and similar risks of disease.

blindness. People who are diabetic are much more likely to be obese and have heart disease, kidney disease, high blood pressure, thromboses, strokes, and Alzheimer's disease.[170] The U.S. Centers for Disease Control predicts that the number of Americans with diabetes will double from 12 million to 24 million in the 25 years from the year 2000.[171]

Diabetes was unknown among hunter-gatherers like the San Bushman and the Australian Aborigines.[172] It used to be a rare disease even in industrialized societies, until recent times. When it did occur, this form of diabetes used to be called "adult onset" because it happened later in life, often around middle age. This name has been dropped because it is now happening at much younger ages. In fact, it is increasing out of control among the young. A study of 10- to 19-year-old diabetics in Cincinnati, Ohio, found that doctors were diagnosing ten times the number of adolescents suffering from diabetes in 1994 compared to 1982.[173]

Eskimos, Aborigines, Polynesians, and American Indians develop high rates of diabetes as soon as they adopt a Western diet.[174] We can take just one example, the Pima tribe of Gila, Arizona: 45% of people over 55 were already suffering diabetes in 1965. Yet, that number could soar even higher—to 80%—by 1996.[175] These peoples have blood sugar control systems that cannot cope with a high-glycemic diet. This is an interesting and rare example of how the bodies of farming peoples, over the millennia, have become slightly better than hunter-gatherer bodies at handling glycemic food, but only to a point. No body on the planet can cope with the extreme high-glycemic diet now commonplace in Western societies.

So, why do our blood sugar control systems go haywire? Because they have caved in to the onslaught of foods that provoke an explosive blood sugar rush. The most important thing a diabetic and pre-diabetic can do is to stop presenting unreasonable demands for insulin. Avoid requiring the body to deal with foods that it was never designed to process, and insulin levels will be kept low all the time. This is how our ancestors operated, and when Aborigines and Polynesians return to their ancestral eating patterns, their diabetic symptoms improve dramatically.[176] Everyone on this planet could avoid type 2 diabetes if they adopted a hunter-gatherer lifestyle.

The essential points about the hunter-gatherer lifestyle and diabetes are that their food supply was low glycemic, they had low body fat levels, and they got regular exercise. Studies demonstrate that these are vital conditions for fighting diabetes. There are further factors of secondary importance: a low omega-6 to high omega-3 ratio, a low-fat diet, the absence of smoking, suitable exposure to sunshine, and a rich intake of plant-food micronutrients are all helpful for diabetes.

Ways to Beat Back Diabetes

1. Consume a low-glycemic diet. This is by far the most important action you

can take. The Savanna Model is not only right for diabetics in this regard, it is right for every human on the planet.

2. Exercise has a restorative effect on glucose tolerance. Read chapter 8 and make sure that you exercise at least to the minimum shown there.

3. Lose weight! Diabetics find that their blood sugar is much better controlled when their body fat percentage is down to hunter-gatherer levels.

4. Studies on Eskimos demonstrate that a high consumption of omega-3 fatty acids (in their case, mainly from fish oils) improve insulin sensitivity and glucose tolerance.[177] These confirm other studies suggesting that insulin sensitivity is improved when omega-3 intake is increased.[178] Follow the Savanna Model and make sure you have the omega-6 to omega-3 intakes in balance.

5. Reduce total consumption of fat and saturated fat. Studies show high levels of fat and of saturated fat are risk factors.[179]

6. Have a good consumption of soluble plant fiber and antioxidants from plant food.[180]

7. Avoid smoking. Studies on smokers show that they have double the risk of developing diabetes compared to non-smokers and former smokers.[181]

8. Get enough sunshine. Studies show that diabetes is aggravated by a deficiency of the sunshine vitamin, vitamin D.[182]

We have seen that obesity and diabetes are closely linked by one major dietary error: a high-glycemic diet. Other common factors are a lack of exercise and consumption of unsuitable fats. Diabetics are often obese and obesity often drives one into diabetes, so it can be a vicious cycle. The Savanna Model can help you control both these conditions.

OSTEOPOROSIS

Bone has many functions, but the chief one is to serve as a structural frame to support the body. Bones are not solid—they are constructed in a dense "lattice" structure something like the Eiffel Tower. This arrangement is light, yet very strong and resistant to forces from all directions. Bones are made of two main materials: the rigid stuff making up the girders of the lattice and the connecting material that glues the girders together. The "rigid stuff" is made from the minerals calcium and phosphorus, while the "glue" is a protein called collagen.

In persons afflicted with osteoporosis, the tiny, rigid girders gradually become thinner and rodlike, and the spaces between them grow larger. The bone thus becomes more porous, less dense, and less strong. These lighter and more fragile bones tend to fracture from even minor knocks and falls. In the spine, tiny fractures accumulate resulting in a stooped posture ("dowager's hump"). The bones of the hip and forearm are especially vulnerable to fractures. To understand why this girder-thinning happens, let's look at how the bone lat-ticework is supposed to be maintained.

Bone is not lifeless matter—it is active living tissue. Special cells are con-stantly at work crawling all over the lattice, removing and replacing bone in a process called bone remodeling. It is rather like workmen repainting the Eiffel Tower. As fast as one team strips the old paint off, they are followed by a sec-ond team that puts on a fresh coat. Bone-building cells are called osteoblasts and bone-dissolving cells are called osteoclasts. In a lifetime, the osteoblasts and osteoclasts will have completely rebuilt the whole skeleton some three times over.

Osteoblasts and osteoclasts are operating according to instructions and sig-nals from all over the body. The cells speed up or slow down in response to instructions delivered by hormones. The kidneys, thyroid gland, and parathy-roid gland communicate with each other and to the bone-remodeling cells. The bone-remodeling cells talk to each other and to other parts of the body. In a process called cross-talk, the osteoblasts might call up osteoclasts to where a demolition job needs doing. Both kinds of cell, just like any other, live and die: they multiply themselves at the right times and die off at the right times.

One of the other functions of bones is to act as a "bank" for calcium. Calci-um is a vital ingredient in a whole range of biochemical operations and the body has to keep the level of calcium in the blood within tight limits. When there is too much calcium in the blood, it asks the osteoblasts to work harder and deposit calcium in the bone bank; when there is too little, the osteoclasts go to the bone bank and draw some calcium out.

We now know a lot more about these processes, but they are so intricate that the details are still being worked out. However, it is quite clear that the effects of any one action are so mind-bogglingly complex that the outcomes are impos-sible to predict. In this sense, it is a "chaotic" system.

So, you might reasonably assume that conventional health doctrine would be cautious about how it suggests interfering with these exquisitely delicate and processes. On the contrary, the advice focuses, to the point of fixation, on one tiny part of the big picture—the supply of just one building material: calcium. Eat more calcium, so the thinking goes, and more of it must end up in your bones, which should be a good thing. At least it should be in the West, where the disease of osteoporosis has reached epidemic proportions. But scientists have known for some time that this doctrine (calcium in your mouth equals calcium in your bones) is simplistic. Worse, by putting itself forward as the solution, it diverts attention from the true causes of osteoporosis.

Contrary to received wisdom, women who drink two or more glasses of milk a day are 40% *more* likely to suffer hip fractures than those who drink no milk.[183] Researchers found no signs of osteoporosis in the San Bushmen, even though they do not drink milk or swallow calcium pills.[184] The populations of

Asia and Africa who, although consuming low levels of calcium, nevertheless do not suffer from bone fractures.[185] Eskimos have poor bone health in spite of a high calcium intake. Finally, just because calcium gets into the bloodstream, it does not mean that the body uses it to build bones. On the contrary, the body is quite capable of laying down calcium just where you do not want it. For example, in the arteries and heart valves (as plaque),[186] in the kidneys (as stones),[187] in the breasts (as nodules triggering cancers), and in the joints (as painful spurs). All this can happen while the bones themselves are losing calcium. Clearly something is very wrong with the conventional doctrine.

There is another important phenomenon. People build up bone mass until the age of about 35. This happens without any particular measures made by the individual, although certain lifestyles are better at building up this bone "capital" than others. After the age of 35, many people in Western societies start to lose bone. Even Eskimo children build bone before they succumb to osteoporosis later in life. The point is this: people do not suddenly reduce their calcium intake at the age of 35; some other, powerful factors are at work.

Osteoporosis is a disease whereby the girders of the lattice become progressively thinner to the point where the structure breaks too easily, but why would the girders become thinner? The fundamental answer is that osteoclasts are destroying bone faster than the osteoblasts are building it. Why does this happen?

Factors in the Development of Osteoporosis

Factor 1—Acid/Alkali Imbalance. A high-protein, acidic diet, commonplace in Western societies, is a factor in osteoporosis. In a diet that is relentlessly acidic, the body compensates by drawing calcium out of the bone bank. Put another way, it instructs the osteoclasts to work harder dissolving bone, thereby putting the released calcium into the bloodstream. This neutralizes the excess acidity and the kidneys then eject the waste products in the urine. Where does this acidity come from? High protein intake is a major reason, a mechanism called "protein-induced calciuria."[188] The consumption of starches causes a smaller, yet significant acidifying effect. They are less acidic than protein, but they contribute nothing to reducing acidity and get in the way of foods that could— fruits, salads, and vegetables. Secondly, protein has a particular effect on the kidneys. Kidneys filter waste matter from the bloodstream and dump it into the urine. The kidneys' filters should not be so porous that they let through "good" substances, but only eliminate waste products. However, the kidneys lose this fine-tuning under the pressure of abnormally high levels of protein, and they start to leak calcium. Here we have a major explanation for why Eskimos suffer osteoporosis—they consume a very high protein, and acidic, diet.

Factor 2—Lack of Micronutrients. Low consumption of fruit, salads, and vegetables is a factor in osteoporosis. Studies show that healthy bone building is dependant on a high intake of fruits.[189] There are over 20,000 active compounds in fruits and they are far from all being identified and evaluated. Certainly, adequate intakes of potassium, zinc, magnesium, fiber, and vitamin C are important, but not sufficient. Other studies show that vegetarians who consume plenty of green plant food have healthier bones.[190] Vitamin K, readily found in leafy vegetables, is a powerful bone-building helper.[191] It is not good enough to take vitamin and mineral supplements. You have to consume the fruits and vegetables themselves to get the benefit of all the bone-building compounds.

Factor 3—Essential Fatty Acids Out of Balance. Domination of omega-6 oils over omega-3 oils is a factor in osteoporosis. The hormones (prostaglandins) made by essential fatty acids have a powerful effect on bone building. Omega-6 oils speed up bone destruction; omega-3 oils speed up bone building.[192] One reason why osteoporosis has become so prevalent since World War II is that the omega-6 vegetable oils (corn oil, peanut oil, and sunflower oil) became commonplace at that time. In parallel, sources of omega-3 oils have dwindled.

Factor 4—Excess Salt. Domination of salt over potassium (instead of the other way around) is a factor in osteoporosis. Excess salt causes the kidneys to raid the calcium bank to show this unwanted mineral, sodium, the back door.[193] The ratio between salt and the mineral potassium should be kept at no more than 1 to 5.[194] Potassium is chiefly found in fruits, salads, and vegetables. The ratio between potassium and sodium in Western diets is not only unbalanced, it is upside-down: instead of 1 to 5, it is 5 to 1.

Factor 5—Excess Phosphorus. Not many people know that they consume phosphorus in large quantities. Why might this be a problem? Bone-remodeling cells listen to the signals carried by the powerful hormone PTH, secreted by the parathyroid gland. They prompt osteoclasts to speed up their bone-destroying efforts. Why would the parathyroid gland send those instructions? An excess of phosphorus in the diet stimulates the parathyroid gland to go into overdrive, churning out instructions to destroy bone. So, how do we let phosphorus into our lives? Consumption of phosphorus-containing cola has increased from near zero to over 48 gallons per American per year just in living memory. Colas contain phosphorus in the form of phosphoric acid, and the consumption of colas promotes bone disease.[195]

Factor 6—Deficiency of Sunshine and the Sunshine Vitamin. Lack of appropriate sunshine is a factor in osteoporosis. One of the major effects of sunshine is to produce vitamin D in the skin. Vitamin D is an essential active ingredient in bone remodeling. In some circumstances, it increases bone building, while in others it increases bone destruction. It is important to get the doses just right at the right times. This is an important example of how it is impossible to micromanage these processes. Yet, if we live the way nature intended, the body sorts it out just right and we grow healthy bones.

Factor 7—Lack of Physical Activity. Lack of suitable physical activity is a factor in osteoporosis. The human organism has come to depend on a certain level of physical activity. The jolting of rhythmic jogging creates microscopic fractures in the bone lattice. This signals the osteoblasts to speed up and build stronger bone. In one study, elderly women benefited from as little as one hour per week of lower-intensity activity—42% lower risk of hip fracture and 33% lower risk of vertebra fracture.[196] In contrast, people who do little activity (astronauts in space are an extreme example) find that their bones start to dissolve.

Factor 8—Grains. The antinutrients in grains and their acidification of the blood can encourage osteoporosis.[197] The effect is particularly marked in those who have acute sensitivity to gluten.[198]

Factor 9—High Blood Sugar. High blood sugar levels, notably in diabetics, can aggravate osteoporosis.[199]

Factor 10—Alcohol Abuse. Chronic alcoholism and even binge drinking destroy bones.[200]

Factor 11—Vitamin C Deficiency. Lack of vitamin C can lead to osteoporosis. This deficiency is surprisingly common in some populations, particularly in inner cities, who eat hardly any fresh fruit, salads, and vegetables.

Factor 12—Iron Overload. An excessive intake of iron leads to osteoporosis. This can happen in some communities that use iron cooking pots, anyone who supplements with iron, or sufferers of the condition called hemochromatosis, whose bodies do not know how to handle iron in the diet.

Factor 13—Calcium Overload. Overdosing on calcium supplements can have a number of drawbacks. The main ones are kidney stones, the depletion of other essential minerals like zinc and magnesium,[201] and toxic levels of blood calcium leading to kidney failure.[202]

Factor 14—Vitamin D Overload. Overdosing on vitamin D either in food or in supplements promotes bone thinning. Vitamin D is such an important compound for bone building that people mistakenly self-medicate with pills and overdo it. Vitamin D in excess is toxic to the bones and promotes the development of osteoporosis.[203]

Some Reassurances About Osteoporosis

Changing the lifestyle factors outlined above can help you maintain good bone health right up to old age. It is not a coincidence that these factors are, without exception, measures that fit into the Savanna Model. There are many misconceptions about what factors might be harmful to bone health. Here we provide some reassurances.

Fluoride. The savannas of east Africa are regions of high fluoride availability, particularly in the water. In such circumstances, we would predict that the human organism came to depend on it. Indeed, tests show that the human skeleton does well on a good fluoride intake.[204] This is not an argument to go out and take fluoride supplements, but rather a reassurance that, if your water is fluoridated or you use fluoridated toothpaste, it is fine to accept it.

Caffeine. Moderate consumption of caffeine, such as two cups of American coffee per day, is harmless to calcium metabolism.[205]

Alcohol. Moderate consumption of alcohol, such as one glass of wine per day, is innocuous and can even be modestly helpful.[206]

Estrogen Therapy. If anyone still needed convincing that osteoporosis is a hormonal problem, just consider this: the only medication prescribed by doctors that is truly helpful is the hormone estrogen. Estrogen is used successfully to slow the deterioration in bone health of menopausal women. But if you get your lifestyle patterns right, osteoporosis will be a non-issue.

Pregnancy and Breastfeeding. We all have the idea that women who are pregnant or breastfeeding have an extra need for calcium. After all, they are building bones in a fetus or making milk for a nursing baby. So, does the mother need to consume more calcium? The San mothers certainly did not do anything special and we can suppose that our Pleistocene ancestors did not either. Humans have no instinct whatsoever to seek out calcium-rich foods. Pregnant and nursing mothers' bodies take no account whatsoever of any increase in calcium intake.

Instead, the mother's body meets the demand for extra calcium by triggering three main activities. First, specialized hormones instruct the intestines to absorb a higher percentage of calcium from the ordinary foods that she eats. Second, the kidneys are instructed to recover a higher percentage of calcium from the urine.[207] Third, specialized hormones instruct the osteoclasts to release calcium from the bone bank. Nothing that the mother eats, supplements, or does changes this process. Whatever she does, her bones lose mass, but as soon as menstruation restarts, the hormones go into reverse. In no time at all, her bones recover their normal density.[208] Even though doctors conventionally prescribe calcium pills during this time, they are ineffective and can even be harmful.[209]

This is a graphic illustration of how little control we can exercise over the way our bodies maintain bone health. Our interventions, albeit well-intentioned, are usually in vain and might make matters worse. Also, we can draw a lesson from our Pleistocene past: our ancestors (quite naturally) spaced their pregnancies by some four years, which gives the bones ample time to recover before the next pregnancy. The good news is that women who have had several pregnancies are at no greater risk for osteoporosis.[210]

THE BOND EFFECT AND YOUR HEALTH

This book has been a quest to discover our human heritage, notably as it applies to our health, both physical and mental. We have used these discoveries to establish the right lifestyle pattern for human beings. On the way, we highlighted how the mismatch between today's lifestyle and our savanna-bred ideal makes us sick in various ways. We've seen how the major health problems that trouble us today are, indeed, "diseases of civilization."

However, there is no "magic bullet" to fix every disease. The human body is an extraordinary collection of incredibly intricate processes whose detail is impossible to comprehend. Fortunately, we do not need to micromanage these processes but rather focus on the big picture. Get that right, and the body, with its savanna programming, does the rest. That is the Bond Effect in action.

All this might sound too good to be true. To deflect any accusations of hubris, we acknowledge that not every condition can be cured by adopting a healthy lifestyle. Nevertheless, whether we are sick or healthy lies largely under our own control. All the evidence points to one simple conclusion: whether you are worried about cancer or heart disease or osteoporosis, the remedy is the same—adopt the Savanna Model.

Conclusion

In this book, I talk about confronting prejudices. I know what that means because I have had to confront my own. I was brought up as a vegetarian. My family conditioned me to believe that it was the "natural" state of affairs and they taught me it was "unnatural" (as well as unkind) to kill and eat animals. Nevertheless, I was sufficiently skeptical to want proof, not just assertions.

I wanted something that set out, in a rational way, just what and how we should be feeding the human organism. We thought we knew, back then in the late 1950s, that our closest cousins, the chimpanzees and other apes, were vegetarians. If nature designed their bodies for a vegetarian diet, then it seemed reasonable it so designed ours too. It would just require a little investigation to put the ideas on a scientific footing, fill in a few gaps, and identify the feeding pattern that was right for humans.

In our family, it was an article of faith that butter, honey, and whole-wheat bread were "good" (because they were "natural"); margarine, sugar and white bread were artificial and inferior. That does not sound uncontroversial, yet I had to abandon every one of these articles of faith, as well as many more.

We were still confused in 1960 about the location of the human birthplace. Although chimpanzees had been kept in zoos for over 100 years, nobody had studied them in the wild. However, for me, these were mere details, ones that were not of fundamental significance. How wrong I was! I imagined that many of the answers would lie in studying the traditional feeding patterns of indigenous, tribal peoples.

Where does one find tribal peoples? Africa seemed to be the most auspicious place to start looking, and so I spent my first post-graduate decade in the late 1960s living with a variety of indigenes: the Fulani cattle herders of Sokoto, the Hausa farmers of Kaduna, the fierce Touareg warriors of the Sahara Desert, the Berbers of Morocco and Algeria. They certainly practiced a wide variety of feeding patterns. Mostly they ate what was available and, of course, what was available was what they had traditionally grown or raised. There was no pattern to it at all. It was not as though they were particularly healthy either: they lived hard lives, often had toothless gums, and succumbed to nasty tropical diseases.

Perhaps my most disconcerting discovery was their universal yearning for meat. Animal flesh was scarce, highly prized, and much fought over. Yet, even though broccoli was scarce, no one fought over that! Moreover, I was taken aback by the sheer blood-thirsty nature of killing animals. They slit sheep's throats and twisted off chicken's heads with excitement and anticipation, not with distaste. The children took part and danced around in glee while the butchery took place. I was in denial that this might be a normal human activity. Influenced by Blank Slate theories, I assumed that these practices were culturally determined.

Science was moving on. Louis Leakey's work seemed to locate the origins of the human race in east Africa. Mildly interesting, but apparently so long ago—at least a million years—as not to be significant for my purposes. But Leakey also encouraged Jane Goodall to live with the chimpanzee and Dian Fossey to live with the gorilla. Both women spent decades in the bush, carefully recording everything they could about their creature's behavior.

Fossey confirmed that gorillas are indeed vegetarian and are shy, mostly gentle creatures. However, another species of great ape, the human ape, was not so gentle. Fossey fought against poachers who were decimating her gorilla families. Tragically, she lost her life, murdered in her Rwandan campsite, probably by the same poachers. Fortunately, she left behind a remarkable book, *Gorillas in the Mist,* and a crusading foundation dedicated to preserving the few gorillas left in the wild.

It was Jane Goodall's work with chimpanzees in Gombe, Tanzania, that produced an earthquake in received ideas. One day in October 1960, she saw chimps strip leaves off twigs to fashion tools for fishing termites from a nest. Scientists thought humans were the only species to make tools, but here was evidence to the contrary. Jane later observed male chimps go on murderous hunting expeditions, where they caught small monkeys and bushpigs. The chimps did not simply catch the creatures—the victims were ripped limb from limb in sadistic ecstasy and consumed with gusto. The raw meat, dripping with blood, was more than a meal, it was a prize. The successful meat owner tore bits off and rewarded his friends and allies. Encouraged by these bribes, females frantically offered their bodies for mating. Here was inescapable evidence that chimpanzees were efficient hunters and enthusiastic meat-eaters. Our nearest cousin was not a gentle vegetarian as I had so fondly imagined.

Until that time, we still assumed that humans, while close to the great apes, belonged nevertheless to a separate family. Then, in 1984, Charles Sibley and Jon Ahlquist studied the DNA of apes and humans. The first shock was that humans are not a separate family, rather they fit squarely within the great ape family. Secondly, humans and chimps are on a descent of their own: they had a common ancestor only 5 million years ago. In other words, humans are on the killer-and-meat-eater branch of the ape family.

The final breakthrough came with the studies by geneticists like L. Luca Cavalli-Sforza. By the early 1990s, they made it clear that humans burst out of Africa not millions of years ago but just 60,000 years ago. In other words, our bodies were just the same as they were back then and designed by nature for life on the savannas of east Africa. The importance of this insight cannot be underestimated. The question was now very simple: what was life like for our ancestors back then and in that place? For it was there that nature forged our bodies and minds.

It dawned on me that I had been looking in the wrong place for the answers to human lifestyle and nutrition. We needed to go back to the savannas and to study peoples who still lived the way of our ancient ancestors. In 1956, Laurens van der Post aired a television series called "The Lost World of the Kalahari," a documentary featuring the San Bushmen. It was probably the last time when African Pleistocene life could still be studied largely uncontaminated by contact with modern civilization. The San were clearly hunters as well as gatherers. As each piece of evidence thudded into place, it was obvious that "animal matter" had played an important role in our naturally adapted diet. I had to confront my last illusion and acknowledge that humans were not naturally either peaceful or vegetarian.

That is the story of how I had to come to terms with a new reality. Anyone who wishes to fully understand what it means to be human in lifestyle terms will experience a similar process. This book has been a journey assembling the pieces of the puzzle—rediscovering the lost Owner's Manual for the human species.

It is still possible to navigate your way through the challenges of modern life—to align the way you live with the way nature intended. However, the modern world is not structured in an ideal fashion. You are under pressure to contort yourself to fit the structure that is offered today. The problem is that science, technology, commerce, and economics are a runaway train rushing us headlong into a future that, if it conforms to human nature, does so only in parts and by accident.

Marketing techniques are all-pervasive, and they manipulate us to behave in ways that serve the interests of the marketplace rather than our own best interests as human beings. The plains of the Midwest produce huge quantities of grain; someone must consume it. Similar observations go for beef, sugar, potato, tobacco, soybean, milk, sunflower oil, and many more. What is on offer, people must be persuaded to want it and buy it. And the best way to persuade them? Make them feel good about it and make them "love their servitude." But it is an illusion—in reality, it makes them sick, obese, neurotic, and, in the longer term, dissatisfied and unhappy.

However, this is ultimately an optimistic book. The main message is this: you can take control of your life and lead it in ways that are in harmony with your savanna-bred nature. We have shown you the way and given you the roadmap. But you must do it for yourself, no one will do it for you. This book has been a quest to discover our humanity. Now go out—confident and proud—and just do it!

Resources

I passionately believe in the insights contained in this work. My driving motivation is to stimulate everyone, no matter what your origins and background, to improve your lives. I hope that this book has inspired and encouraged you to know more. I have created a reservoir of resources to help you put the Savanna Model principles into practice, that is, do the Bond Effect.

The Bond Effect Website • www.TheBondEffect.com
Your first port of call should be my website, www.TheBondEffect.com. There you will find online support, speaking engagements, breaking news, updates, hints and tips, and much more. In addition, you can acquire access to many other support materials. Examples are:

The Bond Effect Newsletter
Everyone serious about adopting the Savanna Model will find the monthly newsletter an indispensable aid to keep focused on the essentials. Editors of mainstream food magazines cannot afford to upset their advertisers, so their editorial matter is at best bland, uncontroversial, and meaningless. The *Bond Effect* newsletter takes no advertising and so it is free to give an honest, straight-from-the-shoulder, Bond Effect viewpoint. It typically contains packed pages of hints, tips, health updates, food/disease connections, readers' questions and answers, recipes, the Bond Effect view of breaking news, survival skills (marketing campaigns debunked); and much more. Subscribe at www.TheBondEffect.com.

The Companion Cookbook
This is my wife Nicole's essential handmaiden to everyone living the Bond Effect way. It contains interesting, tasty, and practical recipes that fit in with the Bond Effect precepts. Available at www.TheBondEffect.com.

An Introductory Guide
Originally produced for the 35,000 employees of American Standard Inc., the Introductory Guide is an easy overview of the Bond Effect. In 32 pages, it contains the distilled essence of the principles and practice. Produced in full color and illustrated with specially commissioned watercolors, it also makes a superb gift.

OTHER RESOURCES

Glycemic Index and Glycemic Load • www.glycemicindex.com
A prime feature of the Savanna Model is to eat a low-glycemic diet. Scientists
have tested a great many foods (most of them processed) and this Website, com-
piled by Jennie Brand-Miller at Sydney University, contains a compendium of
the test results. However, many of the tests need to be interpreted, as we did for
the carrot's glycemic index in chapter 7. Also, we do not agree with the *interpre-
tation* that Brand-Miller puts on the tests. With these caveats, the raw data is a
valuable resource.

Consumer Lobbies

Center for Science in the Public Interest • www.cspinet.org

Physicians' Committee for Responsible Medicine • www.pcrm.org
Many groups are fighting the tidal wave of food industry propaganda. These two
lobbies, although they occasionally take positions on some issues that we do not
agree with, they cast a light on the dark and grubby corners that the food industry wants to keep under wraps.

Government Websites

United States Department of Agriculture (USDA) • www.usda.gov
The USDA is the home of the infamous food pyramids and the Dietary Guidelines for Americans. These jostle for visibility among the USDA's advice to farmers about subsidies for sugar production and how to persuade unwilling
Japanese to import American hormone-treated beef. The USDA's nutrition database at www.nal.usda.gov/fnic/etext/ 000020.html is a useful compendium of
the composition of a wide variety of foods. Most of the foods are processed and
proprietary brands, but this is still invaluable for generic foodstuffs as well.

United States Food and Drug Administration (FDA) • www.fda.gov
Here you can follow how the FDA tries to hold the line against the food industry's pressure to approve all kinds of unsuitable products for human consumption and make health claims to boot.

National Institutes of Health (NIH) • www.nih.gov
The NIH is a part of the U.S. Department of Health and Human Services and is the
primary federal agency for conducting and supporting medical research. Its results
are less likely to be tainted by commercial pressures than from other sources.

FURTHER READING

I have included all the relevant books in the list of references, but here is a selection of the primary sources readily accessible to the interested reader.

The Lost World of the Kalahari by Laurens van der Post (New York: Harcourt Brace Jovanovich, 1977). Written by the South African explorer and guru to Prince Charles, this is an inspiring account of van der Post's expeditions in the 1950s to discover the lives and fate of the disappearing San bushmen. Contains fascinating information on their hunter-gatherer feeding habits.

Triumph of the Nomads: A History of Ancient Australia by Geoffrey Blainey (South Melbourne, Australia: Macmillan, 1982). The Australian Aboriginals were the last major group of hunter-gatherers to come into contact with the West. As such, we have many explorers' accounts of their ancient way of life. Blainey has drawn this knowledge together in a readable and informative book.

Vaka: Saga of a Polynesian Canoe by Thomas R.A.H. Davis (Auckland, New Zealand: Polynesian Press, 1992). A precious and rare account, by the royal chief of the Cook Islands, relating how the seafaring and gardening societies of Polynesia lived their lives before Western contact.

Fiji's Times: History of Fiji by Kim Gravelle (Suva, Fiji: Fiji Times, 1988). A review of the bloodthirsty history of Fiji before and during Western contact. An insight into the natural history of this fishing and gardening, yet warlike, society that made cannibalism an integral part of its dietary habits.

The Natural World of the California Indians by Robert Fleming Heizer and Albert B. Elasser (Berkeley, CA: University of California Press, 1981). Most American Indian tribes were hunter-gatherers until the arrival of Europeans. This book describes the people, how they lived, what they manufactured, and in some cases what they thought, before their traditional aboriginal way of life was destroyed.

Guns, Germs, and Steel: The Fates of Human Societies by Jared Diamond (New York: Vintage, 1998). This broad sweep of human history explains how, where, and why agriculture developed over the last 13,000 years. It describes the types of new plants and creatures that farmers domesticated and how their new lifestyle changed the fortunes of their societies.

The Selfish Gene (3rd edition) by Richard Dawkins (Oxford: Oxford University Press, 1989). This classic work, for the first time, shifted our focus to the level of the gene. Its great insight was to understand that the fundamental force driving the behavior of all living things is that of gene success. In the words of the author: "We are survival machines, robot vehicles blindly programmed to preserve the selfish molecules known as genes."

In the Shadow of Man by Jane Goodall (Boston: Houghton Mifflin, 1988). A classic account of the first studies in the wild on our closest cousin, the chimpanzee. Many insights into how they lived their lives and fed themselves.

Gorillas in the Mist by Dian Fossey (Boston: Houghton Mifflin, 1983). A riveting account of the first studies in the wild on our next closest cousin, the gorilla.

Demonic Males by Richard Wrangham and Dale Peterson (Boston: Houghton Mifflin, 1996). The authors dispel the notion that human males are "depraved because they are deprived." Here, they compare the behavior of human foragers, gorillas, and the most violent of all, the chimpanzee. If we are to channel violence, war, and hatred, we have to understand how these forces came about in our evolutionary past.

The Blank Slate: The Modern Denial of Human Nature by Steven Pinker (New York: Penguin, 2003). Pinker, with surgical precision, slices away the myth of the "noble savage" to replace it with a wide ranging exposé of the deep undercurrents driving human behavior.

References

When more than one source is listed under a single reference number, all of the listed resources provide information for the relevant text.

Chapter 1   What is Nutritional Anthropology?

1. Wilson, Allan, and Rebecca Cann. "The Recent African Genesis of Humans." *Scientific American* 266:4 (1992): 68–73.

2. Cavalli-Sforza, L.L. *The History and Geography of Human Genes.* Princeton, NJ: Princeton University Press, 1994.

3. Tattersall, I. "Out of Africa, Again . . . and Again?" *Sci Am* 276:4 (1997): 60–67.

4. Kappelman, J. "Paleoanthropology: They Might Be Giants." *Nature* 387:6629 (1997): 126–127.

5. Van der Post, L. *The Lost World of the Kalahari.* New York: Harcourt Brace Jovanovich, 1977.

6. Semino, O., A.S. Santachiara-Benerecetti, F. Falaschi, et al. "Ethiopians and Khoisan Share the Deepest Clades of the Human Y-chromosome Phylogeny." *Am J Hum Genet* 70:1 (2002): 265–268.

7. Yellen, J. "Settlement Patterns of the !Kung." In Lee, Richard B., and Irven DeVore (eds.). *Kalahari4000Hunter-Gatherers: Studies of the !Kung San and Their Neighbors.* Cambridge, MA: Harvard University Press, 1976.

8. Tanaka, J. "Subsistence Ecology of Central Kalahari San." In Lee, Richard B., and Irven DeVore (eds.). *Kalahari Hunter-Gatherers: Studies of the !Kung San and Their Neighbors.* Cambridge, MA: Harvard University Press, 1976.

9. Lee, R.B. "Lactation, Ovulation, Infanticide, and Women's Work: A Study of Hunter-Gatherer Population Regulation." In Cohen, Mark N., Roy S. Malpass, and Harold G. Klein (eds.). *Biosocial Mechanisms of Population Regulation.* New Haven, CT: Yale University Press, 1980.

10. *Bauhinia esculenta* from the Food and Agriculture Organization of the United Nations (FAO) plant database (2004).

11. Yellen, J., and R.B. Lee. "The Dobe/-Du/da Environment." In Lee, Richard B., and Irven DeVore (eds.). *Kalahari Hunter-Gatherers: Studies of the !Kung San and Their Neighbors.* Cambridge, MA: Harvard University Press, 1976.

12. Yellen, J., and R.B. Lee. "The Dobe/-Du/da Environment." In Lee, Richard B., and Irven DeVore (eds.). *Kalahari Hunter-Gatherers: Studies of the !Kung San and Their Neighbors*. Cambridge, MA: Harvard University Press, 1976.

13. Tanaka, J. "Subsistence Ecology of Central Kalahari San." In Lee, Richard B., and Irven DeVore (eds.). *Kalahari Hunter-Gatherers: Studies of the !Kung San and Their Neighbors*. Cambridge, MA: Harvard University Press, 1976.

14. Lee, R.B. "What Hunters Do for a Living, or How to Make Out on Scarce Resources." In Lee, Richard B., and Irven DeVore (eds.). *Symposium on Man the Hunter.* Chicago: Aldine Publishing, 1968.

15. Lee, R.B. "What Hunters Do for a Living, or How to Make Out on Scarce Resources." In Lee, Richard B., and Irven DeVore (eds.). *Symposium on Man the Hunter.* (Chicago: Aldine Publishing, 1968).

16. Kirchengast, S. "Weight Status of Adult !Kung San and Kavango People from Northern Namibia." *Ann Human Biol* 25:6 (1998): 541–551.

17. Truswell, S., and J. Hansen. "Medical Research Among the !Kung." In Lee, Richard B., and Irven DeVore (eds.). *Kalahari Hunter-Gatherers: Studies of the !Kung San and Their Neighbors*. Cambridge, MA: Harvard University Press, 1976.

18. Jarvis, J., and H.G. van Heerden. "The Acuity of Hearing in the Kalahari Bushmen." *J Laryngol Otol* 81 (1967): 63.

19. Truswell, S., and J. Hansen. "Medical Research Among the !Kung." In Lee, Richard B., and Irven DeVore (eds.). *Kalahari Hunter-Gatherers: Studies of the !Kung San and Their Neighbors*. Cambridge, MA: Harvard University Press, 1976.

20. Blainey, Geoffrey. *Triumph of the Nomads: A History of Ancient Australia.* (South Melbourne: Macmillan, 1982).

21. Lee, A. "The Transition of Aboriginal Diet and Health." *World Rev Nutr Diet* 79 (1996): 1–52.

22. Chewings, C. *Back in the Stone Age.* Sydney: Angus and Robertson, 1936.

23. Naughton, J.M., K. O'Dea, and A.J. Sinclair. "Animal Foods in Traditional Australian Aboriginal Diets: Polyunsaturated and Low in Fat." *Lipids* 21:11 (1986): 684–690.

24. Elphinstone J.J. "The Health of Australian Aboriginals with No Previous Association with Europeans." *Med J Aust* 2:6 (1971): 293–301.

25. Blumenschine, R.J., and J.A. Cavallo. "Scavenging and Human Evolution." *Sci Am* 267:4 (1992): 90–96.

26. Quoted in Leakey, Richard. *The Origin of Humankind.* London: Phoenix, 1996.

27. Richards, M.P., P.B. Pettitt, M.C. Stiner, and E. Trinkaus. "Stable Isotope Evidence for Increasing Dietary Breadth in the European Mid-Upper Paleolithic." *Proc Natl Acad Sci* 98:11 (2001): 6528–6532.

28. Lucas, P., et al. "Principles of Food Breakdown." In Chivers, David J., Bernard A. Wood, and Alan Bilsborough (eds.). *Food Acquisition and Processing in Primates.* New York: Plenum Press, 1984.

— W. Maier. "Tooth Morphology and Diet." In Chivers, David J., Bernard A. Wood, and Alan Bilsborough (eds.). *Food Acquisition and Processing in Primates.* New York: Plenum Press, 1984.

29. Boyde, A., and L. Martin. "Primate Enamel Microstructure." In Chivers, David J., Bernard A. Wood, and Alan Bilsborough (eds.). *Food Acquisition and Processing in Primates.* New York: Plenum Press, 1984.

30. Lalueza, C., A. Perez-Perez, and D. Turbon. "Dietary Inferences through Buccal Microwear Analysis of Middle and Upper Pleistocene Human Fossils." *Am J Phys Anthropol* 100:3 (1996): 367–387.

31. Kliks, M. "Paleodietetics: A Review of the Role of Dietary Fiber in Preagricultural Human Diets." In Spiller, G.A., and R.J. Amen (eds.). *Topics in Dietary Fiber Research.* New York: Plenum Press, 1978.

32. Sibley, C.G., J.A. Comstock, and J.E. Ahlquist. "DNA Hybridization Evidence of Hominoid Phylogeny: A Reanalysis of the Data." *J Mol Evol* 30:3 (1990): 202–236.

33. Samollow, P.B., L.M. Cherry, S.M. Witte, and J. Rogers. "Interspecific Variation at the Y-linked RPS4Y Locus in Hominoids: Implications for Phylogeny." *Am J Phys Anthropol* 101:3 (1996): 333–343.

34. Goodman, M., D.A. Tagle, D.H. Fitch, et al. "Primate Evolution at DNA Level and a Classification of Hominoids." *J Mol Evol* 30:3 (1990): 260–266.

35. Milton, K. "Primate Diets and Gut Morphology." In Harris, Marvin, and Eric B. Ross (eds.). *Food and Evolution.* Philadelphia: Temple University Press, 1987.

36. Russell, R.M. "Changes in Gastrointestinal Function Attributed to Ageing." *Am J Clin Nutr* 55 (1992): 1203S–1207S.

Chapter 2   The Farming Revolution and Its Consequences

1. Diamond, Jared. *Guns, Germs and Steel.* (New York: Vintage, 1998).

2. United States Department of Agriculture. "The Evolving Food and Agriculture System." Available online at www.usda.gov/news/pubs/farmpolicy01/chapter1.pdf.

3. Chandler, Tertius. *Four Thousand Years of Urban Growth.* Lewiston, NY: Edwin Mellon Press, 1987.

4. Brand-Miller, J., et al. "Evolutionary Aspects of Diet and Insulin Resistance." *World Rev Nutr Diet* 84 (1999): 74–105.

5. Segal, Jerome. "What We Work for Now: Changing Household Patterns in the 20th Century." Institute for Philosophy and Public Policy, University of Maryland, December 2001. Available online at www.redefiningprogress.org.

6. Wiley, Harvey W. *The History of a Crime Against the Pure Food Law.* New York: Ayer Company Publishers, 1976.

Chapter 3   How We Eat and Its Consequences

1. Dibner, J.J., and J.D. Richards. *J Appl Poultry Res* (Spring 2004).

2. Eaton, S.B., and D.A. Nelson. "Calcium in Evolutionary Perspective." *Am J Clin Nutr* 54 (1991): 281S–287S.

— Angel, J.L. "Paleoecology, Paleodemography and Health." In Polgar, S. *Population, Ecology and Social Evolution.* The Hague: Mouton, 1975, pp. 167–190.

— Nickens, P.R. "Stature Reduction as an Adaptive Response to Food Production in Mesoamerica." *J Archaeol Sci* 3 (1976): 31–41.

— Cohen, M.N. "The Significance of Long-term Changes in Human Diet and Food Economy." In Harris, M., and E.B. Ross (eds.). *Food and Evolution: Toward a Theory of Human Food Habits*. Philadelphia: Temple University Press, 1987, pp. 261–283.

3. Cohen, M.N. "The Significance of Long-term Changes in Human Diet and Food Economy." In Harris, M., and E.B. Ross (eds.). *Food and Evolution: Toward a Theory of Human Food Habits*. Philadelphia: Temple University Press, 1987, pp. 261–283.

— Cassidy, C.M. "Nutrition and Health in Agriculturalists and Hunter-gatherers: A Case Study of Two Prehistoric Populations." In Jerome, Norge W., Randy F. Kandel, Gretel H. Pelto (eds.). *Nutritional Anthropology: Contemporary Approaches to Diet and Culture*. Pleasantville, NY: Redgrave Publishing, 1980, pp. 117–145.

4. Cohen, M.N. "The Significance of Long-term Changes in Human Diet and Food Economy." In Harris, M., and E.B. Ross (eds.). *Food and Evolution: Toward a Theory of Human Food Habits*. Philadelphia: Temple University Press, 1987, pp. 261–283.

— Cassidy, C.M. "Nutrition and Health in Agriculturalists and Hunter-gatherers: A Case Study of Two Prehistoric Populations." In Jerome, Norge W., Randy F. Kandel, Gretel H. Pelto (eds.). *Nutritional Anthropology: Contemporary Approaches to Diet and Culture*. Pleasantville, NY: Redgrave Publishing, 1980, pp. 117–145.

5. Cohen, M.N. "The Significance of Long-term Changes in Human Diet and Food Economy." In Harris, M., and E.B. Ross (eds.). *Food and Evolution: Toward a Theory of Human Food Habits*. Philadelphia: Temple University Press, 1987, pp. 261–283.

— Cassidy, C.M. "Nutrition and Health in Agriculturalists and Hunter-gatherers: A Case Study of Two Prehistoric Populations." In Jerome, Norge W., Randy F. Kandel, Gretel H. Pelto (eds.). *Nutritional Anthropology: Contemporary Approaches to Diet and Culture*. Pleasantville, NY: Redgrave Publishing, 1980, pp. 117–145.

— Diamond, J. *The Third Chimpanzee: The Evolution and Future of the Human Animal*. New York: HarperCollins, 1992, pp. 261–291.

— Lallo, J.W., et al. "The Role of Diet, Disease and Physiology in the Origins of Porotic Hyperostosis." *Human Biol* 49 (1977): 471–473.

6. Cohen, M.N. "The Significance of Long-term Changes in Human Diet and Food Economy." In Harris, M., and E.B. Ross (eds.). *Food and Evolution: Toward a Theory of Human Food Habits*. Philadelphia: Temple University Press, 1987, pp. 261–283.

— Cassidy, C.M. "Nutrition and Health in Agriculturalists and Hunter-gatherers: A Case Study of Two Prehistoric Populations." In Jerome, Norge W., Randy F. Kandel, Gretel H. Pelto (eds.). *Nutritional Anthropology: Contemporary Approaches to Diet and Culture*. Pleasantville, NY: Redgrave Publishing, 1980, pp. 117–145.

— Lallo, J.W., et al. "The Role of Diet, Disease and Physiology in the Origins of Porotic Hyperostosis." *Human Biol* 49 (1977): 471–473.

7. Eaton, S.B., and D.A. Nelson. "Calcium in Evolutionary Perspective." *Am J Clin Nutr* 54 (1991): 281S–287S.

— Cohen, M.N. "The Significance of Long-term Changes in Human Diet and Food Economy." In Harris, M., and E.B. Ross (eds.). *Food and Evolution: Toward a Theory of Human Food Habits*. Philadelphia: Temple University Press, 1987, pp. 261–283.

— Cassidy, C.M. "Nutrition and Health in Agriculturalists and Hunter-gatherers: A Case Study of Two Prehistoric Populations." In Jerome, Norge W., Randy F. Kandel,

Gretel H. Pelto (eds.). *Nutritional Anthropology: Contemporary Approaches to Diet and Culture.* Pleasantville, NY: Redgrave Publishing, 1980, pp. 117–145.

— Lallo, J.W., et al. "The Role of Diet, Disease and Physiology in the Origins of Porotic Hyperostosis." *Human Biol* 49 (1977): 471–473.

8. Cohen, M.N. "The Significance of Long-term Changes in Human Diet and Food Economy." In Harris, M., and E.B. Ross (eds.). *Food and Evolution: Toward a Theory of Human Food Habits.* Philadelphia: Temple University Press, 1987, pp. 261–283.

— Cassidy, C.M. "Nutrition and Health in Agriculturalists and Hunter-gatherers: A Case Study of Two Prehistoric Populations." In Jerome, Norge W., Randy F. Kandel, Gretel H. Pelto (eds.). *Nutritional Anthropology: Contemporary Approaches to Diet and Culture.* Pleasantville, NY: Redgrave Publishing, 1980, pp. 117–145.

— Turner, C.G. "Dental Anthropological Indications of Agriculture Among the Jomon People of Central Japan." *Am J Phys Anthropol* 51 (1979): 619–636.

9. Kniker, T. "Dietary Changes May Help Some with Autism." 12th International Conference on Autism, Durham University, England, April 2001.

10. Lorenz, K. "Cereals and Schizophrenia." *Adv Cereal Sci Technol* 10 (1990): 435–469.

11. Gobbi, G., F. Bouquet, L. Greco, et al. "Coeliac Disease, Epilepsy and Cerebral Calcifications." *Lancet* 340:8817 (1992): 439–443.

— Fois, A., et al. "Celiac Disease and Epilepsy in Pediatric Patients." *Childs Nerv Syst* 10 (1994): 450–454.

12. Matheson, N.A. "Multiple Sclerosis and Diet." *Lancet* ii (1974): 1204.

13. Shatin, R. "Report of the Treatment of Rheumatoid Arthritis with High Protein Gluten-free Diet and Supplements." *Med J Aust* 2 (1964): 169–172.

— Lepore, L., et al. "Prevalence of Celiac Disease in Patients with Juvenile Arthritis." *J Pediatr* 129 (1996): 311–313.

14. Andersson, H., and H. Mobacken. "Dietary Treatment of Dermatitis Herpetiformus." *Eur J Clin Nutr* 46:5 (1992): 309–315.

15. Ames, B.N. "Nature's Chemicals and Synthetic Chemicals: Comparative Toxicology." *Proc Natl Acad Sci USA* 87 (1990): 7782–7786.

16. Nöll, Gunter. Personal communication, July 11, 2005.

17. Cordain, L., B.A. Watkins, G.L. Florant, et al. "Fatty Acid Analysis of Wild Ruminant Tissues: Evolutionary Implications for Reducing Diet-related Chronic Disease." *Eur J Clin Nutr* 56:3 (2002): 181–191.

18. United States Department of Agriculture Economic Research Service (ERS/USDA). Food consumption (per capita) data system, 2006. Available online at: http://www.ers.usda.gov/data/foodconsumption.

19. United States Department of Agriculture Economic Research Service (ERS/USDA). Food consumption (per capita) data system, 2006. Available online at: http://www.ers.usda.gov/data/foodconsumption.

20. Broadhurst, C.L., S.C. Cunnane, and M.A. Crawford. "Rift Valley Lake Fish and Shellfish Provided Brain-specific Nutrition for Early *Homo.*" *Br J Nutr* 79:1 (1998): 3–21.

21. Paoletti, M.G., E. Buscardo, D.J. VanderJagt, et al. "Nutrient Content of Earth-

worms Consumed by Ye'Kuana Amerindians of the Alto Orinoco of Venezuela." *Proc Biol Sci* 270:1512 (2003): 249–257.

22. Paoletti, M.G., et al. "Palm Worm (Insecta, Coleoptera, Curculionidae: *Rhynchophorus palmarum*) Traditional Food." *Amazonas, Venezuela: Nutritional Composition, Small Scale Production and Tourist Palatability* (Unpublished paper, 2004).

23. Nagata, C., N. Takatsuka, Y. Kurisu, and H. Shimizu. "Decreased Serum Total Cholesterol Concentration Is Associated with High Intake of Soy Products in Japanese Men and Women." *J Nutr* 128 (1998): 209–213.

24. Hidayaki, Tsuji. "Allergens in Major Crops." *Nutr Res* 21 (2001): 925.

25. Allred, C.D., K.K. Allred, Y.H. Ju, et al. "Soy Diets Containing Varying Amounts of Genistein Stimulate Growth of Estrogen-dependent (MCF-7) Tumors in a Dose-dependent Manner." *Cancer Res* 61:13 (2001): 5045–5050.

— Allred, C.D. "Dietary Genistin Stimulates Growth of Estrogen-dependent Breast Cancer Tumors Similar to that Observed with Genistein." *Carcinogenesis* 22:10 (2001): 1667–1673.

26. White, L.R., et al. "Brain Aging and Midlife Tofu Consumption." *J Am Coll Nutr* 19:2 (2000): 242–255.

27. Divi, R.L., H.C. Chang, and D.R. Doerge. "Anti-thyroid Isoflavones from Soybean: Isolation, Characterization, and Mechanisms of Action." *Biochem Pharm* 54:10 (1997): 1087–1096

28. Shahidi, F. (ed.). *Antinutrients and Phytochemicals in Food.* ACS Symposium Series. Washington, DC: American Chemical Society, 1997.

— Cordain, L. "Humanity's Double Edged Sword." *World Rev Nutr Diet* 84 (1999): 19–73.

29. "Olive." *Britannica Concise Encyclopedia* from Encyclopedia Britannica Premium Service: http://www.britannica.com/ebc/article?eu=399303.

30. Meehan, B. *Shell Bed to Shell Midden.* Canberra: Australian Institute of Aboriginal Studies, 1982.

31. Ransome, H.M. *The Sacred Bee in Ancient Times and Folklore.* London: George Allen and Unwin, 1937.

32. Darby, W.J., P. Ghalioungui, and L. Grivetti. *Food: The Gift of Osiris.* New York: Academic Press, 1977.

33. Best, M.R. *Gervase Markham: The English Housewife* (first published in 1600). Kingston: McGill-Queen's University Press, 1986.

34. Staden, Hans. Published in Marburg 1557; quoted in *Word IQ Encyclopedia,* available online at www.wordiq.com.

35. United States Department of Agriculture Economic Research Service (ERS/USDA). Food consumption (per capita) data system, 2006. Available online at: http://www.ers.usda.gov/data/foodconsumption.

36. "How Much Sodium and How Much Chloride are in a Teaspoon of Salt?" (Data sheet) Alexandria, VA: Salt Institute, 2004.

37. Eaton, S.B., S.B. Eaton 3rd, M.J. Konner, and M. Shostak. "An Evolutionary Perspective Enhances Understanding of Human Nutritional Requirements." *J Nutr* 126:6 (1996): 1732–1740.

38. Zarkadas, M., R. Gougeon-Reyburn, E.B. Marliss, et al. "Sodium Chloride Supplementation and Urinary Calcium Excretion in Postmenopausal Women." *Am J Clin Nutr* 50:5 (1989): 1088–1094.

— Sellmeyer, D.E., M. Schloetter, and A. Sebastian. "Potassium Citrate Prevents Increased Urine Calcium Excretion and Bone Resorption Induced by a High Sodium Chloride Diet." *J Clin Endocrinol Metab* 87:5 (2002): 2008–2012.

— Cirillo, M., C. Ciacci, M. Laurenzi, et al. "Salt Intake, Urinary Sodium and Hypercalciuria." *Miner Electrolyte Metab* 23:3–6 (1997): 265–268.

40. Tobian, L., and S. Hanlon. "High Sodium Chloride Diets Injure Arteries and Raise Mortality Without Changing Blood Pressure." *Hypertension* 15:6 Part 2 (1990): 900–903.

41. Eaton, Boyd. "Evolutionary Aspects of Diet." *World Rev Nutr Diet* 81 (1997): 26–37.

42. "'The Real Thing': Nominal Price Rigidity of the Nickel Coke, 1886–1959." Bar-Ilan University Economics Working Paper No. 2004. Levy, Daniel, and Andrew T. Young (Department of Economics, Emory University, February 4, 2004).

43. United States Department of Agriculture Economic Research Service (ERS/USDA). Food consumption (per capita) data system, 2004. Available online at: http://www.ers.usda.gov/data/foodconsumption.

Chapter 4   The Science I: Population Studies and Biochemical Clues

1. United Nations Statistics Division.

2. United Nations ESCAP. Family Planning Programme, China Population Information and Research Centre (2002).

3. Helsing, E. "Traditional Diets and Disease Patterns of the Mediterranean, Circa 1960." *Am J Clin Nutr* 61:Suppl (1995): 1329S–1337S.

4. Kushi, L.H. "Health Implications of Mediterranean Diets in Light of Contemporary Knowledge. 1. Plant Foods and Dairy Products." *Am J Clin Nutr* 61:Suppl (1995): 1407S–1415S.

5. *WHO Health Statistics Annual.* Geneva: World Health Organization, 1995.

6. Gjonka, A., and M. Bobak. "The Albanian Paradox." *Lancet* 350:9094 (1997): 1815–1817.

7. World Health Organization (WHO) Report, June 5, 2000.

8. Paleonutrition & Modern Nutrition; Connie Phillipson; *World Rev Nutri Diet;* 1997; vol 81; pp 38–48

9. Adams, Ruth. *Eating in Eden.* Emmaus, PA: Rodale Press, 1976.

10. Sinclair. "Diet of Canadian Indians and Eskimos: Unusual Foods for Human Consumption." *Symposium Proc* 12 (1953): 69–82.

11. Keenleyside, A. "Skeletal Evidence of Health and Disease in Pre-contact Alaskan Eskimos and Aleuts." *Am J Phys Anthropol* 107:1 (1998): 51–70.

11. Sinclair. "Diet of Canadian Indians and Eskimos: Unusual Foods for Human Consumption." *Symposium Proc* 12 (1953): 69–82.

12. Mann, et al. "The Health and Nutritional Status of Alaskan Eskimos." *Am J Clin Nutr* 11 (1962): 31–76.

13. Mazes and Mather. "Bone Mineral Content of North Alaskan Eskimos." *Am J Clin Nutr* 27 (1974): 916–925.

14. Booyens, J., C.C. Louwrens, and I.E. Katzeff. "The Eskimo Diet: Prophylactic Effects Ascribed to the Balanced Presence of Natural cis Unsaturated Fatty Acids and to the Absence of Unnatural Trans and cis Isomers of Unsaturated Fatty Acids." *Med Hypotheses* 21:4 (1986): 387–408

15. Ho, K.J., B. Mikkelson, L.A. Lewis, et al. "Alaskan Arctic Eskimos: Responses to a Customary High Fat Diet." *Am J Clin Nutr* 25:8 (1972): 737–745.

16. Bang, H.O., J. Dyerberg, and A.B. Nielsen. "Plasma Lipid and Lipoprotein Pattern in Greenlandic West-coast Eskimos." *Lancet* 1:7710 (1971): 1143–1145.

17. Bang, H.O., J. Dyerberg, and A.B. Nielsen. "Plasma Lipid and Lipoprotein Pattern in Greenlandic West-coast Eskimos." *Lancet* 1:7710 (1971): 1143–1145.

18. Food and Agricultural Organization. *Analysis of the Food Consumption of Japanese Households.* Rome: Food and Agricultural Organization, 2003.

19. Furst, B. "On the Use of Migration Studies in the Explanation of Diseases of Multifactorial Causality: The Risk of Non-Insulin-Dependent Diabetes in Japanese-Americans." *Nutrition Noteworthy* 1 (1998): Article 5.

— Marmot, M.G. "Acculturation and Coronary Heart Disease in Japanese-Americans." *Am J Epidemiol* 104:3 (1976): 225–247.

20. Kagawa, Y., M. Nishizawa, M. Suzuki, et al. "Eicosapolyenoic Acids of Serum Lipids of Japanese Islanders with Low Incidence of Cardiovascular Diseases." *J Nutr Sci Vitaminol* 28:4 (1982): 441–453.

21. Cockerham, W.C., and Y. Yamori. "Okinawa: An Exception to the Social Gradient of Life Expectancy in Japan." *Asia Pac J Clin Nutr* 10:2 (2001): 154–158.

22. Kagawa, Y., M. Nishizawa, M. Suzuki, et al. "Eicosapolyenoic Acids of Serum Lipids of Japanese Islanders with Low Incidence of Cardiovascular Diseases." *J Nutr Sci Vitaminol* 28:4 (1982): 441–453.

23. Keys, A. "Coronary Heart Disease in Seven Countries." *Circulation* 41:4 Suppl (1970): 1–211.

— Keys, A. *How to Eat Well and Stay Well the Mediterranean Way.* New York: Doubleday, 1975.

24. Renaud, S., M. de Lorgeril, J. Delaye, et al. "Cretan Mediterranean Diet for Prevention of Coronary Heart Disease." *Am J Clin Nutr* 61:6 Suppl (1995): 1360S-1367S.

25. Jenkins, D.J., T.M. Wolever, R.H. Taylor, et al. "Glycemic Index of Foods: A Physiological Basis for Carbohydrate Exchange." *Am J Clin Nutr* 34:3 (1981): 362–366.

26. Holt, S.H., J.C. Miller, and P. Petocz. "An Insulin Index of Foods: The Insulin Demand Generated by 1000-kJ Portions of Common Foods.." *Am J Clin Nutr* 66:5 (1997): 1264–1276.

27. Holt, S.H., J.C. Miller, and P. Petocz. "An Insulin Index of Foods: The Insulin Demand Generated by 1000-kJ Portions of Common Foods.." *Am J Clin Nutr* 66:5 (1997): 1264–1276.

28. Brand-Miller, J.C., and S. Colagiuri. "Evolutionary Aspects of Diet and Insulin Resistance." *World Rev Nutr Diet* 84 (1999): 74–105.

29. O'Dea, K. "Marked Improvement in Carbohydrate and Lipid Metabolism in Dia-

betic Australian Aborigines After Temporary Reversion to Traditional Lifestyle." *Diabetes* 33 (1984): 596–603.

30. Gundry, Steven. Personal communication, January 23, 2003.

31. Hayek, et al. "Utilization of n-3 Fatty Acids in Companion Animal Nutrition." *World Rev Nutr Diet* 83 (1998): 176–185.

32. Hayek, M.G., and G.A. Reinhart. "Utilization of n-3 Fatty Acids in Companion Animal Nutrition." *World Rev Nutr Diet* 83 (1998): 176–185.

33. Broadhurst, C.L., Y. Wang, M.A. Crawford, et al. "Brain-specific Lipids from Marine, Lacustrine or Terrestrial Resources: Potential Impact on Early African *Homo sapiens*." *Comp Biochem Physiol B Biochem Mol Biol* 131:4 (2002): 653–673.

34. Broadhurst, C.L., S.C. Cunnane, and M.A. Crawford. "Rift Valley Lake Fish and Shellfish Provided Brain Specific Nutrition for Early *Homo*." *Br J Nutr* 79:1 (1998): 3–21.

35. Renaud, S., M. de Lorgeril, J. Delaye, et al. "Cretan Mediterranean Diet for Prevention of Coronary Heart Disease." *Am J Clin Nutr* 61:6 Suppl (1995): 1360S-1367S.

36. Renaud, S., M. de Lorgeril, J. Delaye, et al. "Cretan Mediterranean Diet for Prevention of Coronary Heart Disease." *Am J Clin Nutr* 61:6 Suppl (1995): 1360S-1367S.
— Renaud, Serge. *Le Régime Santé.* Paris: Éditions Odile Jacob, 1995.

37. Renaud, S. Personal communication, July 22, 1997.

38. Eaton, Boyd. "Evolutionary Aspects of Diet." *World Rev Nutr Diet* 81 (1997): 26–37.

39. Tobian, L., and S. Hanlon. "High Sodium Chloride Diets Injure Arteries and Raise Mortality Without Changing Blood Pressure." *Hypertension* 15:6 Part 2 (1990): 900–903.

40. Zarkadas, M., R. Gougeon-Reyburn, E.B. Marliss, et al. "Sodium Chloride Supplementation and Urinary Calcium Excretion in Postmenopausal Women." *Am J Clin Nutr* 50:5 (1989): 1088–1094.

41. Sellmeyer, D.E., M. Schloetter, and A. Sebastian. "Potassium Citrate Prevents Increased Urine Calcium Excretion and Bone Resorption Induced by a High Sodium Chloride Diet." *J Clin Endocrinol Metab* 87:5 (2002): 2008–2012.
— Cirillo, M., C. Ciacci, M. Laurenzi, et al. "Salt Intake, Urinary Sodium and Hypercalciuria." *Miner Electrolyte Metab* 23:3–6 (1997): 265–268.

42. Sebastian, A., L.A. Frassetto, D.E. Sellmeyer, et al. "Estimation of the Net Acid Load of the Diet of Ancestral Preagricultural *Homo sapiens* and Their Hominid Ancestors." *Am J Clin Nutr* 76:6 (2002): 1308–1316.

43. McCance, R.A., and E.M. Widdowson. *The Composition of Foods.* London: HMSO, 1960.

Chapter 5   The Science II: Digestive System and Dietary Clues

1. Moreau, M.C., and M. Coste. "Immune Responses to Dietary Protein Antigens." *World Rev Nutr Diet* 74 (1993): 22–57.

2. Truswell, A.S. "Dietary Fiber and Health." *World Rev Nutr Diet* 72 (1993): 148–164.

3. Diel, P., S. Olff, S. Schmidt, and H. Michna. "Molecular Identification of Potential Selective Estrogen Receptor Modulator (SERM)–like Properties of Phytoestrogens in the Human Breast Cancer Cell Line MCF-7." *Planta Med* 67:6 (2001): 510–514.

— Fokialakis, N., G. Lambrinidis, D.J. Mitsiou, et al. "A New Class of Phytoestrogens: Evaluation of the Estrogenic Activity of Deoxybenzoins." *Chem Biol* 11:3 (2004): 397–406.

4. Holzer, P. "Sensory Neurone Responses to Mucosal Noxae in the Upper Gut: Relevance to Mucosal Integrity and Gastrointestinal Pain." *Neurogastroenterol Motil* 14:5 (2002): 459–475.

5. Rodriguez-Stanley, S., K.L. Collings, M. Robinson, et al. "The Effects of Capsaicin on Reflux, Gastric Emptying and Dyspepsia." *Aliment Pharmacol Ther* 14:1 (2000): 129–134.

6. Jensen-Jarolim, E., L. Gajdzik, I. Haberl, et al. "Hot Spices Influence Permeability of Human Intestinal Epithelial Monolayers." *J Nutr* 128:3 (1998): 577–581.

7. Vines. G. "A Gut Feeling—Junk Foods Grow Bad Bacteria." *New Scientist* (August 8, 1998): 26–30.

8. Pitcher, M.C., and J.H. Cummings. "Hydrogen Sulphide: A Bacterial Toxin in Ulcerative Colitis?" *Gut* 39:1 (1996): 1–4.

9. Mathias, J.R., R. Franklin, D.C. Quast, et al. "Relation of Endometriosis and Neuromuscular Disease of the Gastrointestinal Tract: New Insights." *Fertil Steril* 70:1 (1998): 81–88.

10. Rothman, S.S. "Regulation of Digestive Reactions by the Pancreas." In Forte, J.G. (ed.). *Handbook of Physiology, Section 6: The Gastrointestinal System.* Bethesda, MD: American Physiological Society, 1989.

11. McCance, R.A., and E.M. Widdowson. *The Composition of Foods,* 5th edition. London: Royal Society of Chemistry, 1995.

12. Milton, K. "Nutritional Characteristics of Wild Primate Foods: Do the Diets of Our Closest Living Relatives Have Lessons for Us?" *Nutrition* 15:6 (1999): 488–498.

13. Cordain, L. "Cereal Grains: Humanity's Double-edged Sword." *World Rev Nutr Diet* 84 (1999): 19–73.

14. Frøkier, H., T.M. Jørgensen, A. Rosendal, et al. "Antinutritional and Allergenic Proteins." In Shahidi, F. (ed.). *Antinutrients and Phytochemicals in Food.* ACS Symposium Series. Washington, DC: American Chemical Society, 1997.

15. Fasano, A., I. Berti, T. Gerarduzzi, et al. "Prevalence of Celiac Disease in At-risk and Not-at-risk Groups in the United States: A Large Multicenter Study." *Arch Intern Med* 163:3 (2003): 286–292.

16. Tsuji, H., M. Kimoto, and Y. Natori. "Allergens in Major Crops." *Nutr Res* 21 (2001): 925–934.

17. Plhak, L.C., and P. Sporns. "Biological Activities of Potato Glycoalkaloids." In Shahidi, F. (ed.). *Antinutrients and Phytochemicals in Food.* ACS Symposium Series. Washington, DC: American Chemical Society, 1997.

18. Anonymous. *Br Med J* (1979): 1458–1459.

19. Morris, S.C., and T.H. Lee. "The Toxicity and Teratogenicity of Solanaceae Glycoalkaloids, Particularly Those of the Potato (*Solanum tuberosum*): A Review." *Food Technol Aust* 36:3 (1984): 118–124.

20. Milton, K. "Nutritional Characteristics of Wild Primate Foods: Do the Diets of Our Closest Living Relatives Have Lessons for Us?" *Nutrition* 15:6 (1999): 488–498.

21. Milton, K. "Primate Diets and Gut Morphology." In Harris, Marvin, and Eric B. Ross (eds.). *Food and Evolution*. Philadelphia: Temple University Press, 1987.

22. Milton, K. "Back to Basics: Why Foods of Primates Have Relevance for Modern Health." *Nutrition* 16:7–8 (2000): 480–483.

23. Simopoulos, A.P., H.A. Norman, and J.E. Gillaspy. "Purslane in Human Nutrition and Its Potential for World Agriculture." *World Rev Nutr Diet* 77 (1995): 47–74.

24. Milton, K. "Nutritional Characteristics of Wild Primate Foods: Do the Diets of Our Closest Living Relatives Have Lessons for Us?" *Nutrition* 15:6 (1999): 488–498.

— Milton, K. "Back to Basics: Why Foods of Primates Have Relevance for Modern Health." *Nutrition* 16:7–8 (2000): 480–483.

25. Milton, K. "Nutritional Characteristics of Wild Primate Foods: Do the Diets of Our Closest Living Relatives Have Lessons for Us?" *Nutrition* 15:6 (1999): 488–498.

26. Anonymous. "Plant Foods and Atherosclerosis." *Nutr Rev* 35:6 (1977): 148–150.

27. Kniker, T. "Dietary Changes May Help Some with Autism." 12th International Conference on Autism, Durham University, England, April 2001.

28. Feskanich, D., W.C. Willett, M.J. Stampfer, and G.A. Colditz. "Milk, Dietary Calcium and Bone Fractures in Women: A 12-year Prospective Study." *Am J Public Health* 87:6 (1997): 992–997.

29. Chan, J.M., M.J. Stampfer, J. Ma, et al. "Dairy Products, Calcium and Prostate Cancer Risk in the Physicians' Health Study." *Am J Clin Nutr* 74:4 (2001): 549–554.

30. De Stefani, E., E.T. Fontham, V. Chen, et al. "Fatty Foods and the Risk of Lung Cancer: A Case-control Study from Uruguay." *Int J Cancer* 71:5 (1997): 760–766.

31. Liljeberg Elmstahl, H., and I. Bjorck. "Milk as a Supplement to Mixed Meals May Elevate Postprandial Insulinaemia." *Eur J Clin Nutr* 55:11 (2001): 994–999.

32. Abraham, G.E. "Nutritional Factors in the Etiology of the Premenstrual Tension Syndromes." *J Reprod Med* 28:7 (1983): 446–464.

33. Chen, H., S.M. Zhang, M.A. Hernan, et al. "Diet and Parkinson's Disease: A Potential Role of Dairy Products in Men." *Ann Neurol* 52:6 (2002): 793–801.

34. Riordan, A.M., J.O. Hunter, R.E. Cowan, et al. "Treatment of Active Crohn's Disease by Exclusion Diet: East Anglian Multicentre Controlled Trial." *Lancet* 342:8880 (1993): 1131–1134.

35. Grant, W. "Milk and Other Dietary Influences on Coronary Heart Disease." *Altern Med Rev* 3:4 (1998): 281–294.

36. Crawford, M.A. "Fatty-acid Ratios in Free-living and Domestic Animals. Possible Implications for Atheroma." *Lancet* 1:7556 (1968): 1329–1333.

37. Koizumi, I., Y. Suzuki, and J.J. Kaneko. "Studies on the Fatty Acid Composition of Intramuscular Lipids of Cattle, Pigs and Birds." *J Nutr Sci Vitaminol* (*Tokyo*) 37:6 (1991): 545–554.

38. Simopoulos, A.P., and N. Salem Jr. "n-3 Fatty Acids in Eggs from Range-fed Greek Chickens." *N Engl J Med* 321:20 (1989): 1412.

39. Simopoulos, A.P. "New Products from the Agri-food Industry: The Return of n-3 Fatty Acids Into the Food Supply." *Lipids* 34:Suppl (1999): S297–S301.

40. Levin, Y., Y. Sherer, H. Bibi, et al. "Rare *Jatropha multifida* Intoxication in Two Children." *J Emerg Med* 19:2 (2000): 173–175.

41. Greenfield, R.A., B.R. Brown, J.B. Hutchins, et al. "Microbiological, Biological, and Chemical Weapons of Warfare and Terrorism." *Am J Med Sci* 323:6 (2002): 326–340.

42. Sharom, F.J., M.P. Lamb, C.C. Kupsh, and S. Head. "Inhibition of Lymphocyte 5′-nucleotidase by Lectins: Effects of Lectin Specificity and Cross-linking Ability." *Biochem Cell Biol* 66:7 (1988): 715–723.

43. Newbold, R.R., E.P. Banks, B. Bullock, and W.N. Jefferson. "Uterine Adenocarcinoma in Mice Treated Neonatally with Genistein." *Cancer Res* 61:11 (2001): 4325–4328.

44. Allred, C.D., Y.H. Ju, K.F. Allred, et al. "Dietary Genistin Stimulates Growth of Estrogen-dependent Breast Cancer Tumors Similar to that Observed with Genistein." *Carcinogenesis* 22:10 (2001): 1667–1673.

— Ju, Y.H., C.D. Allred, K.F. Allred, et al. "Physiological Concentrations of Dietary Genistein Dose-dependently Stimulate Growth of Estrogen-dependent Human Breast Cancer (MCF-7) Tumors Implanted in Athymic Nude Mice." *J Nutr* 131:11 (2001): 2957–2962.

— Allred, C.D., K.F. Allred, Y.H. Ju, et al. "Soy Diets Containing Varying Amounts of Genistein Stimulate Growth of Estrogen-dependent (MCF-7) Tumors in a Dose-dependent Manner." *Cancer Res* 61:13 (2001): 5045–5050.

45. Foucard, T., and I. Malmheden Yman. "A Study on Severe Food Reactions in Sweden—Is Soy Protein an Underestimated Cause of Food Anaphylaxis?" *Allergy* 54:3 (1999): 261–265.

— Tsuji, H., M. Kimoto, and Y. Natori. "Allergens in Major Crops." *Nutr Res* 21 (2001): 925–934.

46. Divi, R.L., H.C. Chang, and D.R. Doerge. "Anti-thyroid Isoflavones from Soybean: Isolation, Characterization, and Mechanisms of Action.." *Biochem Pharm* 54:10 (1997): 1087–1096.

47. White, L.R., H. Petrovitch, G.W. Ross, et al. "Brain Aging and Midlife Tofu Consumption." *J Am Coll Nutr* 19:2 (2000): 242–255.

48. Shahidi, F. (ed.). *Antinutrients and Phytochemicals in Food.* ACS Symposium Series. Washington, DC: American Chemical Society, 1997. Cordain, L. "Cereal Grains: Humanity's Double-edged Sword." *World Rev Nutr Diet* 84 (1999): 19–73.

49. Irvine, C.H.G., M. Fitzpatrick, I. Robertson, and D. Woodhams. "The Potential Adverse Effects of Soybean Isoflavones in Infant Feeding." *NZ Med J* 108 (1995): 218.

50. Irvine, C.H.G., M. Fitzpatrick, I. Robertson, and D. Woodhams. "The Potential Adverse Effects of Soybean Isoflavones in Infant Feeding." *NZ Med J* 108 (1995): 218.

— Freni-Titulaer, L.W., J.F. Cordero, L. Haddock, et al. "Premature Thelarche in Puerto Rico. A Search for Environmental Factors." *Am J Dis Child* 140:12 (1986): 1263–1267.

51. Freni-Titulaer, L.W., J.F. Cordero, L. Haddock, et al. "Premature Thelarche in

Puerto Rico. A Search for Environmental Factors." *Am J Dis Child* 140:12 (1986): 1263–1267.

52. Lack, G., D. Fox, K. Northstone, et al. "Factors Associated with the Development of Peanut Allergy in Childhood." *N Engl J Med* 348:11 (2003): 977–985.

53. Food Standards Agency. *Report on Phytoestrogens and Health.* London: Food Standards Agency, May 2003.

54. Sicherer, S.H. "Clinical Update on Peanut Allergy." *Ann Allergy Asthma Immunol* 88:4 (2002): 350–361.

55. Sampson, H.A. "Food Allergy, Part 1: Immunopathogenesis and Clinical Disorders." *J Allergy Clin Immunol* 103:5 Part 1 (1999): 717–728.

— Sampson, H.A. "Clinical Practice. Peanut Allergy." *N Engl J Med* 346:17 (2002): 1294–1299.

— Sicherer, S.H., J.A. Forman, and S.A. Noone. "Use Assessment of Self-administered Epinephrine Among Food-allergic Children and Pediatricians." *Pediatrics* 105 (2000): 359–362.

56. Grant, W. "Reassessing the Role of Sugar in the Etiology of Heart Disease." *J Orthomol Med* 13 (1998): 95–104.

57. Morselli, Mariafranca, and M. Lynn Whalen. "Maple Chemistry and Quality." In Koelling, M.R., and R.B. Heiligmann (eds.). *North American Maple Syrup Producers Manual,* Bulletin 856, Appendix 2. Columbus, OH: Ohio State University, 1996.

58. Jenkins, D.J., T.M. Wolever, R.H. Taylor, et al. "Glycemic Index of Foods: A Physiological Basis for Carbohydrate Exchange." *Am J Clin Nutr* 34:3 (1981): 362–366.

59. Arcot, J., and J. Brand-Miller. *A Preliminary Assessment of the Glycemic Index of Honey: A Report for the Rural Industries Research and Development Corporation.* RIRDC Publication No 05/027. Barton, Australia: RIRDC, 2005. Available online at: www.rirdc.gov.au.

60. Katiyar, S.K., and H. Mukhtar. "Tea Consumption and Cancer." *World Rev Nutr Diet* 79 (1996): 154–184.

— Arts, I.C., P.C. Hollman, H.B. Bueno De Mesquita, et al. "Dietary Catechins and Epithelial Cancer Incidence: The Zutphen Elderly Study." *Int J Cancer* 92:2 (2001): 298–302.

61. Ishikawa, T., M. Suzukawa, T. Ito, et al. "Effect of Tea Flavonoid Supplementation on the Susceptibility of Low-density Lipoprotein to Oxidative Modification." *Am J Clin Nutr* 66:2 (1997): 261–266.

62. Sesso, H.D., J.M. Gaziano, J.E. Buring, and C.H. Hennekens. "Coffee and Tea Intake and the Risk of Myocardial Infarction." *Am J Epidemiol* 149:2 (1999): 162–167.

63. Geleijnse, J.M., L.J. Launer, A. Hofman A, et al. "Tea Flavonoids May Protect Against Atherosclerosis: The Rotterdam Study." *Arch Intern Med* 159:18 (1999): 2170–2174.

Chapter 6   The Owner's Manual

1. Bray, G.A., S.J. Nielsen, and B.M. Popkin. "Consumption of High-fructose Corn

Syrup in Beverages May Play a Role in the Epidemic of Obesity." *Am J Clin Nutr* 79:4 (2004): 537–543.

2. Singleton, M.J., C.Heiser, K. Jamesen, and R.D. Mattes. "Sweetener Augmentation of Serum Triacylglycerol During a Fat Challenge Test in Humans." *J Am College Nutr* 18:2 (1999): 179–185.

— Elliott, S.S., N.L. Keim, J.S. Stern, et al. "Fructose, Weight Gain, and the Insulin Resistance Syndrome." *Am J Clin Nutr* 76:5 (2002): 911–922.

3. Popkin, B.M. "A New Proposed Guidance System for Beverage Consumption in the United States." *Am J Clin Nutr* 83:3 (2006): 529–542.

Chapter 7 Eating the "Savanna Model" Way

1. Worthington, V. "Nutritional Quality of Organic versus Conventional Fruits, Vegetables, and Grains." *J Altern Complement Med* 7:2 (2001): 161–173.

2. Petrie, H.J., S.E. Chown, L.M. Belfie, et al. "Caffeine Ingestion Increases the Insulin Response to an Oral-glucose-tolerance Test in Obese Men Before and After Weight Loss." *Am J Clin Nutr* 80:1 (2004): 22–28.

— Lane, J.D., C.E. Barkauskas, R.S. Surwit, and M.N. Feinglos. "Caffeine Impairs Glucose Metabolism in Type 2 Diabetes." *Diabetes Care* 27:8 (2004): 2047–2048.

3. Tuomilehto, J., G. Hu, S. Bidel, et al. "Coffee Consumption and Risk of Type 2 Diabetes Mellitus Among Middle-aged Finnish Men and Women." *JAMA* 291:10 (2004): 1213–1219.

— Salazar-Martinez. "Coffee Consumption and Risk for Type 2 Diabetes Mellitus." *Ann Intern Med* 140:1 (2004): 1–8.

4. Nawrot, P., S. Jordan, J. Eastwood, et al. "Effects of Caffeine on Human Health." *Food Addit Contam* 20:1 (2003): 1–30.

5. Food Standards Agency. *Report on Phytoestrogens and Health.* London: Food Standards Agency, May 2003.

6. Allen, Lindsay E. "Women's Dietary Calcium Requirements are Not Increased by Pregnancy or Lactation." *Am J Clin Nutr* 67:4 (1998): 591–592.

— Laskey, M.A., A. Prentice, L.A. Hanratty, et al. "Bone Changes after Three Months of Lactation: Influence of Calcium Intake, Breast-milk Output, and Vitamin D-receptor Genotype.." *Am J Clin Nutr* 67:4 (1998): 685–692.

— Ritchie, L.D., E.B. Fung, B.P. Halloran, et al. "A Longitudinal Study of Calcium Homeostasis During Human Pregnancy and Lactation and After Resumption of Menses." *Am J Clin Nutr* 67:4 (1998): 693–701.

7. Holloway, Marguerite, and Marjorie Profet. "A Profile: Evolutionary Theories for Everyday Life." *Sci Am* (April 1996).

Chapter 8 The Savanna Model Lifestyle

1. Gregg, E.W., J.A. Cauley, D.G. Seeley, et al. "Physical Activity and Osteoporotic Fracture Risk in Older Women. The Study of Osteoporotic Fractures Research Group." *Ann Intern Med* 129 (1998): 81–88.

2. Kujala, U.M., J. Kaprio, S. Sarna, and M. Koskenvuo. "Relationship of Leisure-time

Physical Activity and Mortality: The Finnish Twin Cohort." *JAMA* 279:6 (1998): 440–444.

3. Daly M., and M. Wilson. "Human Behavior as Animal Behavior." In Bolhuis, J.J., and L.A. Giraldeau, eds. *The Behavior of Animals. Mechanisms, Function, and Evolution.* Oxford: Blackwell Publishing, 2005, pp. 393–408.

4. Freeman, D. *Margaret Mead and the Heretic.* New York: Penguin, 1997.

5. Brown, D.E. "Human Universals and Their Implications." In *Being Humans: Anthropological Universality and Particularity in Transdisciplinary Perspectives.* New York: Walter de Gruyter; 2000.

6. Damasio, Antonio. *Looking For Spinoza: Joy, Sorrow and the Feeling Brain.* Harvest Books, 2003.

7. Dawkins, R. *The Selfish Gene.* Oxford: Oxford University Press, 1989.

8. Dawkins, R. *The Selfish Gene.* Oxford: Oxford University Press, 1989.

9. John, E.M., G.G. Schwartz, D.M. Dreon, and J. Koo. "Vitamin D and Breast Cancer Risk: The NHANES I Epidemiologic Follow-up Study, 1971–1975 to 1992. National Health and Nutrition Examination Survey." *Cancer Epid Biomarkers Prev* 8:5 (1999): 399–406.

10. Grant, W. "An Estimate of Premature Cancer Mortality in the U.S. Due to Inadequate Doses of Solar Ultraviolet-B Radiation." *Cancer* 94:6 (2002): 1867–1875.

11. Calhoun, J. "Population Density and Social Pathology." *Sci Am* 206 (1962): 139–148.

12. Diamond, Jared. *Guns, Germs, and Steel.* New York: Vintage, 1998, p. 171.

13. Davis, Thomas. *Vaka: Saga of a Polynesian Canoe.* Auckland, New Zealand: Polynesian Press, 1992.

14. Marshall, Lorna. "Sharing Talking and Giving." In Lee, Richard B., and Irven DeVore (eds.). *Kalahari Hunter-Gatherers.* Cambridge, MA: Harvard University Press, 1998.

15. Trivers, R. "The Evolution of Reciprocal Altruism." *Qtr Rev Biol* 46 (1971): 35–47.

— Trivers, R. "Parent-Offspring Conflict." *Am Zoologist* 14 (1974): 249–264.

— Trivers, R. "Parental Investment and Sexual Selection." In Campbell, B. (ed). *Sexual Selection and the Descent of Man.* Chicago: Aldine.

— Trivers, R. *Social Evolution.* Reading, MA: Benjamin-Cummings, 1985.

16. Chagnon, N. "Life Histories, Blood Revenge and Warfare in a Tribal Population." *Science* 239 (1992): 985–992.

— Chagnon, N. *Yanomam: The Last Days of Eden.* New York: Harcourt Brace, 1992.

— Daly and Wilson. *Homicide.* Hawthorne, NY: Aldine de Gruyter, 1988.

— Gaulin, S., and D. McBurney. *Psychology: An Evolutionary Approach.* Upper Saddle River, NJ: Prentice Hall, 2004.

17. Manson, J. "Intergroup Aggression in Chimpanzees." *Curr Anthropol* 32 (1991): 369–390.

18. de Waal, F. "A Century of Getting to Know the Chimpanzee." *Nature* 437 (2005): 56–59.

19. Hauser, M. "Our Chimpanzee Mind." *Nature* 437 (2005): 60–63.

20. Taylor, S.E., L.C. Klein, B.P. Lewis, et al. "Biobehavioral Responses to Stress in Females: Tend-and-Befriend, Not Fight-or-Flight." *Psychol Rev* 107:3 (2000): 411–429.

21. Diamond, Jared. *Guns, Germs, and Steel.* New York: Vintage, 1998, p. 173.

22. Wrangham, R., and D. Petersen. *Demonic Males.* Boston: Houghton Mifflin, 1996.

23. Warner, W.L. *A Black Civilization.* New York: Harper, 1937.

24. Keeley, L. *War Before Civilization: The Myth of the Peaceful Savage.* New York: Oxford University Press, 1996.

25. Van der Post, L. *The Lost World of the Kalahari.* New York: Harvest/Harcourt Brace, 1977.

26. Silverman, I. "Evolved Mechanisms Underlying Wayfinding—Further Studies on the Hunter-gatherer Theory of Spatial Sex Differences." *Evol Hum Behav* 21:3 (2000): 201–213.

27. Cook, P., and G. Sachs. *Abuse Your Illusions: The Disinformation Guide to Media Mirages and Establishment Lies.* The Disinformation Company, 2003.

28. Sommers, C. *The War Against Boys: How Misguided Feminism is Harming Our Young Men.* New York: Simon & Schuster, 2001.

29. Kanazawa, S. "Is 'Discrimination' Necessary to Explain the Sex Gap in Earnings?" *J Econ Psychol* 26 (2005): 269–287.

30. Marshall, L. "Sharing, Talking and Giving." In Lee, Richard B., and Irven DeVore (eds.). *Kalahari Hunter-Gatherers.* Cambridge, MA: Harvard University Press, 1998.

31. Marshall, L. "Sharing, Talking and Giving." In Lee, Richard B., and Irven DeVore (eds.). *Kalahari Hunter-Gatherers.* Cambridge, MA: Harvard University Press, 1998.

32. Nelson, David A., Clyde C. Robinson, and Craig H. Hart. "Relational and Physical Aggression of Preschool-Age Children: Peer Status Linkages Across Informants." *Early Educ Develop* 16:2 (April 2005).

33. Zerjal, T. "The Genetic Legacy of the Mongols." *Am J Human Genetics* 72:3 (2003): 717–721.

34. Farthing, W. "Attitudes Toward Heroic and Nonheroic Physical Risk Takers as Mates and as Friends." *Evol Human Behav* 26:2 (2005): 171–185.

35. Zahavi, A. "Mate Selection—A Selection for a Handicap." *J Theor Biol* 53:1 (1975): 205–214.

36. Shostak, M. "A !Kung Woman's Memories of Childhood." In Lee, Richard B., and Irven DeVore (eds.). *Kalahari Hunter-Gatherers.* Harvard University Press, 1998.

37. Lee, R.B. "Lactation, Ovulation, Infanticide, and Women's Work: A Study of Hunter-Gatherer Population Regulation." In Cohen, Mark N., Roy S. Malpass, and Harold G. Klein (eds.). *Biosocial Mechanisms of Population Regulation.* New Haven, CT: Yale University Press, 1980.

38. Howell, F. Clark, and the Editors of *Life. Early Man.* Life Nature Library. New York: Time, 1965.

39. Geary, D. "Evolution of Human Mate Choice." *J Sex Res* (February 2004).

40. Lee, R. "Male-Female Residence Arrangements and Political Power in Human Hunter Gatherers." *Arch Sex Behav* 3 (1974): 167–173.

41. Schmitt, D.P., and D.M. Buss. "Human Mate Poaching: Tactics and Temptations for Infiltrating Existing Mateships." *J Pers Soc Psych* 80:6 (2001): 894–917.

42. Peters, J. "Understanding Domestic Violence Against Women—Using Evolutionary Psychology to Extend the Feminist Analysis." *Violence Vict* 17:2 (2002): 255–264.

43. Geary, D.C., J. Vigil, and J. Byrd-Craven. "Evolution of Human Mate Choice." *J Sex Res* 41:1 (2004): 27–42.

44. Buss, D.M. *Evolution of Desire: Strategies of Human Mating.* New York: Basic Books, 1994.

— MacDonald, K. "Warmth as a Developmental Construct: An Evolutionary Analysis." *Child Develop* 63 (1992): 753–773.

45. Li, N.P., J.M. Bailey, D.T. Kenrick, and J.A. Linsenmeier. "The Necessities and Luxuries of Mate Preferences: Testing the Tradeoffs." *J Pers Soc Psych* 82:6 (2002): 947–955.

46. Geary, D.C., and M.V. Flinn. "Evolution of Human Parental Behavior and the Human Family." *Parent Sci Pract* 1 (2001): 5–61.

— Hill, K., and A.M. Hurtado. *Ache Life History: The Ecology and Demography of a Foraging People.* New York: Aldine de Gruyter, 1996.

— Surbey, M.K., and C.D. Conohan. "Willingness to Engage in Casual Sex: The Role of Parental Qualities and Perceived Risk of Aggression." *Human Nature* 11 (2000): 367–386.

47. Clutton-Brock, T.H. "Mammalian Mating Systems." *Proc Royal Soc London B* 236:1285 (1989): 339–372.

48. Jasienska, G., A. Ziomkiewicz, P.T. Ellison, et al. "Large Breasts and Narrow Waists Indicate High Reproductive Potential in Women." *Proc Royal Soc Biol Sci* 271:1545 (2004): 1213–1217.

49. Smith, M.J., D.I. Perrett, B.C. Jones, et al. "Facial Appearance is a Cue to Oestrogen Levels in Women." *Proc Biol Sci* 273:1583 (2006): 135–140.

50. Abitbol, J., P. Abitbol, and B. Abitbol. "Sex Hormones and the Female Voice." *J Voice* 13:3 (1999): 424–446.

51. Grammer, K., B. Fink, and N. Neave. "Human Pheromones and Sexual Attraction." *Eur J Obstet Gynecol Reprod Biol* 118:2 (2005): 135–142.

52. Shostak, M. "A !Kung Woman's Memories of Childhood." In Lee, Richard B., and Irven DeVore (eds.). *Kalahari Hunter-Gatherers.* Cambridge, MA: Harvard University Press, 1998.

53. Blainey, G. *Triumph of the Nomads: A History of Ancient Australia.* South Melbourne: Macmillan, 1985.

54. Howell, N. "The Population of the Dobe! Area Kung." In Lee, Richard B., and Irven DeVore (eds.). *Kalahari Hunter-Gatherers.* Cambridge, MA: Harvard University Press, 1998.

55. Blainey, G. *Triumph of the Nomads: A History of Ancient Australia.* South Melbourne: Macmillan, 1985.

56. Kippley, S. *Breast Feeding and Natural Child Spacing.* New York: Penguin Books, 1975.

57. Lee, R.B. "Lactation, Ovulation, Infanticide, and Women's Work: A Study of Hunter-Gatherer Population Regulation." In Cohen, Mark N., Roy S. Malpass, and Harold G. Klein (eds.). *Biosocial Mechanisms of Population Regulation*. New Haven, CT: Yale University Press, 1980.

58. Konner, M.J. "Maternal Care, Infant Behavior and Development." In Lee, Richard B., and Irven DeVore (eds.). *Kalahari Hunter-Gatherers*. Cambridge, MA: Harvard University Press, 1998.

59. Hawkes, K. "Grandmothering and Evolution." *Proc Natl Acad Sci USA* 95 (1998): 1336–1339.

60. Draper, P. "Social and Economic Restraints on Child Life." In Lee, Richard B., and Irven DeVore (eds.). *Kalahari Hunter-Gatherers*. Cambridge, MA: Harvard University Press, 1998.

61. Draper, P. "Social and Economic Restraints on Child Life." In Lee, Richard B., and Irven DeVore (eds.). *Kalahari Hunter-Gatherers*. Cambridge, MA: Harvard University Press, 1998.

62. Shostak, M. "A !Kung Woman's Memories of Childhood." In Lee, Richard B., and Irven DeVore (eds.). *Kalahari Hunter-Gatherers*. Cambridge, MA: Harvard University Press, 1998.

63. Marshall, Lorna. "Sharing, Talking and Giving." In Lee, Richard B., and Irven DeVore (eds.). *Kalahari Hunter-Gatherers*. Cambridge, MA: Harvard University Press, 1998.

64. Shostak, M. "A !Kung Woman's Memories of Childhood." In Lee, Richard B., and Irven DeVore (eds.). *Kalahari Hunter-Gatherers*. Cambridge, MA: Harvard University Press, 1998.

65. Orians, G., and J. Heerwgen. "Evolved Responses to Landscapes." In Barkow, J.H., L. Cosmides, and J. Tooby (eds.). *The Adapted Mind: Evolutionary Psychology and the Generation of Culture*. New York: Oxford University Press, 1992.

66. Kuo, F.E., and A.F. Taylor. "A Potential Natural Treatment for Attention-deficit/Hyperactivity Disorder: Evidence From a National Study." *Am J Public Health* 94:9 (2004): 1580–1586.

67. Katz, R. "Education for Transcendence." In Lee, Richard B., and Irven DeVore (eds.). *Kalahari Hunter-Gatherers*. Cambridge, MA: Harvard University Press, 1998.

68. Van der Post, Laurens. *The Lost World of the Kalahari*. New York: Harcourt Brace, 1998.

69. Van der Post, Laurens. *The Lost World of the Kalahari*. New York: Harcourt Brace, 1998.

70. Harris, Judith. *The Nurture Assumption: Why Children Turn Out the Way They Do*. New York: Free Press, 1998.

71. Koenig, L.B., M. McGue, R.F. Krueger, and T.J. Bouchard Jr. "Genetic and Environmental Influences on Religiousness: Findings for Retrospective and Current Religiousness Ratings." *J Pers* 73:2 (2005): 471–488.

72. Pinker, S. *The Blank Slate: The Modern Denial of Human Nature*. New York: Viking, 2002.

73. Gray, J. *Men Are From Mars, Women Are From Venus*. New York: HarperCollins, 1993.

Chapter 9   Disease and the Bond Effect

1. Wilson, Allan, and Rebecca Cann. "Recent African Genesis of Humans." *Sci Am* (April 1992).

2. Gibbs, W.W. "Untangling the Roots of Cancer." *Sci Am* 289:1 (2003): 56–65.

3. National Institutes of Health. *Understanding the Immune System: How It Works.* NIH Publication 03-5423. Bethesda, MD: National Institutes of Health, 2003.

4. Gibbs, W.W. "Untangling the Roots of Cancer." *Sci Am* 289:1 (2003): 56–65.

5. John, E.M., G.G. Schwartz, D.M. Dreon, and J. Koo. "Vitamin D and Breast Cancer Risk: The NHANES I Epidemiologic Follow-up Study, 1971–1975 to 1992. National Health and Nutrition Examination Survey." *Cancer Epidemiol Biomarkers Prev* 8:5 (1999): 399–406.

6. John, Esther. "Sun Exposure, Vitamin D Receptor Gene Polymorphisms, and Risk of Advanced Prostate Cancer." *Cancer Res* 65:12 (2005): 5470–5479.

7. Garland, C.F., G.W. Comstock, F.C. Garland, et al. "Serum 25-hydroxyvitamin D and Colon Cancer: Eight-year Prospective Study." *Lancet* 2:8673 (1989): 1176–1178.

8. Berwick, M., B.K. Armstrong, L. Ben-Porat, et al. "Sun Exposure and Mortality From Melanoma." *J Natl Cancer Inst* 97:3 (2005): 195–199.

— Smedby, K.E., H. Hjalgrim, M. Melbye, et al. "Ultraviolet Radiation Exposure and Risk of Malignant Lymphomas." *J Natl Cancer Inst* 97:3 (2005): 199–209.

9. Grant, W.B. "An Estimate of Premature Cancer Mortality in the U.S. Due to Inadequate Doses of Solar Ultraviolet-B Radiation." *Cancer* 94:6 (2002): 1867–1875.

10. Segerstrom, S.C., and G.E. Miller. "Psychological Stress and the Human Immune System: A Meta-analytic Study of 30 Years of Inquiry." *Psychol Bull* 130:4 (2004): 601–630.

11. Sapolsky, R.M. *Why Zebras Don't Get Ulcers.* New York: Owl Books, 2004.

12. Cho, E. "Premenopausal Fat Intake and Risk of Breast Cancer." *J Natl Cancer Inst* 95:14 (2003): 1079–1085.

— Kohlmeier, L. "Adipose Tissue Trans Fatty Acids and Breast Cancer in the European Community Multicenter Study on Antioxidants, Myocardial Infarction, and Breast Cancer." *Cancer Epidemiol Biomarkers Prev* 6 (1997): 705–710.

13. Bagga, D., S. Capone, H.J. Wang, et al. "Dietary Modulation of Omega-3/Omega-6 Polyunsaturated Fatty Acid Ratios in Patients with Breast Cancer." *J Natl Cancer Inst* 89:15 (1997): 1123–1131.

— Klein, V., V. Chajes, E. Germain, et al. "Low Alpha-linolenic Acid Content of Adipose Breast Tissue is Associated with an Increased Risk of Breast Cancer." *Eur J Cancer* 36:3 (2000): 335–340.

14. Knutson, V. "Insulin, Estrogen Linked With Breast Cancer." Experimental Biology '98 conference, San Francisco, California, June 15, 2004.

15. Berkey, C.S., A.L. Frazier, J.D. Gardner, and G.A. Colditz. "Adolescence and Breast Carcinoma Risk." *Cancer* 85:11 (1999): 2400–2409.

— Key, T.J. "Epidemiology of breast cancer." *Lancet Oncol* 2:3 (2001): 133–140.

16. Ju, Y.H., C.D. Allred, K.F. Allred, et al. "Physiological Concentrations of Dietary

Genistein Dose-dependently Stimulate Growth of Estrogen-dependent Human Breast Cancer (MCF-7) Tumors Implanted in Athymic Nude Mice." *J Nutr* 131:11 (2001): 2957–2962.

— Allred, C.D., Y.H. Ju, K.F. Allred, et al. "Dietary Genistin Stimulates Growth of Estrogen-dependent Breast Cancer Tumors Similar to that Observed with Genistein." *Carcinogenesis* 22:10 (2001): 1667–1673.

— Allred, C.D., K.F. Allred, Y.H. Ju, et al. "Soy Diets Containing Varying Amounts of Genistein Stimulate Growth of Estrogen-dependent (MCF-7) Tumors in a Dose-dependent Manner." *Cancer Res* 61:13 (2001): 5045–5050.

17. Trichopoulos, D., F.P. Li, and D.J. Hunter. "What Causes Cancer?" *Sci Am* 275:3 (1996): 80–87.

18. Takezaki, T., K. Hirose, M. Inoue, et al. "Dietary Factors and Lung Cancer Risk in Japanese: With Special Reference to Fish Consumption and Adenocarcinomas." *Br J Cancer* 84:9 (2001): 1199–1206.

19. Tavani, A., and C. La Vecchia. "Fruit and Vegetable Consumption and Cancer Risk in a Mediterranean Population." *Am J Clin Nutr* 61:6 Suppl (1995): 1374S–1377S.

— Knekt, P., R. Jarvinen, R. Seppanen, et al. "Dietary Flavonoids and the Risk of Lung Cancer and Other Malignant Neoplasms." *Am J Epidemiol* 146:3 (1997): 223–230.

— Axelsson, G., and R. Rylander. "Diet as Risk for Lung Cancer—A Swedish Case-Control Study." *Nutr Canc* 44:2 (2002): 145–151.

— Voorrips, L.E., R.A. Goldbohm, D.T. Verhoeven, et al. "Vegetable and Fruit Consumption and Lung Cancer Risk in the Netherlands Cohort Study on Diet and Cancer." *Cancer Causes Control* 11:2 (2000): 101–115.

20. Kaaks, R., P. Toniolo, A. Akhmedkhanov, et al. "Serum C-peptide, Insulin-like Growth Factor (IGF)-I, IGF-binding Proteins, and Colorectal Cancer Risk in Women." *J Natl Cancer Inst* 92:19 (2000): 1592–1600.

21. Slattery, M.L., J. Benson, K.N. Ma, et al. "Trans-fatty Acids and Colon Cancer." *Nutr Cancer* 39:2 (2001): 170–175.

22. Denis, L., M.S. Morton, and K. Griffiths. "Diet and Its Preventive Role in Prostatic Disease." *Eur Urol* 35:5–6 (1999): 377–387.

23. Chan, J.M., M.J. Stampfer, J. Ma, et al. "Dairy Products, Calcium and Prostate Cancer Risk in the Physicians' Health Study." *Am J Clin Nutr* 74:4 (2001): 549–554.

— Rose, D.P. "Dietary Fatty Acids and Prevention of Hormone Responsive Prostate Cancer." *Proc Soc Exp Biol Med* 216:2 (1997): 224–233.

— Denis, L., M.S. Morton, and K. Griffiths. "Diet and Its Preventive Role in Prostatic Disease." *Eur Urol* 35:5–6 (1999): 377–387.

24. Hughes-Fulford, M., C.F. Li, J. Boonyaratanakornkit, and S. Sayyah. "Arachidonic Acid Activates Phosphatidylinositol 3-kinase Signaling and Induces Gene Expression in Prostate Cancer." *Cancer Res* 66:3 (2006): 1427–1433.

25. Demark-Wahnefried, W., D.T. Price, T.J. Polascik, et al. "Pilot Study of Dietary Fat Restriction and Flaxseed Supplementation in Men with Prostate Cancer Before Surgery: Exploring the Effects on Hormonal Levels, Prostate-specific Antigen, and Histopathologic Features." *Urology* 58:1 (2001): 47–52.

26. John, Esther. "Sun Exposure, Vitamin D Receptor Gene Polymorphisms, and Risk of Advanced Prostate Cancer." *Cancer Res* 65:12 (2005): 5470–5479.

27. Giles, G.G., G. Severi, D.R. English, and J.L. Hopper. "Frequency of Ejaculation and Risk of Prostate Cancer." *JAMA* 292:3 (2004): 329.

28. Fleming, P.R. *A Short History of Cardiology*. Atlanta, GA: Rodopi, 1997.

29. Naughton, J.M., K. O'Dea, and A.J. Sinclair. "Animal Foods in Traditional Australian Aboriginal Diets: Polyunsaturated and Low in Fat." *Lipids* 21:11 (1986): 684–690.

— Groom, D. "Cardiovascular Observations on Tarahumara Indian Runners—The Modern Spartans." *Am Heart J* 81:3 (1971): 304–314.

— Booyens, J., C.C. Louwrens, and I.E. Katzeff. "The Eskimo Diet: Prophylactic Effects Ascribed to the Balanced Presence of Natural Cis Unsaturated Fatty Acids and to the Absence of Unnatural Trans and Cis Isomers of Unsaturated Fatty Acids." *Med Hypotheses* 21:4 (1986): 387–408.

— Truswell, S., and J. Hansen. "Medical Research Among the !Kung." In Lee, Richard B., and Irven DeVore (eds.). *Kalahari Hunter-Gatherers: Studies of the !Kung San and Their Neighbors*. Cambridge, MA: Harvard University Press, 1976.

30. Leaf, A. "Observations of a Peripatetic Gerontologist." *Nutr Today* (September/October 1973).

31. Eaton, S.B., M. Konner, and M. Shostak. "Stone Agers in the Fast Lane: Chronic Degenerative Diseases in Evolutionary Perspective." *Am J Med* 84:4 (1988): 739–749.

32. Engler, M.M., and M.B. Engler. "Omega-3 Fatty Acids: Role in Cardiovascular Health and Disease." *J Cardiovasc Nurs* 21:1 (2006): 17–24.

33. Pyorala, M., H. Miettinen, M. Laakso, and K. Pyorala. "Hyperinsulinemia Predicts Coronary Heart Disease Risk in Healthy Middle-aged Men: The 22-year Follow-up Results of the Helsinki Policemen Study." *Circulation* 98:5 (1998): 398–404.

— Sowers, J.R., P.R. Standley, J.L. Ram, et al. "Hyperinsulinemia, Insulin Resistance, and Hyperglycemia: Contributing Factors in the Pathogenesis of Hypertension and Atherosclerosis." *Am J Hypertens* 6:7 Part 2 (1993): 260S–270S.

— Stout, R.W. "Overview of the Association between Insulin and Atherosclerosis." *Metabolism* 34:12 Suppl 1 (1985): 7–12.

34. Institute of Medicine. "Letter Report on Dietary Reference Intakes for Trans Fatty Acids." July 10, 2002.

35. Tobian, L., and S. Hanlon. "High Sodium Chloride Diets Injure Arteries and Raise Mortality without Changing Blood Pressure." *Hypertension* 15:6 Part 2 (1990): 900–903.

36. Appel, L.J., T.J. Moore, E. Obarzanek, et al. "A Clinical Trial of the Effects of Dietary Patterns on Blood Pressure. DASH Collaborative Research Group." *N Engl J Med* 336:16 (1997): 1117–1124.

37. Richardson, M., E.M. Kurowska, and K.K. Carroll. "Early Lesion Development in the Aortas of Rabbits Fed Low-fat, Cholesterol-free, Semipurified Casein Diet." *Atherosclerosis* 107:2 (1994): 165–178.

— Tailford, K.A., C.L. Berry, A.C. Thomas, and J.H. Campbell. "A Casein Variant in Cow's Milk is Atherogenic." *Atherosclerosis* 170:1 (2003): 13–19.

38. Samman, S., G. Sivarajah, J.C. Man, et al. "A Mixed Fruit and Vegetable Concen-

trate Increases Plasma Antioxidant Vitamins and Folate and Lowers Plasma Homocysteine in Men." *J Nutr* 133:7 (2003): 2188–2193.

39. Rostand, S.G. "Ultraviolet Light May Contribute to Geographic and Racial Blood Pressure Differences." *Hypertension* 30:2 Part 1 (1997): 150–156.

40. McCarty, M.F. "Vegan Proteins May Reduce Risk of Cancer, Obesity, and Cardiovascular Disease by Promoting Increased Glucagon Activity." *Med Hypotheses* 53:6 (1999): 459–485.

— Zino, S., M. Skeaff, S. Williams, and J. Mann. "Randomised Controlled Trial of Effect of Fruit and Vegetable Consumption on Plasma Concentrations of Lipids and Antioxidants." *Br Med J* 314:7097 (1997): 1787–1791.

— Mavri, A., M. Stegnar, J.T. Sentocnik, and V. Videcnik. "Impact of Weight Reduction on Early Carotid Atherosclerosis in Obese Premenopausal Women." *Obesity Res* 9:9 (2001): 511–516.

41. Min, James K. "Prediction of Coronary Heart Disease by Erectile Dysfunction in Men Referred for Nuclear Stress Testing." *Arch Intern Med* 166 (2006): 201–206.

42. Truswell, S., and J. Hansen. "Medical Research Among the !Kung." In Lee, Richard B., and Irven DeVore (eds.). *Kalahari Hunter-Gatherers: Studies of the !Kung San and Their Neighbors.* Cambridge, MA: Harvard University Press, 1976.

43. Eaton, S.B., M. Konner, and M. Shostak. "Stone Agers in the Fast Lane: Chronic Degenerative Diseases in Evolutionary Perspective." *Am J Med* 84:4 (1988): 739–749.

44. Brown, L., B. Rosner, W.W. Willett, and F.M. Sacks. "Cholesterol-lowering Effects of Dietary Fiber: A Meta-analysis." *Am J Clin Nutr* 69:1 (1999): 30–42.

— Truswell, A.S. "Dietary Fiber and Health." *World Rev Nutr Diet* 72 (1993): 148–164.

45. Greene, C.M., et al. "Plasma LDL and HDL Characteristics and Carotenoid Content are Positively Influenced by Egg Consumption in an Elderly Population." *Nutr Metab (London)* 3 (2006): 6.

— Vorster, H.H., N. Silvis, C.S. Venter, et al. "Serum Cholesterol, Lipoproteins, and Plasma Coagulation factors in South Africa Blacks on a High-egg but Low-fat Intake." *Am J Clin Nutr* 46:1 (1987): 52–57.

46. Eaton, S.B., M. Konner, and M. Shostak. "Stone Agers in the Fast Lane: Chronic Degenerative Diseases in Evolutionary Perspective." *Am J Med* 84:4 (1988): 739–749.

47. Ravnskov, U. *The Cholesterol Myths.* Washington, DC: New Trends Publishing, 2000.

— Bradford, R.H., C.L. Shear, A.N. Chremos, et al. "Expanded Clinical Evaluation of Lovastatin (EXCEL) Study Results. I. Efficacy in Modifying Plasma Lipoproteins and Adverse Event Profile in 8245 Patients with Moderate Hypercholesterolemia." *Arch Intern Med* 151:1 (1991): 43–49.

48. Pfizer, Inc. Lipitor package insert. Available online at http://www.pfizer.com-download/uspi_lipitor.pdf.

49. Cantorna, M.T., C. Munsick, C. Bemiss, and B.D. Mahon. "1,25-dihydroxycholecalciferol Prevents and Ameliorates Symptoms of Experimental Murine Inflammatory Bowel Disease." *J Nutr* 130:11 (2000): 2648–2652.

50. Rigas, Basil. Private communication, May 31, 1998.

51. Fass, R., S.F. Quan, G.T. O'Connor, et al. "Predictors of Heartburn During Sleep in a Large Prospective Cohort Study." *Chest* 127:5 (2005): 1658–1666.

52. American Academy of Allergy, Asthma and Immunology. http://www.aaaai.org.

53. Foucard, T., and I. Malmheden Yman. "A Study on Severe Food Reactions in Sweden—Is Soy Protein an Underestimated Cause of Food Anaphylaxis?" *Allergy* 54:3 (1999): 261–265.

54. Hoff, S., H. Seiler, J. Heinrich, et al. "Allergic Sensitisation and Allergic Rhinitis are Associated with n-3 Polyunsaturated Fatty Acids in the Diet and in Red Blood Cell Membranes." *Eur J Clin Nutr* 59:9 (2005): 1071–1080.

55. Jensen-Jarolim, E., L. Gajdzik, I. Haberl I, et al. "Hot Spices Influence Permeability of Human Intestinal Epithelial Monolayers." *J Nutr* 128:3 (1998): 577–581.

56. Elenkov, I.J., D.G. Iezzoni, A. Daly, et al. "Cytokine Dysregulation, Inflammation and Well-being." *Neuroimmunomodulation* 12:5 (2005): 255–269.

57. Svanes, C., D. Jarvis, S. Chinn, and P. Burney. "Childhood Environment and Adult Atopy: Results from the European Community Respiratory Health Survey." *J Allergy Clin Immunol* 103:3 part 1 (1999): 415–420.

58. Gibson, P.G., J.W. Wlodarczyk, M.J. Hensley, et al. "Epidemiological Association of Airway Inflammation with Asthma Symptoms and Airway Hyperresponsiveness in Childhood." *Am J Respir Crit Care Med* 158:1 (1998): 36–41.

59. Broughton, K.S., C.S. Johnson, B.K. Pace, et al. "Reduced Asthma Symptoms with n-3 Fatty Acid Ingestion are Related to 5-series Leukotriene Production." *Am J Clin Nutr* 65:4 (1997): 1011–1017.

— Mickleborough, T.D. "Dietary Omega-3 Polyunsaturated Fatty Acid Supplementation and Airway Hyperresponsiveness in Asthma." *J Asthma* 42:5 (2005): 305–314.

60. Hijazi, Z., A.M. Molla, H. Al-Habashi, et al. "Intestinal Permeability is Increased in Bronchial Asthma." *Arch Dis Child* 89:3 (2004): 227–229.

61. Ratner, D., E. Shoshani, and B. Dubnov. "Milk Protein–free Diet for Nonseasonal Asthma and Migraine in Lactase-deficient Patients." *Isr J Med Sci* 19:9 (1983): 806–809.

62. Cook, D.G., I.M. Carey, P.H. Whincup, et al. "Effect of Fresh Fruit Consumption on Lung Function and Wheeze in Children." *Thorax* 52:7 (1997): 628–633.

63. Butland, B.K., A.M. Fehily, and P.C. Elwood. "Diet, Lung Function, and Lung Function Decline in a Cohort of 2512 Middle-aged Men." *Thorax* 55:2 (2000): 102–108.

64. Tabak, C., H.A. Smit, L. Rasanen, et al. "Dietary Factors and Pulmonary Function: A Cross-sectional Study in Middle-aged Men from Three European Countries." *Thorax* 54:11 (1999): 1021–1026.

65. Black, P.N., and R. Scragg. "Relationship Between Serum 25-hydroxyvitamin D and Pulmonary Function in the Third National Health and Nutrition Examination Survey." *Chest* 128:6 (2005): 3792–3798.

66. Gabrielli, M. "Association Between Migraine and Celiac Disease: Results from a Preliminary Case-control and Therapeutic Study. *Am J Gastroenterol* 98:3 (2003): 625–629.

— Serratrice, J. "Migraine and Coeliac Disease." *Headache* 38:8 (1998): 627–628.

67. Ratner, D. "Milk Protein–free Diet for Nonseasonal Asthma and Migraine in Lactase-deficient Patients." *Isr J Med Sci* 19:9 (1983): 806–809.

68. Baldwin, A.L. "Pharmacological Food Reactions." In Metcalfe, D.D., H.A. Sampson, and R.A. Simon (eds.). *Food Allergy: Adverse Reactions to Food and Food Additives,* 2nd ed. Oxford: Blackwell Scientific, 1991.

69. Goksel, B.K. "Is Low Blood Magnesium Level Associated with Hemodialysis Headache?" *Headache* 46:1 (2006): 40–45.

— Peikert, A. "Prophylaxis of Migraine with Oral Magnesium: Results from a Prospective Multi-centre, Placebo-controlled, Double-blind, Randomised Study." *Cephalalgia* 16 (1996): 257–263.

— Welch, K.M., and N.M. Ramadan. "Mitochondria, Magnesium and Migraine." *J Neurol Sci* 134 (1995): 9–14.

70. Schoenen, J., J. Jacquy, and M. Lenaerts. "Effectiveness of High-dose Riboflavin in Migraine Prophylaxis: A Randomised Controlled Trial." *Neurology* 50 (1998): 466–470.

— Boehnke, C., U. Reuter, U. Flach, et al. "High-dose Riboflavin Treatment is Efficacious in Migraine Prophylaxis: An Open Study in a Tertiary Care Centre." *Eur J Neurol* 11 (2004): 475–477.

— Breen, C. "High-dose Riboflavin for Prophylaxis of Migraine." *Can Fam Physician* 49 (2003): 1291–1293.

71. Jacome, D.E. "Hypoglycemia Rebound Migraine." *Headache* 41:9 (2001): 895–898.

72. Kong, Y.Y., U. Feige, I. Sarosi, et al. "Activated T Cells Regulate Bone Loss and Joint Destruction in Adjuvant Arthritis Through Osteoprotegerin Ligand." *Nature* 402:6759 (1999): 304–309.

73. Kremer, J.M., D.A. Lawrence, G.F. Petrillo, et al. "Effects of High-dose Fish Oil on Rheumatoid Arthritis After Stopping Nonsteroidal Antiinflammatory Drugs. Clinical and Immune Correlates." *Arth Rheum* 38:8 (1995): 1107–1114.

74. Han, S.N., L.S. Leka, A.H. Lichtenstein, et al. "Effect of Hydrogenated and Saturated, Relative to Polyunsaturated, Fat on Immune and Inflammatory Responses of Adults with Moderate Hypercholesterolemia." *J Lipid Res* 43:3 (2002): 445–452.

75. Comstock, G.W., A.E. Burke, S.C. Hoffman, et al. "Serum Concentrations of Alpha Tocopherol, Beta Carotene, and Retinol Preceding the Diagnosis of Rheumatoid Arthritis and Systemic Lupus Erythematosus." *Ann Rheum Dis* 56:5 (1997): 323–325.

76. Linos, A., V.G. Kaklamani, E. Kaklamani, et al. "Dietary Factors in Relation to Rheumatoid Arthritis: A Role for Olive Oil and Cooked Vegetables?" *Am J Clin Nutr* 70:6 (1999): 1077–1082.

77. Hafstrom, I., B. Ringertz, A. Spangberg A, et al. "A Vegan Diet Free of Gluten Improves the Signs and Symptoms of Rheumatoid Arthritis: The Effects on Arthritis Correlate with a Reduction in Antibodies to Food Antigens." *Rheumatology (Oxford)* 40:10 (2001): 1175–1179.

— Carli, P., A. Chagnon, J.R. Harle, et al. "Inflammatory Rheumatism and Celiac Disease in Adults: Coincidence or Pathogenic Relationship?" *Presse Med* 24:13 (1995): 606–610.

78. Ratner, D., E. Eshel, and K. Vigder. "Juvenile Rheumatoid Arthritis and Milk Allergy." *J R Soc Med* 78:5 (1985): 410–413.

79. Molleson, T. "Eloquent Bones of Abu Hureyra." *Sci Am* 271:2 (1994): 70–75.

80. Kurtz, S., F. Mowat, K. Ong, et al. "Prevalence of Primary and Revision Total Hip

and Knee Arthroplasty in the United States from 1990 Through 2002." *J Bone Joint Surg Am* 87:7 (2005): 1487–1497.

81. Curtis, C.L., S.G. Rees, J. Cramp, et al. "Effects of n-3 Fatty Acids on Cartilage Metabolism." *Proc Nutr Soc* 61:3 (2002): 381–389.

— James, M.J., S.M. Proudman, and L.G. Cleland. "Dietary n-3 Fats as Adjunctive Therapy in a Prototypic Inflammatory Disease: Issues and Obstacles for Use in Rheumatoid Arthritis." *Prostaglandins Leukot Essent Fatty Acids* 68:6 (2003): 399–405.

82. Wucherpfennig, K.W., and J.L. Strominger. "Molecular Mimicry in T Cell–mediated Autoimmunity: Viral Peptides Activate Human T Cell Clones Specific for Myelin Basic Protein." *Cell* 80:5 (1995): 695–705.

83. Matheson, N.A. "Letter: Multiple Sclerosis and Diet." *Lancet* 2:7884 (1974): 831.

84. Hartung, H.P., and P. Rieckmann. "Pathogenesis of Immune-mediated Demyelination in the CNS." *J Neural Transm Suppl* 50 (1997): 173–181.

85. Lange, L.S., and M. Shiner. "Small-bowel Abnormalities in Multiple Sclerosis." *Lancet* 2:7999 (1976): 1319–1322.

86. Bernsohn, J., and L.M. Stephanides. "Aetiology of Multiple Sclerosis." *Nature* 215:103 (1967): 821–823.

— Kishimoto, Y., N.S. Radin, W.W. Tourtellotte, et al. "Gangliosides and Glycerophospholipids in Multiple Sclerosis White Matter." *Arch Neurol* 16:1 (1967): 41–54.

87. Kromann, N., and A. Green. "Epidemiological Studies in the Upernavik District, Greenland. Incidence of Some Chronic Diseases 1950–1974." *Acta Med Scand* 208 (1980): 401–406.

88. Simopoulos, A.P. "Omega-3 Fatty Acids in Inflammation and Autoimmune Diseases." *J Am Coll Nutr* 21:6 (2002): 495–505.

89. Ghadirian, P., R. Morisset, and M. Jain. "Nutritional Factors in the Aetiology of Multiple Sclerosis: A Case-control Study in Montreal, Canada." *Intl J Epidemiol* 27:5 (1998): 845–852.

— Nordvik, I., K.M. Myhr, H. Nyland, et al. "Effect of Dietary Advice and n-3 Supplementation in Newly Diagnosed MS Patients." *Acta Neurol Scand* 102:3 (2000): 143–149.

— Cendrowski, W. "Multiple Sclerosis and MaxEPA." *Br J Clin Pract* 40:9 (1986): 365–367.

90. Munger, K.L., S.M. Zhang, E. O'Reilly, et al. "Vitamin D Intake and Incidence of Multiple Sclerosis." *Neurology* 62:1 (2004): 60–65.

91. Cantorna, M.T. "Vitamin D and Autoimmunity: Is Vitamin D Status an Environmental Factor Affecting Autoimmune Disease?" *Proc Soc Exp Biol Med* 223:3 (2000): 230–233.

92. World Health Organization. *Mental Health: New Understanding, New Hope. The World Health Report 2001.* Geneva: World Health Organization, 2001.

93. World Health Organization. *Mental Health: New Understanding, New Hope. The World Health Report 2001.* Geneva: World Health Organization, 2001.

94. Bennet, C.N., and D.F. Horrobin. "Gene Targets Related to Phospholipid and

Fatty Acid Metabolism in Schizophrenia and Other Psychiatric Disorders: An Update." *Prostaglandins Leukot Essent Fatty Acids* 63:1–2 (2000): 47–59.

— Horrobin, David, and Crispin N. Bennett. "The Phospholipid Concept of Psychiatric Disorders." In Peet, M., I. Glen, and D. Horrobin (eds.). *Phospholipid Spectrum Disorders in Psychiatry and Neurology*, 2nd edition. Carnforth: Marius Press, 2003.

95. Mann, J., and A.S. Truswell. *Essentials of Human Nutrition*, 2nd edition. Oxford: Oxford University Press, 2002

96. Chafetz, M.D. *Nutrition and Neurotransmitters: The Nutrient Bases of Behaviour.* Englewood Cliffs, NJ: Prentice Hall, 1990.

97. Casadesus, G. "Caloric Restriction Versus a Diet High in Antioxidants: Are They Equipotent in Altering or Reversing the Course of Aging?" In Mattson, Mark P. (ed.). *Diet-Brain Connections: Impact on Memory, Mood, Aging and Disease.* Dordrecht: Kluwer Academic Publishers, 2002.

98. Crawford, M., and D. Marsh. *The Driving Force: Food, Evolution and the Future.* New York: Harper & Row, 1989.

99. Benton, D. "Diet and Mood." In Mattson, Mark P. (ed.). *Diet-Brain Connections: Impact on Memory, Mood, Aging and Disease.* Dordrecht: Kluwer Academic Publishers, 2002.

100. Richardson, A.J., and B.K. Puri. "The Potential Role of Fatty Acids in Attention-Deficit/Hyperactivity Disorder." *Prostaglandins Leukot Essent Fatty Acids* 63:1–2 (2000): 79–87.

101. Hull, M., K. Lieb, and B.L. Fiebich. "Pathways of Inflammatory Activation in Alzheimer's Disease: Potential Targets for Disease-modifying Drugs." *Curr Med Chem* 9:1 (2002): 83–88.

102. Hendrie, H.C., B.O. Osuntokun, K.S. Hall, et al. "Prevalence of Alzheimer's Disease and Dementia in Two Communities: Nigerian Africans and African Americans." *Am J Psychiatry* 152:10 (1995): 1485–1492.

— White, L., H. Petrovitch, G.W. Ross, et al. "Prevalence of Dementia in Older Japanese-American Men in Hawaii: The Honolulu-Asia Aging Study." *JAMA* 276:12 (1996): 955–960.

103. Grant, W.B. "Dietary Links to Alzheimer's Disease." *Alzheimer's Dis Rev* 2 (1997): 42–55.

— Kalmijn, S. "Dietary Fatty Acids and Cognitive Function." In Mattson, Mark P. (ed.). *Diet-Brain Connections: Impact on Memory, Mood, Aging and Disease.* Dordrecht: Kluwer Academic Publishers, 2002.

— Kalmijn, S., L.J. Launer, A. Ott, et al. "Dietary Fat Intake and the Risk of Incident Dementia in the Rotterdam Study." *Ann Neurol* 42:5 (1997): 776–782.

— Morris, M.C., D.A. Evans, J.L. Bienias, et al. "Dietary Fats and the Risk of Incident Alzheimer Disease." *Arch Neurol* 60:2 (2003): 194200.

104. Kalmijn, S. "Dietary Fatty Acids and Cognitive Function." In Mattson, Mark P. (ed.). *Diet-Brain Connections: Impact on Memory, Mood, Aging and Disease.* Dordrecht: Kluwer Academic Publishers, 2002.

— Conquer, J.A., M.C. Tierney, J. Zecevic, et al. "Fatty Acid Analysis of Blood Plasma of Patients with Alzheimer's Disease, Other Types of Dementia, and Cognitive Impairment." *Lipids* 35:12 (2000): 1305–1312.

— Tully, A.M., H.M. Roche, R. Doyle, et al. "Low Serum Cholesteryl Ester-Docosa-hexaenoic Acid Levels in Alzheimer's Disease: A Case-Control Study." *Br J Nutr* 89:4 (2003): 483–489.

— Soderberg, M., C. Edlund, K. Kristensson, and G. Dallner. "Fatty Acid Composition of Brain Phospholipids in Aging and in Alzheimer's Disease." *Lipids* 26:6 (1991): 421–425.

105. Arvanitakis, Z., R.S. Wilson, J.L. Bienias, et al. "Diabetes Mellitus and Risk of Alzheimer Disease and Decline in Cognitive Function." *Arch Neurol* 61:5 (2004): 661–666.

106. Convit, A., O.T. Wolf, C. Tarshish, and M.J. de Leon. "Reduced Glucose Tolerance is Associated with Poor Memory Performance and Hippocampal Atrophy Among Normal Elderly." *Proc Natl Acad Sci USA* 100:4 (2003): 2019–2022.

107. Gustafson, D., L. Lissner, C. Bengtsson, et al. "A 24-year Follow-up of Body Mass Index and Cerebral Atrophy." *Neurology* 63 (2004): 1876–1881.

— Whitmer, R.A., E.P. Gunderson, E. Barrett-Connor, et al. "Obesity in Middle Age and Future Risk of Dementia: A 27-year Longitudinal Population-based Study." *Br Med J* 330:7504 (2005): 1360.

108. White, L.R., H. Petrovitch, G.W. Ross, et al. "Brain Aging and Midlife Tofu Consumption." *J Am Coll Nutr* 19:2 (2000): 242–255.

109. Seshadri, S., A. Beiser, J. Selhub, et al. "Plasma Homocysteine as a Risk Factor for Dementia and Alzheimer's Disease." *N Engl J Med* 346:7 (2002): 476–483.

— Clarke, R., A.D. Smith, K.A. Jobst, et al. "Folate, Vitamin B_{12}, and Serum Total Homocysteine Levels in Confirmed Alzheimer Disease." *Arch Neurol* 55:11 (1998): 1449–1455.

— Polidori, M.C., P. Mattioli, S. Aldred S, et al. "Plasma Antioxidant Status, Immunoglobulin G Oxidation and Lipid Peroxidation in Demented Patients: Relevance to Alzheimer Disease and Vascular Dementia." *Dement Geriatr Cogn Disord* 18:3–4 (2004): 265–270.

110. Broadhurst, C.L., S.C. Cunnane, and M.A. Crawford. "Rift Valley Lake Fish and Shellfish Provided Brain-specific Nutrition for Early *Homo*." *Br J Nutr* 79:1 (1998): 3–21.

111. Panza, F., V. Solfrizzi, A.M. Colacicco, et al. "Mediterranean Diet and Cognitive Decline." *Public Health Nutr* 7:7 (2004): 959–963.

— Kalmijn, S., L.J. Launer, A. Ott, et al. "Dietary Fat Intake and the Risk of Incident Dementia in the Rotterdam Study." *Ann Neurol* 42:5 (1997): 776–782.

— Barberger-Gateau, P., L. Letenneur, V. Deschamps, et al. "Fish, Meat, and Risk of Dementia: Cohort Study." *Br Med J* 325:7370 (2002): 932–933.

— Morris, M.C., D.A. Evans, J.L. Bienias, et al. "Consumption of Fish and n-3 Fatty Acids and Risk of Incident Alzheimer Disease." *Arch Neurol* 60:7 (2003): 940–946.

— Kalmijn, S. "Dietary Fatty Acids and Cognitive Function." In Mattson, Mark P.

(ed.). *Diet-Brain Connections: Impact on Memory, Mood, Aging and Disease.* Dordrecht: Kluwer Academic Publishers, 2002.

— Calon, F., G.P. Lim, F. Yang, et al. "Docosahexaenoic Acid Protects from Dendritic Pathology in an Alzheimer's Disease Mouse Model." *Neuron* 43:5 (2004): 633–645.

112. Solfrizzi, V., F. Panza, F. Torres, et al. "High Monounsaturated Fatty Acids Intake Protects against Age-Related Cognitive Decline." *Neurology* 52:8 (1999): 1563–1569.

113. Mattson, M.P., W. Duan, and Z. Guo. "Meal Size and Frequency Affect Neuronal Plasticity and Vulnerability to Disease: Cellular and Molecular Mechanisms." *J Neurochem* 84:3 (2003): 417–431.

114. Mattson, M.P., S.L. Chan, and W. Duan. "Modification of Brain Aging and Neurodegenerative Disorders by Genes, Diet, and Behavior." *Neurobiol Aging* 23:5 (2002): 695–705.

115. Engelhart, M.J., M.I. Geerlings, A. Ruitenberg, et al. "Dietary Intake of Antioxidants and Risk of Alzheimer Disease." *JAMA* 287:24 (2002): 3223–3229.

— Morris, M.C., D.A. Evans, J.L. Bienias, et al. "Dietary Intake of Antioxidant Nutrients and the Risk of Incident Alzheimer Disease in a Biracial Community Study." *JAMA* 287:24 (2002): 3230–3237.

— Corrada, M., C. Kawas, et al. "Reduced Risk of Alzheimer's Disease with High Folate Intake: The Baltimore Longitudinal Study of Aging." *Alzheimer's Dement* 1:1 (2005): 11–18.

— Wang, H.X., A. Wahlin, H. Basun H, et al. "Vitamin B(12) and Folate in Relation to the Development of Alzheimer's Disease." *Neurology* 56:9 (2001): 1188–1194.

— Marambaud, P., H. Zhao, and P. Davies. "Resveratrol Promotes Clearance of Alzheimer's Disease Amyloid-beta Peptides." *J Biol Chem* 280:45 (2005): 37377–37382.

— Savaskan, E., G. Olivieri, F. Meier, et al. "Red Wine Ingredient Resveratrol Protects from Beta-amyloid Neurotoxicity." *Gerontology* 49:6 (2003): 380–383.

— Heo, H.J., and C.Y. Lee. "Protective Effects of Quercetin and Vitamin C Against Oxidative Stress-induced Neurodegeneration." *J Agric Food Chem* 52:25 (2004): 7514–7517.

116. Polidori, M.C., P. Mattioli, S. Aldred S, et al. "Plasma Antioxidant Status, Immunoglobulin G Oxidation and Lipid Peroxidation in Demented Patients: Relevance to Alzheimer Disease and Vascular Dementia." *Dement Geriatr Cogn Disord* 18:3–4 (2004): 265–270.

117. Clarke, R., A.D. Smith, K.A. Jobst, et al. "Folate, Vitamin B_{12}, and Serum Total Homocysteine Levels in Confirmed Alzheimer Disease." *Arch Neurol* 55:11 (1998): 1449–1455.

118. Giem, P., W.L. Beeson, and G.E. Fraser. "The Incidence of Dementia and Intake of Animal Products: Preliminary Findings from the Adventist Health Study." *Neuroepidemiology* 12:1 (1993): 28–36.

119. Abbott, R., L.R. White, G.W. Ross, et al. "Walking and Dementia in Physically Capable Elderly Men." *JAMA* 292:12 (2004): 1447–1453.

120. Eriksson, P.S., E. Perfilieva, T. Bjork-Eriksson, et al. "Neurogenesis in the Adult Human Hippocampus." *Nature Med* 4:11 (1998): 1313–1317.

121. Zelnik, N., A. Pacht, R. Obeid, and A. Lerner. "Range of Neurological Disorders in Patients with Celiac Disease." *Pediatrics* 113:6 (2004): 1672–1676.

122. Goldman, J., R.H. Lerman, J.H. Contois, and J.N. Udall Jr. "Behavioral Effects of Sucrose on Preschool Children." *J Abnormal Child Psychol* 14:4 (1986): 565–577.

— Jones, T.W., W.P. Borg, S.D. Boulware, et al. "Enhanced Adrenomedullary Response and Increased Susceptibility to Neuroglygopenia: Mechanisms Underlying the Adverse Effect of Sugar Ingestion in Children." *J Pediatrics* 126:2 (1995): 171–177.

123. Millstone, E. "Adverse Reactions to Food Additives: The Extent and Severity of the Problem." *J Nutr Environ Med* 7:4 (1997): 323–332.

— Bateman, B., J.O. Warner, E. Hutchinson, et al. "The Effects of a Double-blind, Placebo-controlled, Artificial Food Colourings and Benzoate Preservative Challenge on Hyperactivity in a General Population Sample of Preschool Children." *Arch Dis Child* 89:6 (2004): 506–511.

— Eigenmann, P.A., and C.A. Haenggeli. "Food Colourings and Preservatives—Allergy and Hyperactivity." *Lancet* 364:9437 (2004): 823–824.

124. Bateman, B., J.O. Warner, E. Hutchinson, et al. "The Effects of a Double-blind, Placebo-controlled, Artificial Food Colourings and Benzoate Preservative Challenge on Hyperactivity in a General Population Sample of Preschool Children." *Arch Dis Child* 89:6 (2004): 506–511.

125. Keeley, J. "Case Study: Appleton Central Alternative Charter High School's Nutrition and Wellness Program." *Better Food, Better Behavior.* Michael Fields Agricultural Institute, 2004. Available online at http://www.michaelfieldsaginst.org.

126. Mitchell, E.A., M.G. Aman, S.H. Turbott, and M. Manku. "Clinical Characteristics and Serum Essential Fatty Acid Levels in Hyperactive Children." *Clin Pediatr* (*Philadelphia*) 26:8 (1987): 406–411.

— Richardson, A.J., and B.K. Puri. "The Potential Role of Fatty Acids in Attention-Deficit/Hyperactivity Disorder." *Prostaglandins Leukot Essent Fatty Acids* 63:1–2 (2000): 79–87.

127. Stevens, L.J., S.S. Zentall, M.L. Abate, et al. "Omega-3 Fatty Acids in Boys with Behavior, Learning, and Health Problems." *Physiol Behav* 59:4–5 (1996): 915–920.

128. Little, J. "Epidemiology of Neurodevelopmental Disorders in Children." *Prostaglandins Leukot Essent Fatty Acids* 63:1–2 (2000): 11–20.

— Stevens, L.J., S.S. Zentall, J.L. Deck, et al. "Essential Fatty Acid Metabolism in Boys with Attention-Deficit Hyperactivity Disorder." *Am J Clin Nutr* 62:4 (1995): 761–768.

— Colquhoun, I., and S. Bunday. "A Lack of Essential Fatty Acids as a Possible Cause of Hyperactivity in Children." *Med Hypotheses* 7:5 (1981): 673–679.

— Richardson, A.J., and B.K. Puri. "The Potential Role of Fatty Acids in Attention-Deficit/Hyperactivity Disorder." *Prostaglandins Leukot Essent Fatty Acids* 63:1–2 (2000): 79–87.

129. Bilici, M., F. Yildirim, S. Kandil, et al. "Double-Blind, Placebo-Controlled Study

of Zinc Sulfate in the Treatment of Attention Deficit Hyperactivity Disorder." *Prog Neuropsychopharmacol Biol Psych* 28:1 (2004): 181–190.

— Konofal, E., M. Lecendreux, I. Arnulf, and M.C. Mouren. "Iron Deficiency in Children with Attention-Deficit/Hyperactivity Disorder." *Arch Pediatr Adolesc Med* 158:12 (2004): 1113–1115.

— Kozielec, T., and B. Starobrat-Hermelin. "Assessment of Magnesium Levels in Children with Attention Deficit Hyperactivity Disorder (ADHD)." *Magnes Res* 10:2 (1997): 143–148.

130. Kuo, F.E., and A.F. Taylor. "A Potential Natural Treatment for Attention-deficit/Hyperactivity Disorder: Evidence from a National Study." *Am J Public Health* 94:9 (2004): 1580–1586.

131. Logan, A.C. "Omega-3 Fatty Acids and Major Depression: A Primer for the Mental Health Professional." *Lipids Health Dis* 3 (2004): 25.

132. Klerman, G.L. "The Current Age of Youthful Melancholia. Evidence for Increase in Depression among Adolescents and Young Adults." *Br J Psychiatry* 152 (1988): 4–14.

133. Klerman, G.L., and M.M. Weissman. "Increasing Rates of Depression." *JAMA* 261:15 (1989): 2229–2235.

134. Noaghiul, S.F., J.R. Hibbeln, and M.M. Weissman. "Seafood Consumption and Cross-national Prevalence Rates of Bipolar Disorders and Schizophrenia." *Biol Psychiatr* 49:8 Suppl S (2001): 110S.

135. McGrath-Hanna, N.K., D.M. Greene, R.J. Tavernier, and A. Bult-Ito. "Diet and Mental Health in the Arctic: Is Diet an Important Risk Factor for Mental Health in Circumpolar Peoples?—A Review." *Int J Circumpolar Health* 62:3 (2003): 228–241.

136. Tanskanen, A., J.R. Hibbeln, J. Tuomilehto, et al. "Fish Consumption and Depressive Symptoms in the General Population in Finland." *Psychiatr Serv* 52:4 (2001): 529–531.

137. Noaghiul, S.F., J.R. Hibbeln, and M.M. Weissman. "Seafood Consumption and Cross-national Prevalence Rates of Bipolar Disorders and Schizophrenia." *Biol Psychiatr* 49:8 Suppl S (2001): 110S.

138. Maes, M., R. Smith, A. Christophe A, et al. "Fatty Acid Composition in Major Depression: Decreased Omega-3 Ratio Fractions in Cholesteryl Esters and Increased C20: 4 Omega-6/C20:5 Omega-3 Ration in Choleseteryl Esters and Phospholipids." *J Affective Disord* 38:1 (1996): 35–46.

— Hibbeln, Joseph, and Norman Salem Jr. "Omega-3 Fatty Acids and Psychiatric Disorders: Current Status of the Field." In Holick, M.F. (ed.). *Vitamin D: Molecular Biology, Physiology, and Clinical Applications.* Totowa, NJ: Humana Press, 1999.

139. Tolmunen, T., J. Hintikka, A. Ruusunen, et al. "Dietary Folate and the Risk of Depression in Finnish Middle-Aged Men: A Prospective Follow-up Study." *Psychother Psychosom* 73:6 (2004): 334–339.

— Ramos, M.I., L.H. Allen, M.N. Haan, et al. "Plasma Folate Concentrations are Associated with Depressive Symptoms in Elderly Latina Women Despite Folic Acid Fortification." *Am J Clin Nutr* 80:4 (2004): 1024–1028.

— Carney, M.W., A. Ravindran, M.G. Rinsler, and D.G. Williams. "Thiamine, Riboflavin and Pyridoxine Deficiency in Psychiatric In-Patients." *Br J Psychiatry* 141 (1982): 271–272.

— Hintikka, J., T. Tolmunen, A. Tanskanen, and H. Viinamaki. "High Vitamin B_{12} Level and Good Treatment Outcome May Be Associated in Major Depressive Disorder." *BMC Psychiatry* 3:1 (2003): 17.

140. Wehr, T.A., W.C. Duncan Jr, L. Sher, et al. "A Circadian Signal of Change of Season in Patients with Seasonal Affective Disorder." *Arch Gen Psychiatry* 58:12 (2001): 1108–1114.

141. Lane, A.M., and D.J. Lovejoy. "The Effects of Exercise on Mood Changes: The Moderating Effect of Depressed Mood." *J Sports Med Phys Fitness* 41:4 (2001): 539–545.

142. Jablensky, A., N. Sartorius, G. Ernberg, et al. "Schizophrenia: Manifestations, Incidence and Course in Different Cultures. A World Health Organization Ten-Country Study." *Psychol Med Monogr Suppl* 20 (1992): 1–97.

143. Barbato, A. *Schizophrenia and Public Health.* Geneva: the World Health Organization, 1998.

144. Puri, B.K., A.J. Richardson, D.F. Horrobin, et al. "Eicosapentaenoic Acid Treatment in Schizophrenia Associated with Symptom Remission, Normalisation of Blood Fatty Acids, Reduced Neuronal Membrane Phospholipid Turnover and Structural Brain Changes." *Int J Clin Pract* 54:1 (2000): 57–63.

145. Peet, M. "Eicosapentaenoic Acid in the Treatment of Schizophrenia and Depression: Rationale and Preliminary Double-Blind Clinical Trial Results." *Prostaglandins Leukot Essent Fatty Acids* 69:6 (2003): 477–485.

— Peet, M., J. Brind, C.N. Ramchand, et al. "Two Double-Blind Placebo-Controlled Pilot Studies of Eicosapentaenoic Acid in the Treatment of Schizophrenia." *Schizophr Res* 49:3 (2001): 243–251.

146. Christensen, O., and E. Christensen. "Fat Consumption and Schizophrenia." *Acta Psychiatr Scand* 78:5 (1988): 587–591.

147. Peet, M. "International Variations in the Outcome of Schizophrenia and the Prevalence of Depression in Relation to National Dietary Practices: An Ecological Analysis." *Br J Psychiatry* 184 (2004): 404–408.

148. Eaton, W., P.B. Mortensen, E. Agerbo, et al. "Coeliac Disease and Schizophrenia: Population-based Case-control Study with Linkage of Danish National Registers." *Br Med J* 328:7437 (2004): 438–439.

— Lorenz, K. "Cereals and Schizophrenia." *Adv Cereal Sci Technol* 10 (1990): 435–469.

149. Lorenz, K. "Cereals and Schizophrenia." *Adv Cereal Sci Technol* 10 (1990): 435–469.

150. Peet, M. "International Variations in the Outcome of Schizophrenia and the Prevalence of Depression in Relation to National Dietary Practices: An Ecological Analysis." *Br J Psychiatry* 184 (2004): 404–408.

151. Dohan, F.C., and J.C. Grasberger. "Relapsed Schizophrenics: Early Discharge

from the Hospital after Cereal-free, Milk-free Diet." *Am J Psychiatry* 130:6 (1973): 658–688.

152. Chen, H., S.M. Zhang, M.A. Hernan, et al. "Diet and Parkinson's Disease: A Potential Role of Dairy Products in Men." *Ann Neurol* 52:6 (2002): 793–801.

153. Park, M. "Consumption of Milk and Calcium in Midlife and the Future Risk of Parkinson Disease." *Neurology* 64:6 (2005): 1047–1051.

154. Duan, W., B. Ladenheim, R.G. Cutler, et al. "Dietary Folate Deficiency and Elevated Homocysteine Levels Endanger Dopaminergic Neurons in Models of Parkinson's Disease." *J Neurochem* 80:1 (2002): 101–110.

155. Abbott, R.D., H. Petrovitch, L.R. White, et al. "Frequency of Bowel Movements and the Future Risk of Parkinson's Disease." *Neurology* 57:3 (2001): 456–462.

156. McCarty, M.F. "Does a Vegan Diet Reduce Risk for Parkinson's Disease?" *Med Hypotheses* 57:3 (2001): 318–323.

— Johnson, C.C., J.M. Gorell, B.A. Rybicki, et al. "Adult Nutrient Intake as a Risk Factor for Parkinson's Disease." *Intl J Epidemiol* 28:6 (1999): 1102–1109.

157. Ross, G.W., R.D. Abbott, H. Petrovitch, et al. "Association of Coffee and Caffeine Intake with the Risk of Parkinson Disease." *JAMA* 283:20 (2000): 2674–2679.

158. Kniker, T. "Dietary Changes Improve Autistic Symptoms in Some Patients." 12th International Conference on Autism, Durham University, April 5, 2001.

159. Sun, Z. "Beta-casomorphin Induces Fos-like Immunoreactivity in Discrete Brain Regions Relevant to Schizophrenia and Autism." *Autism* 3 (1999): 67–83.

160. Sun, Z. "A Peptide Found in Schizophrenia and Autism Causes Behavioral Changes in Rats." *Autism* 3 (1999): 85–95.

— Kniker, T. "Dietary Changes Improve Autistic Symptoms in Some Patients." 12th International Conference on Autism, Durham University, April 5, 2001.

161. Dunne, C. "Adaptation of Bacteria to the Intestinal Niche: Probiotics and Gut Disorder." *Inflamm Bowel Dis* 7:2 (2001): 136–145.

162. Knickmeyer, R., S. Baron-Cohen, P. Raggatt, and K. Taylor. "Foetal Testosterone, Social Relationships, and Restricted Interests in Children." *J Child Psychol Psychiatry* 46:2 (2005): 198–210.

— Baron-Cohen, S., R.C. Knickmeyer, and M.K. Belmonte. "Sex Differences in the Brain: Implications for Explaining Autism." *Science* 310:5749 (2005): 819–823.

163. Konturek, P.C., J.W. Konturek, M. Czesnikiewicz-Guzik, et al. "Neuro-hormonal Control of Food Intake: Basic Mechanisms and Clinical Implications." *J Physiol Pharmacol* 56:Suppl 6 (2005): 5–25.

164. le Roux, C.W., M. Patterson, R.P. Vincent, et al. "Postprandial Plasma Ghrelin is Suppressed Proportional to Meal Calorie Content in Normal-weight but Not Obese Subjects." *J Clin Endocrinol Metab* 90:2 (2005): 1068–1071.

165. Flier, J.S., and J.K. Elmquist. "A Good Night's Sleep: Future Antidote to the Obesity Epidemic?" *Ann Intern Med* 141:11 (2004): 885–886.

166. Rothenberg, R. "Is Growth Hormone Replacement for Normal Aging Safe?" *Anti-Aging Therapeutics*, vol. 6. Chicago: American Academy of Anti-Aging Medicine, 2004, Chapter 3.

167. Estrich, D., A. Ravnik, G. Schlierf G, et al. "Effects of Co-ingestion of Fat and Protein upon Carbohydrate-induced Hyperglycemia." *Diabetes* 16:4 (1967): 232–237.

168. Chen, J.D. "Evolutionary Aspects of Exercise." *World Rev Nutr Diet* 84 (1999): 106–117.

— Cordain, L., R.W. Gotshall, and S.B. Eaton. "Evolutionary Aspects of Exercise." *World Rev Nutr Diet* 81 (1997): 49–60.

169. Long, S.J., K. Hart, and L.M. Morgan. "The Ability of Habitual Exercise to Influence Appetite and Food Intake in Response to High- and Low-energy Preloads in Man." *Br J Nutr* 87:5 (2002): 517–523.

— Tsofliou, F., Y.P. Pitsiladis, D. Malkova, et al. "Moderate Physical Activity Permits Acute Coupling Between Serum Leptin and Appetite–Satiety Measures in Obese Women." *Int J Obes Relat Metab Disord* 27:11 (2003): 1332–1339.

170. Arvanitakis, Z., R.S. Wilson, J.L. Bienias, et al. "Diabetes Mellitus and Risk of Alzheimer Disease and Decline in Cognitive Function." *Arch Neurol* 61:5 (2004): 661–666.

171. Boyle, J.P. "Projection of Diabetes Burden Through 2050: Impact of Changing Demography and Disease Prevalence in the U.S." *Diabetes Care* 24 (2001): 1936–1940.

172. Brand-Miller, J.C., and S. Colagiuri. "Evolutionary Aspects of Diet and Insulin Resistance." *World Rev Nutr Diet* 84 (1999): 74–105.

173. Pinhas-Hamiel, O., L.M. Dolan, S.R. Daniels, et al. "Increased Incidence of Non-insulin-dependent Diabetes Mellitus among Adolescents." *J Pediatr* 128:5 Part 1 (1996): 608–615.

174. Zimmet, P., G. Dowse, C. Finch, et al. "The Epidemiology and Natural History of NIDDM—Lessons from the South Pacific." *Diabetes Metab Rev* 6:2 (1990): 91–124.

175. National Institutes of Health (NIH) statistics.

176. O'Dea, K. "Marked Improvement in Carbohydrate and Lipid Metabolism in Diabetic Australian Aborigines after Temporary Reversion to Traditional Lifestyle." *Diabetes* 33:6 (1984): 596–603.

177. Ebbesson, S.O., P.M. Risica, L.O. Ebbesson, et al. "Omega-3 Fatty Acids Improve Glucose Tolerance and Components of the Metabolic Syndrome in Alaskan Eskimos: The Alaska Siberia Project." *Int J Circumpolar Health* 64:4 (2005): 396–408.

178. Nettleton, J.A., and R. Katz. "n-3 Long-chain Polyunsaturated Fatty Acids in Type 2 Diabetes: A Review." *J Am Diet Assoc* 105:3 (2005): 428–440.

— Denkins, Y. "DHA Might Decrease Insulin Resistance in Overweight Individuals." Experimental Biology Conference 2002, New Orleans, Louisiana.

— Ghafoorunissa, A. Ibrahim, and S. Natarajan. "Substituting Dietary Linoleic Acid with Alpha-linolenic Acid Improves Insulin Sensitivity in Sucrose Fed Rats." *Biochim Biophys Acta* 1733:1 (2005): 67–75.

179. van Dam, R.M. "Dietary Fat and Meat Intake in Relation to Risk of Type 2 Diabetes in Men." *Diabetes Care* 25:3 (2002): 417–424.

180. Katsilambros, N.L. "Nutrition in Diabetes Mellitus." *Exp Clin Endocrinol Diabetes* 109:Suppl 2 (2001): S250–S258.

181. Foy, C.G., R.A. Bell, D.F. Farmer, et al. "Smoking and Incidence of Diabetes

among U.S. Adults: Findings from the Insulin Resistance Atherosclerosis Study." *Diabetes Care* 28:10 (2005): 2501–2507.

182. Chiu, K.C., A. Chu, V.L. Go, and M.F. Saad. "Hypovitaminosis D is Associated with Insulin Resistance and Beta Cell Dysfunction." *Am J Clin Nutr* 79:5 (2004): 820–825.

183. Feskanich, D., W.C. Willett, M.J. Stampfer, and G.A. Colditz GA. "Milk, Dietary Calcium, and Bone Fractures in Women: A 12-year Prospective Study." *Am J Public Health* 87:6 (1997): 992–997.

184. Truswell, S., and J. Hansen. "Medical Research Among the !Kung." In Lee, Richard B., and Irven DeVore (eds.). *Kalahari Hunter-Gatherers: Studies of the !Kung San and Their Neighbors.* Cambridge, MA: Harvard University Press, 1976.

185. Nilas, L. "Calcium Intake and Osteoporosis." *World Rev Nutr Diet* 73 (1993): 1–26.

186. Srivatsa, S.S., P.J. Harrity, P.B. Maercklein, et al. "Increased Cellular Expression of Matrix Proteins that Regulate Mineralization is Associated with Calcification of Native Human and Porcine Xenograft Bioprosthetic Heart Valves." *J Clin Invest* 99:5 (1997): 996–1009.

187. Jackson, R.D., A.Z. LaCroix, M. Gass, et al. "Calcium Plus Vitamin D Supplementation and the Risk of Fractures." *New Engl J Med* 354:7 (2006): 669–683.

188. Allen, L.H., E.A. Oddoye, and S. Margen, et al. "Protein Induced Hypercalciuria—A Longer Term Study." *Am J Clin Nutr* 32:4 (1979): 741–749.

— Barzel, U.S., and L.K. Massey. "Excess Dietary Protein Can Adversely Affect Bone." *J Nutr* 128:6 (1998): 1051–1053.

— Linkswiler, H.M., M.B. Zemel, M. Hegsted, and S. Schuette. "Protein-induced Hypercalciuria." *Fed Proc* 40:9 (1981): 2429–2433.

— Lutz, J. "Calcium Balance and Acid-base Status of Women as Affected by Increased Protein Intake and by Sodium Bicarbonate Ingestion." *Am J Clin Nutr* 39:2 (1984): 281–288.

— Johnson, N.E., E.N. Alcantara, and H. Linkswiler. "Effect of Level of Protein Intake on Urinary and Fecal Calcium and Calcium Retention of Young Adult Males." *J Nutr* 100:12 (1970): 1425–1430.

189. New, S.A., C. Bolton-Smith, D.A. Grubb, and D.M. Reid. "Nutritional Influences on Bone Density: A Cross-sectional Study in Premenopausal Women." *Am J Clin Nutr* 65:6 (1997): 1831–1839.

190. Ellis, F., S. Holesh, and J.W. Ellis. "Incidence of Osteoporosis in Vegetarians and Omnivores." *Am J Clin Nutr* 25:6 (1972): 555–558.

191. Weber, P. "Vitamin K and Bone Health." *Nutrition* 17:10 (2001): 880–887.

192. Watkins. "Regulatory Effects of Polyunsaturates on Bone Modeling and Cartilage Function." *World Rev Nutr Diet* 83 (1998): 38–51.

— Das, U.N. "Essential Fatty Acids and Osteoporosis." *Nutrition* 16:5 (2000): 386–390.

193. Zarkadas, M., R. Gougeon-Reyburn, E.B. Marliss, et al. "Sodium Chloride Supplementation and Urinary Calcium Excretion in Postmenopausal Women." *Am J Clin Nutr* 50:5 (1989): 1088–1094.

— Cirillo, M., C. Ciacci, M. Laurenzi, et al. "Salt Intake, Urinary Sodium and Hypercalciuria." *Miner Electrolyte Metab* 23:3–6 (1997): 265–268.

194. Sellmeyer, D.E., M. Schloetter, and A. Sebastian. "Potassium Citrate Prevents Increased Urine Calcium Excretion and Bone Resorption Induced by a High Sodium Chloride Diet." *J Clin Endocrinol Metab* 87:5 (2002): 2008–2012.

195. Calvo, M.S., R. Kumar, and H. Heath. "Persistently Elevated Parathyroid Hormone Secretion and Action in Young Women after Four Weeks of Ingesting High Phosphorus, Low Calcium Diets." *J Clin Endocrinol Metab* 70:5 (1990): 1334–1340.

— Wyshak, G. "Teenaged Girls, Carbonated Beverage Consumption and Bone Fractures." *Arch Pediatr Adolesc Med* 154:6 (2000): 610–613.

— Wyshak, G., and R.E. Frisch. "Carbonated Beverages, Dietary Calcium, the Dietary Calcium/Phosphorus Ratio, and Bone Fractures in Girls and Boys." *J Adolesc Health* 15:3 (1994): 210–215.

196. Gregg, E.W., J.A. Cauley, D.G. Seeley, et al. "Physical Activity and Osteoporotic Fracture Risk in Older Women. Study of Osteoporotic Fractures Research Group." *Ann Intern Med* 129:2 (1998): 81–88.

197. Remer, T., and F. Manz. "Potential Renal Acid Load of Foods and Its Influence on Urine pH." *J Am Diet Assoc* 95:7 (1995): 791–797.

198. McGough, N., and J.H. Cummings. "Coeliac Disease: A Diverse Clinical Syndrome Caused by Intolerance of Wheat, Barley and Rye." *Proc Nutr Soc* 64:4 (2005): 434–450.

— Alaedini, A., and P.H. Green. "Narrative Review: Celiac Disease: Understanding a Complex Autoimmune Disorder." *Ann Intern Med* 142:4 (2005): 289–298.

199. Raska, I. Jr., and P. Broulik. "The Impact of Diabetes Mellitus on Skeletal Health: An Established Phenomenon with Inestablished Causes?" *Prague Med Rep* 106:2 (2005): 137–148.

— Tjaderhane, L., and M. Larmas. "A High Sucrose Diet Decreases the Mechanical Strength of Bones in Growing Rats." *J Nutr* 128:10 (1998): 1807–1810.

200. Bikle, D.D. "Alcohol Induced Bone Disease." *World Rev Nutr Diet* 73 (1993): 53–79.

201. Wood, R.J., and J.J. Zheng. "High Dietary Calcium Intakes Reduce Zinc Absorption and Balance in Humans." *Am J Clin Nutr* 65:6 (1997): 1803–1809.

202. Food and Nutrition Board, Institute of Medicine. *A Risk Assessment Model for Establishing Upper Intake Levels for Nutrients*. Washington, DC: National Academy of Sciences, 1998.

203. Adams, J.S., and G. Lee. "Gains in Bone Mineral Density with Resolution of Vitamin D Intoxication." *Ann Intern Med* 127:3 (1997): 203–206.

204. Boivin, G., J. Dupuis, and P.J. Meunier. "Fluoride and Osteoporosis" *World Rev Nutr Diet* 73 (1993): 80–103.

205. Lloyd, T., N. Rollings, D.F. Eggli, et al. "Dietary Caffeine Intake and Bone Status of Postmenopausal Women." *Am J Clin Nutr* 65:6 (1997): 1826–1830.

206. New, S.A., C. Bolton-Smith, D.A. Grubb, and D.M. Reid. "Nutritional Influences on Bone Density: A Cross-sectional Study in Premenopausal Women." *Am J Clin Nutr* 65:6 (1997): 1831–1839.

207. King, J.C. "Effect of Reproduction on the Bioavailability of Calcium, Zinc and Selenium." *J Nutr* 131:4 Suppl (2001): 1355S–1358S.

208. Ritchie, L.D., E.B. Fung, B.P. Halloran, et al. "A Longitudinal Study of Calcium Homeostasis during Human Pregnancy and Lactation and After Resumption of Menses." *Am J Clin Nutr* 67:4 (1998): 693–701.

209. Laskey, M.A., A. Prentice, L.A. Hanratty, et al. "Bone Changes after 3 Months of Lactation: Influence of Calcium Intake, Breast-milk Output, and Vitamin D-receptor Genotype." *Am J Clin Nutr* 67:4 (1998): 685–692.

— Ritchie, L.D., E.B. Fung, B.P. Halloran, et al. "A Longitudinal Study of Calcium Homeostasis during Human Pregnancy and Lactation and After Resumption of Menses." *Am J Clin Nutr* 67:4 (1998): 693–701.

— Kalkwarf, H.J., B.L. Specker, D.C. Bianchi, et al. "The Effect of Calcium Supplementation on Bone Density during Lactation and After Weaning." *N Engl J Med* 337:8 (1997): 523–528.

210. Kalkwarf, H.J. "Lactation and Maternal Bone Health." *Adv Exp Med Biol* 554 (2004): 101–114.

Index

EAT SMART, EAT RAW

Creative Vegetarian Recipes for a Healthier Life

Kate Wood

As the popularity of raw vegetarian cuisine continues to soar, so does the mounting scientific evidence that uncooked food is amazingly good for you. From healing diseases to detoxifying your body, from lowering cholesterol to eliminating excess weight, the many important health benefits derived from such a diet are too important to ignore. However, now there is another compelling reason to go raw—taste! In her new book *Eat Smart, Eat Raw,* cook and health writer Kate Wood not only explains how to get started, but also provides delicious kitchen-tested recipes guaranteed to surprise and delight even the fussiest of eaters.

$15.95 US / $21.95 CAN • 184 Pages • 7.5 x 9-inch quality paperback • ISBN 0-7570-0261-7

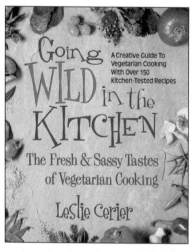

GOING WILD IN THE KITCHEN

The Fresh & Sassy Tastes of Vegetarian Cooking

Leslie Cerier

Go wild in the kitchen! Be creative! Venture beyond the usual beans, grains, and vegetables to include an exciting variety of organic vegetarian fare in your meals. Step outside the box and prepare dishes with beautiful edible flowers; flavorful wild mushrooms, herbs, and berries; tangy sheep and goat cheeses; tasty sea vegetables; and exotic ancient grains like teff, quinoa, and Chinese "forbidden" black rice. Author and expert chef Leslie Cerier is crazy about the great taste and goodness of organically grown foods. In this exciting cookbook, she shares scores of her favorite recipes that spotlight these fresh, wholesome ingredients.

$16.95 US / $25.50 CAN • 240 Pages • 7.5 x 9-inch quality paperback • ISBN 0-7570-0091-6

TRANSITIONS LIFESTYLE SYSTEM
GLYCEMIC FOOD
INDEX GUIDE

For Weight Loss, Cardiovascular
Health, Diabetic Management, and
Maximum Energy

Dr. Shari Lieberman

From one of America's leading nutritionists
comes an easy-to-use guide to the glycemic
index of a wide range of common foods and
beverages. Designed to be used at home or
on the go, this will quickly become the first
resource you turn to whenever you want to
select a food that can help you reach your
health and dietary goals. This book:

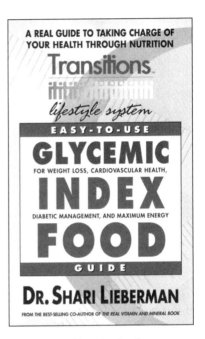

■ Provides both the glycemic index and the glycemic load of hundreds of
foods and beverages, including raw foods, cooked foods, and popular
combination and prepared foods.

■ Makes foods easy to find by listing them both singly and under helpful
categories.

■ Includes tips within the listings to guide you towards the best food choices.

■ Provides lists of ethnic foods for use at your favorite restaurants.

■ Presents easy-to-understand explanations of glycemic index, glycemic
load, and other important terms.

■ Expands your food choices by helping you integrate high-glycemic index
foods into your diet.

■ Explains how the glycemic index can help you manage a range of disorders,
from diabetes to cardiovascular disease.

■ Answers commonly asked questions about carbohydrates, blood glucose,
and the glycemic index.

Whether you are interested in controlling your glucose levels to manage your
diabetes, lose weight, increase your heart health, boost your energy level, or
simply improve your overall well-being, *Transition Lifestyle System Easy-to-Use
Glycemic Index Food Guide* is the best place to start.

$7.95 US / $9.95 CAN • 160 Pages • 4 x 7-inch quality paperback • ISBN 0-7570-0245-5

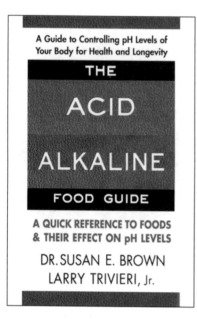

A Guide to Controlling pH Levels of
Your Body for Health and Longevity

THE

ACID

ALKALINE

FOOD GUIDE

**A QUICK REFERENCE TO FOODS
& THEIR EFFECT ON pH LEVELS**

DR. SUSAN E. BROWN
LARRY TRIVIERI, Jr.

THE ACID-ALKALINE FOOD GUIDE

A Quick Reference to Foods & Their Effect on pH Levels

Susan E. Brown, PhD, CCN
and Larry Trivieri, Jr.

In the last few years, researchers around the world have reported the importance of acid-alkaline balance. When the body enjoys pH balance, you experience radiant good health. When the body is not in balance, the disease process begins, resulting in problems ranging from bone loss to premature aging and more. The key to a healthy pH is proper diet, but for a long time, acid-alkaline food guides have included only a small number of foods. Or they did, until now.

The Acid-Alkaline Food Guide is a complete resource for people who want to widen their food choices. The book begins by explaining how the acid-alkaline environment of the body is influenced by foods. It then presents a list of thousands of foods and their acid-alkaline effects. Included are not only single foods, such as fruits and vegetables, but also popular combination and even fast foods, like burgers and fries. In each case, you'll not only discover whether a food is acidifying or alkalizing, but you'll learn the *degree* to which that food affects the body. Informative insets guide you in choosing the food that's right for you.

The first book of its kind, The Acid-Alkaline Food Guide will quickly become the resource you turn to at home, in restaurants, and whenever you want to select a food that can help you reach your health and dietary goals.

ABOUT THE AUTHORS

Susan E. Brown, PhD, CCN, is a medical anthropologist and New York State Certified Nutritionist. A clinician, researcher, and author, she has over twenty years experience in clinical nutrition and lay and professional health education. Dr. Brown directs the Osteoporosis Education Project and the Nutrition Education and Consulting Service in East Syracuse, New York.

Larry Trivieri, Jr. is a professional writer in the field of holistic health. His articles on health have appeared in numerous magazines and newspapers throughout North America, and he served as coauthor of the bestseller *Alternative Medicine: The Definitive Guide.*

$7.95 • 208 pages • 4 x 7-inch paperback • ISBN 0-7570-0280-3